Is Your Parent in
Good Hands?

Is Your Parent in
Good Hands?

Protecting Your Aging Parent from Financial Abuse and Neglect

Edward J. Carnot, Esq.

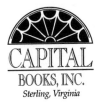

CAPITAL
BOOKS, INC.
Sterling, Virginia

Capital Books, Inc.
P.O. Box 605
Herndon, Virginia 20172-0605

ISBN 1-931868-37-9 (alk.paper)

Library of Congress Cataloging-in-Publication Data
Carnot, Edward J., 1947–

Is your parent in good hands? : protecting your aging parent from
abuse—financial, emotional, legal, and physical / Edward J. Carnot—
1st ed.
    p. cm.
Includes bibliographical references and index.
  ISBN 1–931868–37–9 (alk. paper)
  1. Aged—Crimes against—United States—Prevention.   2. Aging parents—
Care—United States.   3. Aging parents—Legal status, laws, etc.—United States.
4. Adult children—Legal status, laws, etc.—United States.   5. Caregivers—Legal
status, laws, etc.—United States.   I. Title
  HV6250.4A34C37 2003
  362.6'0973—dc21

2003012140

Printed in the United States of America on acid-free paper that meets the American National Standards Institute Z39-48 Standard.

First Edition

10 9 8 7 6 5 4 3 2

The events described in these pages are factual. Some names and places have been changed to protect the identity of persons who may not want to be mentioned in connection with these events.

This book is dedicated to my wonderful family,
Pamela, Brett, and Kimberly, who I love dearly,
and to the "baby boomers" who have the responsibility
of caring for an elderly parent.
I hope my personal story
and the suggestions contained in this book
ease your burden.

Contents

Acknowledgments

Writing this book has been an incredible learning experience. I have new respect for the dedication of those who choose to write. While working in my law firm, writing was a collegial effort. If I had a mental block on an issue, it was natural to walk down the hall to discuss the issue and get guidance from my colleagues. Writing a book is totally different. It is a singular, often lonely, endeavor. I have spent countless solitary hours in my office writing, editing and revising what I already edited. This does not mean that no one was available for support. Quite the contrary. It is just that the people who helped make this book possible were not down the hall, though in a larger sense they were always there when I needed them.

My thanks go to Myrna Wohl, who was kind enough to read the first chapters and encourage me to continue. She was always positive about the merits of my story and she wanted it published as much as I did. Whenever I had self doubts, she was my cheerleader.

Many thanks to Ralph Mittelberger, who was kind enough to offer me expert legal advice in the morass of publishers' contracts.

Our Maryland travel group, Terry and Linda Vann, Lew and Lynn Cohen, Art and Marlene Hartstein, and Myrna and Ron Wohl, were always willing to spend time with me while we were on vacations to learn about the progress of this book and to offer meaningful suggestions.

Donald A. Berlin, Carol Mills R.N.M.A. and Robert Eringer, a successful author in his own right, who were willing to drop everything they were doing and give me guidance regardless of the issue.

Last, but not least, are the three most important people in this effort: my wife, Pamela; my sister, K.C.; and my editor, Jacquelyn Landis. Pamela was my touchstone for reality and my strongest supporter. Whatever the issue, she was always willing to listen and willing to help. It was Pamela who on countless occasions had to endure a long background explanation before I could describe my mental block. As a participant in the story, she also offered her insights on its presentation. I know that I was a bit of a bore, constantly charging Pam with the duty of being my sounding board. She took it all in good stride and was always the voice of encouragement.

K.C. and I were at the front line of the ordeal together. She was as hurt by what happened to Dad as I was. I know it was difficult for her to dredge up the memories of the events that I recount here. She was, in a word, incredible. Despite the pain of reliving this experience again with me, K.C. was always willing to discuss what had happened, even though it sometimes brought her to tears. Her help and guidance were much appreciated. I am a better person for having learned from K.C. about dealing with our mutual loss, and it has brought us closer together.

Last but not least is Jacquelyn Landis, my editor. Without Jackie, this task would have been impossible to complete. Jackie, an experienced editor and published author, was always there to keep me focused. She was much more than an editor. She did extraordinary research, made wonderful suggestions regarding content and approach, and, when I was worn out and ready to throw in the towel, was there to prop me up and keep me going. We had many discussions about approach and content, often covering the same ground because of my naïveté as a rookie author and success as a lawyer in getting my way if I tenaciously pressed the same issue over and over. This tactic usually led to capitulation by the other side. Not with Jackie. She always kept her cool and kept me focused on the task at hand. I would approach our power coffee-breakfast meetings with anticipation and some trepidation because I knew my agenda covered issues we had discussed previously, but I wanted to raise them again. Jackie treated all of my issues with due consideration, and she would explain her response to my suggestion in the kindest and clearest terms. It took a while for me to get the message without her ever saying we had talked about that before. She is the professional; she has the concept; she has the experience; listen to Jackie. Jackie, you are wonderful. Thank you for everything.

I am sure I have missed others who deserve mention. For all of you, please do not be offended. In my heart I sincerely appreciate all who have contributed to this book.

Introduction

This is not a happy story. It is a factual recounting of my elderly father's victimization by an unscrupulous caregiver. Those circumstances alone were disturbing enough. However, compounding an already bad situation was the inability of our legal system to protect him. The resulting chaos turned my family inside out and ultimately threatened the dignity and independence my father so tenaciously clung to.

When I first set out to write Dad's story, my goal was somewhat vague. Part of me wanted to record the details to preserve them as lessons for future generations. Another part was looking for an outlet for the anger and frustration that have barely abated since the time of my father's victimization. Then, as I began to write, I realized that what I had learned about protecting the elderly from abuse needed to be shared with the millions of Americans whose parents are aging and in need of assistance with their daily lives. My goal shifted to providing proven techniques for both identifying abusive situations and protecting the elderly from abuse.

The rapid increase in the numbers of America's aging citizens has resulted in a demand for an entire new level of services and protection. As a lawyer, I had always believed that the law would be the ultimate safety net should my father or anyone else ever fall victim to abuse, neglect, or exploitation. What I have learned, both since the time of my father's story and while conducting research for this book, is that the law falls short of the kind of protection adult children want—and often mistakenly assume exists—for their elderly parents.

Although legislators in every state are working hard to bring existing laws in line with the realities of aging, the burden of protecting our senior citizens still falls on their adult children. The good news is that, with the many available resources, children can do a lot to make sure their parents receive quality care without being vulnerable to victimization. As you read these pages, you'll soon discover that you need to invest substantial time and effort to arrange for the safety and well-being of your parents. The time spent will be negligible, however, when compared to the peace of mind you will gain from knowing your parents are protected from the many predators who are making a career out of abusing and exploiting the elderly.

This book contains the information you need to start your own plan to care for and protect your elderly parent or parents. My hope is that after reading this book, you will be well equipped to evaluate your own parents' situation and make appropriate plans before problems start to arise. I assure you, reacting to events after they have happened, as I did with my father, is the worst way to proceed.

After assessing my different motivations for writing this book, I have decided that the one I like best surfaced toward the end of the endeavor. I realized there could be no greater tribute to my father than having his story be an instrument of change. If this book is only a tiny step toward this goal, it will be a fitting tribute to a special man who taught his family well the meaning of love and the importance of values. Dad has influenced my life in so many positive ways, and I like the notion of sharing his insights with others.

CHAPTER 1

The Phone Call

"You are free to move around the cabin." The words barely penetrated my consciousness as I stared out the window at the heavy cloud layer below. My mind, filled with a jumble of unsettling thoughts, was traveling a million miles an hour faster than the airplane taking me from Maryland to California.

Of all the problems in life that deserved worry, my 82-year-old father was relatively low on my list. Even though we lived on opposite coasts, I knew Dad was secure. Income from his investment portfolio and Social Security provided him with financial security and a trusted caregiver was in charge of his physical well-being.

Just by chance, though, on some unexplained whim, I had picked up the telephone three days earlier and called my father's stockbroker in California. I didn't use Dad's stockbroker; I had never even met him. But once in a blue moon I would call him, just to talk about stock ideas.

To this day, I still cannot explain why I chose that particular time to call. But that telephone call touched off a series of cataclysmic events that would profoundly change my life, my sister's life and, most of all, my father's life.

The call started so innocently. After the usual hello, how-are-you, and what's-new pleasantries had been exchanged, Arthur, the stockbroker, dropped a bomb. "Ed, I'm glad you called. Your father called me yesterday and instructed me to liquidate all of his holdings and issue a check made payable to cash, which he said he would come by to pick up."

"What do you mean?" I asked in a voice at least an octave higher than normal.

"Right," Arthur said, "your father asked me to sell everything and issue a check payable to cash. In fact, Ben just left me a message, asking when he could pick up the check."

It felt like a knife had been driven into my stomach and turned for good measure. My father, Ben Carnot, was in the salad days of his retirement. For the last ten years or so, all of his assets, around a half-million dollars, had been invested in a conservative stock-and-bond portfolio so that he could live comfortably on the interest income combined with his Social Security.

"Arthur, why didn't you call me?" I asked.

"Ed, I just didn't want to get involved."

My hand holding the telephone was shaking, as anger joined the dread that had already settled in. "Arthur, you have been my father's investment advisor for the last twenty years. You know that he's living off the money you're managing. Did you ask him why he wanted everything sold or why he requested a check payable to cash?"

"No," said Arthur, "I just didn't want to get involved." Arthur did add that Dad had already cashed in about $65,000 from his portfolio in recent months.

I bit my tongue and stopped myself from telling Arthur how I felt about his taking the steps to liquidate all of my father's holdings without calling me, and, instead, reminded him that I had my father's power of attorney. I instructed him not to do anything with my father's portfolio without express instructions from me. Arthur asked, "What should I do if your father calls about the check?"

"Tell him that there's a delay in processing his request, and then call me right away," I said. I hung up the telephone and wondered what was happening to my father in California. I didn't have a clue.

Ben and Bernice, my father and mother, were married in 1946 and the next year moved from Elizabeth, New Jersey, to San Diego. I was born in 1947, and my sister, Kate, whom everyone called K.C., was born in 1950. Ben loved his Bernice dearly. Their happy life together took a downturn when she was stricken with multiple sclerosis in 1962. By 1965, the year I left for college, she could barely walk, even with a walker. As she deteriorated more over the years, Dad refused to put Mom in a nursing home. He wanted the love of his life to have the best care possible at home, where they could be together. So he hired care providers to take care of her at home, around the clock.

Before her illness, my father and mother had been on an upward rise in San Diego. He was a successful businessman; she, the perfect hostess. The phone never stopped ringing. Friends were important to them because, as my father would say, "We are a small family. Friends are a substitute for the family we left on the East Coast." So life for us revolved around the few family members who lived nearby and many good friends.

As Mom's illness progressed, she lost the ability to use her hands and, ultimately, the ability to walk. While she was becoming progressively more disabled, the inside of the house took on the appearance and the smell of a hospital. As more hospital equipment was added to accommodate Mom's illness, friends visited less and less often, and eventually they visited hardly at all. For years it was just my father and his sick wife, holed up in the house with the care providers. Watching Mom deteriorate before his eyes while living in forced isolation was heart wrenching for a previously active, vibrant man who had relied so heavily on his wife and friends for his happiness. Ultimately, as Mom's condition worsened, Dad became increasingly cynical about the people he had called his friends.

Despite his bitterness, Dad lovingly cared for Mom until her death in 1986. Within two years, much to the delight of K.C. and me, Dad found love again with a woman ten years his junior. Sue was a hard-talking, hard-drinking, no-nonsense woman who showered my father with love. Dad had been lucky enough to find another soul mate, and once they were married, it was Ben and Sue against the world. Dad was again the happy-go-lucky man I remembered from my youth, a man who now greeted each new day with a smile because of his love for Sue and her love for him.

Together they traveled near and far, it didn't matter where, as long as they were together. Car trips from their home in San Diego to Las Vegas, Los Angeles, and Palm Springs were common. More extensive trips to Sue's hometown of Dallas and visits to Dad's sisters and brothers in New Jersey and New York were frequent. It seemed they were always on a cruise to somewhere. His life was good.

Dad never imagined he would have to bury another wife, until tests showed that Sue had cancer and not much time left to live. Once she was gone, in 1993, Dad was a lonely, broken man once again.

Immediately after my call to Arthur, I called my father. Dad could offer no plausible explanation for his request to Arthur to liquidate his holdings. He said something about his need to pay off someone he owed money, which didn't make sense. Dad was always conservative with his money. He never owed anyone a dime. What was even more distressing about the conversation was that my father did not seem "right." He seemed distant, out of it.

Since leaving California twenty-four years earlier and moving east, I had tried to speak to my dad every week or so. I usually called him on Sundays, and I pretty much knew what to expect from our conversations. This day's conversation was dramatically different, though. Dad asked none of the usual questions about my law practice; my wife, Pamela; or my two children, twenty-three-year-old Brett, and Kimberly, who was twenty-one.

When I asked my usual questions, I received monosyllabic replies, not the rich details my father had always shared with me in the past. His health was "fine." "Yes," he was taking his meds and seeing his doctors. He described his life as "boring, just staying at home with Grace and watching TV." It was clear that Dad did not want to talk. The stilted conversation notwithstanding, my father also sounded different in a way I could not describe, and I felt certain that something was wrong.

I asked to speak to Grace, a longtime housekeeper for the family whom Dad had promoted to home healthcare provider. Grace must have been close by, maybe even listening in, because she was on the phone in an instant. Grace was as cheery and upbeat as ever. She confirmed that Dad was doing fine and that I should not worry.

How could he be fine, I wondered, when he had made a most bizarre, out-of-character request to his stockbroker and now sounded like he was in the depths of depression? I decided not to discuss this with Grace anymore. It wasn't that I distrusted her, just that I now doubted her ability to make sound judgments about the mental and physical health of my father, since she had just told me that Dad was fine. In my mind the evidence pointed strongly in the opposite direction. I wanted the insight of someone I knew really cared about Dad and whose opinion I truly valued. I thanked Grace for taking care of Dad and asked her to watch him closely. She said that she would and we both said goodbye.

This telephone conversation, on top of the conversation I had just had with Arthur, only added more acid to my already churning stomach.

I next called my sister in San Diego. K.C. lived near Dad, and I knew she checked on him regularly. If anyone would know what was going on, it would be K.C. Luckily, I reached her at home. I told her what I had learned from Arthur, and then I repeated the disturbing conversation I'd had with Dad and Grace. K.C. was as dumbfounded as I, and she couldn't offer any insight into why Dad had ordered the liquidation of his portfolio nor what he intended to do with his entire net worth.

Even over the telephone, I could tell that K.C. was as upset as I was about this disturbing news. She had reason to be upset—even more than I. K.C. was a single parent, working as a real estate agent. I knew that she relied on Dad to help her out financially from time to time. I didn't know the extent of the help Dad provided to K.C., nor did I care. But if Dad was dissipating his entire estate, then there would be no more checks for K.C., and she would be in a difficult situation.

Nonetheless, rather than talk about her own potential financial problems, she said, "Ed, it's his money. But is there something we can do to make sure that he knows what he's doing?" I told K.C. I didn't know what our options were, but I intended to find out. I then asked how Dad had seemed the last time she had seen him. K.C. said, "I've been visiting him at the house or calling him almost every day. For the past few weeks or so," she confessed, "he seems to have been changing—in a bad way."

Dad and K.C. had always been close. He adored his little girl. Since her marriage in 1971, K.C. had lived just a few miles away from Dad, and she visited him frequently. So she was in a good position to pick up on any change in his character. What she told me was not good news.

"I can no longer talk to Dad at the house without Grace being within earshot. And just recently, he refuses to go in the car with me unless Grace comes with us." She continued by saying she was sure that Grace was listening in on her telephone conversations with Dad. "What's particularly strange," said K.C., "is that Dad is now deferring to Grace to make all his decisions." We both knew that Dad was strong willed, even headstrong, and it was completely out of character for him to let someone decide anything for him.

K.C. said it didn't matter if the issue was as mundane as when she should pick Dad up to go to the bank, when she should come by to take him to dinner, or when she should take him to the market, Dad would always defer to Grace and insist that she come with them. "It's as though he has lost the ability to think for himself," said K.C.

Grace had a long history with our family. Before my mother became ill, Grace had been our housekeeper, coming in a few days a week to clean the family house, which was located in Point Loma, a suburb of San Diego. When Mom was stricken with multiple sclerosis, Dad needed more help caring for her. He asked Grace to assist him. From that point on, Grace worked five days a week at the house, caring for Mom. Although my memory of Grace wasn't sharp, I recalled her being somewhat heavyset and extremely pleasant. By now, I thought, she must be in her mid- to late fifties. She had always been nice to me when I visited, and from what I saw, she seemed genuinely concerned about my mother's welfare. I had a distinct memory of Grace feeding my mother a spoonful of food at a time while she lay at a 45-degree angle in the hospital bed Dad had purchased for her comfort.

Grace also had helped care for Sue when she became ill. After Sue died, about three years earlier, Grace stayed on to care for Dad, moving into the house so she could be there on a full-time basis. When Grace had a day off, one of her children, usually an older son, would substitute for her.

K.C. told me that she didn't like the current environment, with Grace and her children having unimpeded access to our father, twenty-fours hours a day; however, Dad would blow up and get extremely angry at any suggestion that someone else be hired in place of Grace and her sons.

K.C. paused for a few seconds. Thinking that she was finished, I asked her, "Is there anything else I should know about?" There was silence on the other end of the phone for a long moment. Then, K.C. told me a story of a confrontation she'd had with Grace just a few days earlier, which stunned me into near speechlessness. "Dad's lost a lot of weight, Ed," K.C. told me, "and I wanted to take him to see his doctor. I was concerned that he wasn't eating a well-balanced diet and that his health was being jeopardized. Dad got belligerent, though, and refused to go. Then Grace interrupted, saying that Dad was okay and that I should 'stop bothering him.'" K.C.'s voice was trembling, and I could tell that the tears were beginning to fall. She continued, "I couldn't believe my ears. All I cared about was Dad's well-being, and here was this outsider, with no medical credentials, putting herself between Dad and me."

Once she started talking, it was like a cork had popped from a bottle and the contents were gushing out. "In the past, Grace would go to her bedroom when I would visit, and she would discreetly close the door behind her so that Dad and I could speak in private. This routine has gone on for years."

Apparently, within the last month or so, there had been a change in this etiquette pattern. Without explanation, instead of going to her bedroom when K.C. arrived, Grace was now remaining in the living room, which was adjacent to the family room where K.C. and Dad would sit talking. As soon as the conversation indicated that K.C. was about to leave, Grace would come uninvited into the family room to say good-bye. So there was no question that she was listening to the conversation between father and daughter.

On this day, however, the new routine had taken a dramatic turn.

As K.C. was trying to persuade Dad to go see his doctor, Grace actually walked into the family room and remonstrated with K.C. in front of Dad. The conversation quickly became heated, with K.C. insisting that Dad go to the doctor and Grace insisting that he was "fine" and K.C. should "mind her own business."

"Ed," K.C. said between sobs, "she pushed me. Not hard, but enough to force me to take a few steps backward to regain my balance." Unbelievably, K.C. who probably weighs 105 pounds sopping wet, had been physically pushed, in her father's presence, by his employee. Even worse, our father did nothing in her defense. K.C. and Grace were screaming at one another when Dad finally stepped in. He ordered them both to sit down and make peace.

K.C. felt that she had no choice in the matter. Clearly, Grace's position in the household had shifted dramatically. K.C. realized that her continued access to Dad might be seriously jeopardized unless she made peace with this woman. So she and Grace both apologized to one another for letting things get out of hand. Dad said that he wanted everyone to get along. He emphasized that Grace had been a good friend of the family for many years and that K.C. was his daughter who cared about his welfare. In the future he did not want another scene like the one he had just witnessed.

I couldn't have been more shocked. I realized that K.C. was releasing a lot of pent-up anxiety about Dad that had been building over the last few months.

K.C. was always Dad's "little dove" or "little bird," which is what he called her when we were growing up. He absolutely adored her. The idea that Dad would allow anyone to touch his little bird was beyond belief. Under normal circumstances, the Ben Carnot I knew would have been provoked to immediate action to defend K.C., despite his age. At a minimum, he surely would have fired Grace on the spot and told her to get packing. Curiously, none of the reactions K.C. or I would have expected from Dad occurred. For Dad not to jump to K.C.'s defense when his pride and joy had been physically shoved in front of him was incomprehensible. The only explanation was that something was seriously wrong with our father.

For Dad, it was unthinkable that adults would engage in physical combat to settle differences. We were a civilized family, trained to resolve disputes using logic and words. The idea of adults in a shoving match of any kind was totally foreign to the way K.C. and I had been brought up. Further, that the caregiver could be so brazen as to push Dad's daughter, right in front of him, without fear of immediate termination of her employment, convinced me that something was going on with Dad and Grace that neither of us understood. I wondered if Dad's bizarre instructions to Arthur were in some way connected to this incident, given that they had both happened within the past few days.

When I asked why she had not told me about this confrontation earlier, K.C. rationalized that there was nothing I could do from three thousand miles away, and she did not want to upset Dad, figuring that I would call to question him about what had happened. She reasonably assumed that I might even suggest that Dad fire Grace and her supporting cast of children, and she already knew Dad's reaction to any such suggestion.

Until my phone call, K.C. had been willing to let bygones be bygones because all had been patched up at the house, but these incidents, combined with Dad's request to liquidate his holdings, elevated our concerns about Grace and Dad.

Although I wished K.C. had shared these incidents with me, I could appreciate her reluctance to do so because I was so far away. But now the critical question was, What could we do about Dad's situation? I knew I needed time to think through everything I had heard and learned in the past few hours. I hung up with a promise to get back to K.C. when I had some ideas.

After the telephone conversation with Arthur, and then hearing K.C. vent about Grace and her concern over Dad, I was feeling drained and numb. I needed some time to let my head clear. I knew, however, that I had to do something—and soon. I was in Rockville, Maryland, far from my sister and father in San Diego. I felt that I just didn't understand enough about why Dad was acting so erratically. The more I thought about what I had learned from Arthur and K.C., the more I realized that there was really only one course of action. I needed to fly to San Diego in the next few days, visit my father and sister, and see firsthand what was going on with my dad. As I calmed down and started to think more rationally, I remembered two other incidents K.C. had told me about not long ago, which now seemed to add more evidence that my concerns about Dad were warranted.

K.C.'s housekeeper, Maria, had been doing double duty until just recently. She worked part time for K.C. and the rest of her time was spent working for Dad. K.C. liked having Maria at Dad's house because she was eyes and ears for K.C. According to K.C., Grace didn't like having someone watching her and reporting to K.C., so Grace made life difficult for Maria at the house. K.C. said they would fight like cats and dogs whenever they were out of Dad's sight. Eventually the situation became so bad that Maria refused to work for Dad any longer.

The other incident now caused me far more worry than when I had first heard about it. For many years, K.C. was a signatory on Dad's checking account and had been helping him write checks and pay bills. After Maria hung up her mop, Dad closed that checking account and opened one on which he was the sole signatory. When K.C. originally told me about this, she believed that Grace had convinced Dad that K.C. should not be writing checks for him. At that time, we agreed not to confront Dad about this decision, believing that he had the right to spend his money without K.C.'s oversight. Still, K.C. felt bad about having been removed from this position of trust. In hindsight, this could have been an early warning sign that trouble was on the horizon.

I cleared my schedule and immediately made reservations to fly out two days later. I called my father to tell him about my plans. Dad seemed excited about his son coming to visit. Typical of his generous nature, he asked me if I wanted to stay at the house. I had hoped he would ask because I wanted to spend as much time with him as possible. As soon as I accepted his offer, I heard words that seemed to be delivered directly from heaven. Dad said, "Grace has just left for China, on a well-deserved three-week vacation. You know, Ed, she works so hard, and she is such a fine, upstanding person." In her absence, Grace's son Thomas was staying at the house, acting as Dad's principal caregiver, with Grace's other sons filling in as necessary.

This was great! My timing couldn't have been better. I wouldn't have to talk to my dad with Grace in the wings. I'd be able to speak frankly to him about my concerns. I suggested that Dad tell Thomas and the others that their services would not be needed for a few days, because his son would be staying with him at the house. Dad said that he would deliver the message as soon as we hung up. Dad sounded so upbeat and "with it" that I momentarily wondered whether there really was a problem that needed my immediate attention. After some reflection and remembering the call to Arthur, however, I was convinced it was best for me to spend some time with Dad as soon as possible.

I then called K.C. to tell her about my telephone conversation with Dad. The relief was palpable in her voice when I told her I was coming to help. For the first time, I realized how much stress she was under, being a single parent of two wonderful but demanding children, trying to balance her responsibilities to them with the ever-increasing demands of our father. K.C. asked me what we could do. I told her that I had a lot of ideas, but before discussing them with her I wanted to consult with one of my law school colleagues.

Before leaving Maryland, I was able to connect with a friend, who was practicing elder law in San Diego. I wanted to find out if I could be appointed Dad's guardian so that he wouldn't be able to unilaterally liquidate his holdings in the future. I knew my power of attorney was good only until Dad revoked it, which he could do with a simple letter. Without the power of attorney, I couldn't legally direct Arthur to ignore Dad's instructions, so my father would be free to do whatever he wanted with his portfolio.

The next step up from a power of attorney is an appointment of guardianship. I knew generally that a guardianship can be ordered by the court after a hearing in which witnesses, usually psychiatrists, testify about the competency of the person for whom guardianship is being sought. If the testimony convinces the judge that the person is incompetent, the judge issues an order appointing another person, usually a family member, as guardian, which means that person has complete control over the incompetent person's assets. Unlike the power of attorney, which can be revoked with a letter, the appointment of the guardian can be revoked only by a judge, which would require another hearing and the judge's determination that the incompetent person is now competent.

Fearing that Dad could act at any time to revoke the power of attorney he had given me, I wanted to learn more from the attorney about the process for quickly getting appointed my father's guardian. I believed my father was still competent, so I was most interested in standards for guardianship besides incompetency. The information that my friend provided was encouraging, at first.

I learned that in California, there are two ways to become the guardian for a person who is competent. First, the person voluntarily agrees that another person can act as his guardian. I ruled this out right away because I did not believe my father would give up control of his assets willingly. The second path to guardianship is to establish in court that the person is a "harm to himself or a harm to others." This was good news, I thought. My father had instructed his stockbroker to liquidate his entire estate, and if I could establish that he intended to give everything he owned to someone else, wouldn't this qualify at least as "harm to himself"? My friend dashed this analysis. "Harm to himself" meant physical harm, not economic harm. So long as Dad was semi-competent—a very low standard—he could give away everything he owned and become a pauper, and there was nothing anyone could do.

My friend then delivered more distressing news. "The law is going to favor your dad, who has all of the cards if he wants to play them." Theoretically, Dad could take all of his worldly possessions, and throw them into the Pacific Ocean, and the law would back him to the hilt. The law was not going to help K.C. and me. It didn't make sense to me that the law could be so deaf to the pleas of children who were trying to protect their father from irrational behavior.

Armed with this knowledge, I prepared some papers whereby my father would voluntarily appoint me as guardian of his property and person. I doubted if Dad would agree, but I wanted to be prepared if the opportunity presented itself.

While I was learning about the guardianship laws in California, my sister had been rooting out some interesting information. K.C., it seems, was friendly with the branch manager of the bank where both she and Dad had accounts. With the manager's cooperation (and because she had been an additional signatory on Dad's account), she had obtained copies of Dad's canceled checks for the last year. The story the checks told was almost unbelievable.

For her services, Grace was supposed to receive room and board and a salary of $400 per week, or $20,800 per year. The checks K.C. had obtained from the bank for the previous year showed stunning abuse. Grace had written paychecks to herself which Dad had signed, often twice and sometimes three times a week. Even worse, there were dozens of checks made out by Grace to "cash" and signed by Dad. In one month alone, Dad's account had been depleted by almost $30,000, with no indication of where the money had gone. I remembered that Arthur had told me Dad had already liquidated $65,000 from his investment portfolio. Doing some quick mental calculations, I realized Dad had gone through more than $100,000 in the past year, with most of it undoubtedly going to Grace. Obviously, Dad was giving Grace virtually free access to his accounts. Why was he doing this, and why was Grace draining his funds? I was seething with anger at Grace. She had taken advantage of my father and deserved to be punished for her actions.

The financial exploitation wasn't limited to just Grace. In addition, there were checks totaling several thousand dollars payable to a church I had never heard of. K.C. thought she had some information about Dad's involvement with this church. Several months earlier, before Dad had insisted on always traveling in the company of Grace, he had been talking to K.C. in the car while she was driving him to his doctor's appointment. Dad was telling K.C. about the fine person Grace was, which was not unusual. As long as we both could remember, he had talked about Grace in the most glowing terms: how smart she was, how she had taken such good care of Bernice and Sue, how she took such good care of him, how well-educated she was, what a good family she came from. The list of positive traits possessed by Grace was never-ending, or so it seemed.

During this conversation, Dad mentioned in passing that one of Grace's sons was the minister of a local church, which, he told her, was located in a community well south of San Diego—a lengthy drive from the house. The church was quite poor because of its small, low-income congregation. Dad told K.C. that occasionally he would go to the church on Sunday with Grace and make a "small donation" after the service.

K.C. was tempted to remind Dad that he had been Jewish for the past eighty-two years. He even had been an officer and board member of his local temple for many years—a temple that had probably the largest congregation in the city—and he had brought up his children in a Jewish household. But K.C. didn't want to get into an argument with him when, from his description, he seemed to be deriving some enjoyment from these occasional visits to church. She did ask, in passing, how much he had donated.

He responded in his typical manner when he didn't want to answer questions that invaded his private domain by saying, "Not much, maybe a few dollars." She could tell by the tone of his voice that he did not want further discussion of the subject. K.C. also understood that it was none of her business how much Dad donated to the church, or what he did with his money. After all, the money was his.

A few dollars, however, was an enormous understatement. Dad was not rolling in cash, so the thousands of dollars he had donated was a lot of money. Also, it seemed strange that a Jewish man would donate a large amount of money to a Christian church.

The situation had now moved beyond merely disturbing. This was serious money and serious abuse of my father. I knew now that Grace had to go. I asked K.C. to work with an agency to line up some care-givers who were bonded. I also asked her if she would fax to me the copies of the canceled checks. I needed to see them with my own eyes.

I told my sister that I was looking forward to seeing her and that things would work out. As I hung up the telephone, I believed in my heart that I had told her the truth.

Now that I had this new knowledge about Grace's receiving nearly three times her agreed-upon salary, combined with the unusually large dona-tions to the church, I again called the San Diego lawyer to discuss the possibility of my being appointed Ben's guardian and Grace being pros-ecuted for her actions. This was no longer a hypothetical situation. Now I had hard facts of serious abuse by Grace. I was loaded for bear.

Unfortunately, I had no ammunition in my rifle. All of my father's bizarre behavior, combined with the unexplained directive to his stock-broker, simply did not rise to the legal standard of "harm to himself or harm to others." In plain English I was told, "As long as Ben is mental-ly competent, don't look to the law for help unless your dad will testify against Grace."

While disheartened to hear the same advice as before from the lawyer, I felt I still had the only arrow in my quiver I really needed to put an end to this horrible nightmare. I was confident that once my father saw the hard evidence of how he had been bilked by Grace, he would fire her on the spot. He might even press criminal charges against her.

Dad was an honorable man. He had taught K.C. and me to believe in the golden rule: Treat others as you want to be treated. We were also taught that what goes around comes around. In other words, if you hurt someone, you will be hurt yourself. I was willing to bet the ranch that Dad would not take this obvious abuse by Grace passively. The Ben Carnot I knew would get mad as hell once he learned about how he had been manipulated over the last year by someone he trusted. He would want to take decisive action to protect others from Grace. This was the kind of man he was. For Grace, I knew it was about to "come around."

As I sat buckled into my seat, flying high over the clouds below, drawing ever closer to San Diego, I thought how wonderful it would be if Dad would sign the guardianship papers I was carrying in my briefcase. I knew I had an advantage over Grace, who was in China and would not be present to comment on the mountain of evidence K.C. had accumulated. I really didn't feel I needed any advantage, under the circumstances. The canceled checks made a compelling case of embezzlement, fraud, fraudulent inducement, and who knew what else, if Dad was willing to testify against Grace. Still, the task of presenting the evidence would be easier without Grace nearby. I hoped that Dad would get so mad for letting himself be duped into paying her and her son's church more than $100,000 over the last year that he would realize he would be better off signing the guardianship papers and letting me manage his financial affairs.

My plan was simple: Show Dad the evidence, get rid of Grace and her kids, retain new, reliable care providers, and maybe even get Dad to agree that I could act as his guardian. If I could do all this it would be a grand slam. Even if I accomplished only a few of these goals, I was confident that the game was over for Grace.

Legal Remedies: What You Can Do

The suggestions and legal remedies presented in this section and in the rest of this book have been generalized so that they apply in all states. You might find some slight differences in your state's law, but those differences will be minimal.

POWERS OF ATTORNEY

As you learned in this chapter, the only legal tool I had to prevent immediate financial disaster from befalling my father and K.C. was the power of attorney he had signed many years ago. With this document, I was able to thwart Dad's order to his stockbroker to liquidate his portfolio. Simply defined, a power of attorney is an authorization for someone else (known as the "attorney-in-fact") to act on behalf of another person (known as the "principal").

In all my years as an attorney working with clients on wealth-preservation issues, I have never failed to recommend that they sign a power of attorney naming someone they trusted as their attorney-in-fact. In fact, I consider a power of attorney one of the most important documents of every wealth-preservation plan. A power of attorney can be very narrow, such as giving the attorney-in-fact the right to sign checks while the principal is on vacation, or a power of attorney can grant much broader authority.

These broader powers of attorney generally fall into two categories:

1. General durable power of attorney
2. Power of attorney subject to a disability

General Durable Power of Attorney

A general durable power of attorney, commonly called a power of attorney, gives immediate authority to the attorney-in-fact to act on behalf of the principal. As soon as your parent signs a general durable power of attorney, if you are the person appointed as the attorney-in-fact, you have the authority to make financial decisions and sign documents on your parent's behalf. These documents might include checks, real estate listing agreements, change of address forms, deeds, mortgage applications, tax returns, charitable pledges, and many more. Obviously, this can be a valuable tool to help you protect your parent, as it was for me.

Another benefit of a general durable power of attorney is that it survives the mental incapacity of the principal. What this means is that if you have your parent's power of attorney and your parent becomes mentally incompetent, the power of attorney will remain in effect. That's the "durable" part of the document-the language within the power of attorney that specifies that even if your parent becomes incompetent, the power of attorney will not automatically be revoked by law.

This form of power of attorney is not without drawbacks, however. From your parent's perspective, a power of attorney has the effect of entrusting another person with control over all his or her assets. Should there be more than one child involved in the care of an aging parent, family disputes may arise when one sibling is chosen over another, or one sibling disagrees with the way the other sibling is managing the parent's assets. And, needless to say, the potential for abuse is large. If an unscrupulous or careless attorney-in-fact embezzles or fritters away the principal's assets, there is little that can be done to recover them. Obviously, parents must be careful and judicious in deciding to whom they should grant a general durable power of attorney.

The principle drawback from the child's perspective is that a general durable power of attorney can be revoked any time by a letter from the parent informing the attorney in fact that the power of attorney is revoked. All my father had to do was revoke my power of attorney, and I would have been powerless to prevent him from liquidating his portfolio.

Power of Attorney Subject to Disability

A power of attorney subject to a disability is the same as the general durable power of attorney except that the principal appoints the attorney-in-fact to act on his or her behalf only when the principal becomes incompetent. To activate this power of attorney, the principal's personal or attending physician must prepare a letter in which the doctor certifies—under penalty of perjury—that the patient is incompetent and incapable of managing his or her affairs. The benefit of this type of power of attorney is that it avoids a guardianship hearing, a complex, expensive procedure that is almost guaranteed to stir up ill will within a family. (Guardianships are discussed in detail in chapter 5.)

If you are named as the attorney-in-fact in your parent's power of attorney subject to disability, and the doctor certifies that your parent is incompetent, you need only attach the doctor's letter to the power of attorney, and you are then empowered to make decisions for your parent. In order words, at that point, the power of attorney subject to a disability operates in the same manner as the general durable power of attorney. On the surface, you might think that this form of power of attorney is all you need to protect your parent. Don't be deceived. If you suddenly discover that your parent is in the hands of an unscrupulous or abusive caregiver, you are powerless to act until you have the doctor's certification. Valuable time (and assets) can be lost while you pursue certification of mental incompetence.

REVOCABLE TRUSTS

Another common method to protect your parent from financial exploitation is a revocable trust. Don't be put off by the word "trust." The concept of a trust is simple, if you think about your basic knowledge of a corporation. A trust is similar, but different terms are used. As you know, the person who runs a corporation is the president, and the people who get distributions from the corporation are the shareholders. A trust is the same. The president of a trust is the "trustee," and the shareholders of a trust are called the "beneficiaries."

There are many different kinds of trusts, and most are not relevant for protecting an aging parent. But a revocable trust can be used for this purpose. A revocable trust is simply a trust in which the trustee (your parent) can change the terms or even end the trust, should he or she wish to.

Here's how it works. A revocable trust is prepared by an attorney for one parent or both parents. Let's assume here that only your father is alive when the revocable trust is prepared. Your father would transfer all of his assets to the trust. This can be as simple as your father going to the bank and changing the name on his savings and checking accounts from his name alone to his name as the trustee of the Revocable Trust. So, in my father's case, his savings and checking accounts would have read "Ben Carnot as Trustee of the Ben Carnot Revocable Trust." (There is no tax associated with this transfer or any other transfer of your parent's assets to a revocable trust.) According to the trust document, your father manages the trust as the trustee and is the sole beneficiary of the trust. This means that all distributions from the trust are made by the parent. For your parent, life is no different, because control over assets is not shifted to another person.

The way a revocable trust can help prevent financial exploitation is that in the revocable trust document your parent has to name a back-up trustee or a co-trustee. The person named as back-up or co-trustee should be someone the parent can trust, such as you or a sibling. A back-up trustee manages the trust assets for the benefit of the parent if the parent becomes incompetent or resigns as trustee. As a co-trustee, you and your parent would have to agree on all distributions from the trust, a situation similar to having a joint checking account with your parent in which both of your signatures are required on checks. The advantages to the co-trustee arrangement are obvious. The co-trustee would be in a position to prevent financial abuse when its earliest signs appear.

Your parent's estate-planning attorney will strongly endorse a revocable trust because it eliminates all probate costs. Further, once a parent moves his or her assets into a revocable trust, purely for estate-planning purposes, he or she soon decides to let the children come in as sole trustees and take over the management of the trust's assets for the parent's benefit. I wish I could explain why this happens, but it involves psychology that is well beyond my expertise. I can assure you, though, it happens all the time.

The drawback to the revocable trust is no different from the powers of attorney discussed earlier. The parent can dismiss the back-up trustee or co-trustee or cancel the revocable trust as easily as a power of attorney can be revoked. However, after having gone through the process of transferring assets to a revocable trust and paying an attorney for preparing the trust documents, your parent is less likely to dismiss you as a trustee. Your parent is simply too invested in the process to demand a change once the revocable trust has been funded.

Keep in mind that when you broach the subject of a power of attorney or a revocable trust, it should be done within the context of a family discussion about your parent's healthcare issues in general. Parents are often resistant initially to what they might perceive as interference by their children. Suggestions for a discussion of this type are detailed in chapter 2.

CHAPTER 2

The Confrontation

San Diego is especially beautiful at night, and landing there is always a breathtaking event. The final approach to the airport takes the plane right over the center of the city, past a few high-rise buildings, coming so close to them that from above it looks as if the wheels might touch their roofs. As we descended, I could see lights everywhere, showing off the city at its best, with the lights on the boats in the bay adding to the spectacular panoramic view. Even though I had not lived in San Diego for the last twenty-four years, when the wheels touched down, I felt I was home.

After claiming my bags and signing for a rental car, I used my cell phone to leave a message on my sister's answering machine to meet me at the house. By a little after eight, I was on my way to see my dad.

It wasn't far from the airport to my father's home in Point Loma, an older community in San Diego that occupies a peninsula bisecting the Pacific Ocean on the west side and San Diego Bay on the east. The drive is picturesque—alongside San Diego Bay, past the historic Naval Training Center, and then up a short, winding road through a canyon gorge to the top of the hill. Only fifteen minutes had passed since I left the airport, and I was just a few blocks from the house where I grew up.

Dad loved San Diego. He always referred to it as God's Country. He loved his house, too. The house was modest, built in the mid-1940s, and not big by anyone's standards. But it was comfortable, with a one-story floor plan comprising three bedrooms, two baths, a living room, dining room, family room, and kitchen. Out in back was a small yard. My father and mother were the original owners, having purchased it during the post-World War II building boom. K.C. and I had grown up in this house, and I always felt a special warmth when I returned for visits. As my childhood home came into view, memories of the many good times I spent there with my family were tugging at my heart.

I parked in the driveway and didn't bother retrieving the suitcase from the trunk because I couldn't wait to see Dad. I grabbed my briefcase from the passenger's seat and walked quickly to the front door. I didn't even have to knock. As I approached, the door opened and there stood my father, the man who had influenced my life so much and whom I loved so dearly.

Dad greeted me at the door in his usual style: a wide grin, a big bear hug and a kiss on the cheek. But his appearance was shocking. He was "dressed" in his undershorts, had open-toed bedroom slippers on his feet, and wore a loose-fitting sport shirt with only the second and third buttons fastened, not completely covering his torso. The few articles of clothing he wore were literally hanging on him. Even worse than his inappropriate attire, his face was gaunt, his hair was unkempt and well past gray, and he wasn't even standing erect but was listing forward and wobbling on his feet. This was only a shadow of the man I had last seen eleven months ago. He now looked heartbreakingly frail.

In spite of his appearance, Dad said he "felt great" and was "happy to see" me. I was sick inside at the way Dad looked but tried not to let my concern show on my face as I entered the house.

We walked together from the front door past the living room to the family room, where I put down my briefcase and asked to use the bathroom. Dad said he would get me a soda while I went to the "little boys' room." I headed for the bathroom I had used as a kid, walking from the family room to the hall and making a right. The bathroom was the second door down.

As I walked into the bathroom, I saw on the counter a large assortment of prescription drug bottles, maybe fifteen containers. This didn't concern me too much. Dad was eighty-two, after all, and I knew he had some heart problems, was diabetic, and had a few other medical conditions that would require lots of different medicines.

What did alarm me, however, was the cracking I felt beneath my feet as I crossed the threshold from the carpet on the hallway floor to the bare tile of the bathroom. I looked down to see that the floor where I was standing was literally covered with pills or their fragments. The cracking sound was my grinding the pills into powder as I stepped on them.

This discovery was troubling for a couple of reasons. First, it just seemed so out of character to find any disorder in Dad's house. Both my mother and Sue had insisted on a spotless house, and after their passing, my father had continued to employ Grace and other housekeepers to keep the house to their high standards. More troubling, though, was the clear evidence that Dad was not taking his medication properly. In addition to light housecleaning, Grace's responsibilities were to make sure that Dad ate well and took his medicine as prescribed by his doctors. Simple. Nothing more was required. And for this she had probably pulled down more than $100,000 last year! Again I started to seethe with anger as a result of this latest discovery. My hatred of Grace for abusing my dad was growing.

After I finished in the bathroom, I returned to the family room, anxious to talk with Dad. I wanted to determine whether he was capable of having an intelligent conversation with me. This was important if he was going to understand the information I had prepared about Grace.

I settled in, took a sip of soda, and didn't have to wait long before Dad started with his usual questions. "How are the kids, Ed, and how is Pamela?" I was relieved to hear him sound so normal. I relaxed a bit and told Dad about the family. Then he asked about my law practice. This would be the real test, I thought. He had always had a keen business mind, and I was interested to see if he would show his normal interest in a merger case I was involved in. I told him that I was working on a merger in which the acquiring company wanted to finance the acquisition with an increase in its line of credit. "In order to agree to the increase in the line," I explained, "the bank wants a lien on all of the inventory, equipment, and raw materials, which I think is excessive."

To my great relief, Dad jumped right in. "How much security is the bank asking for?" This was an astute question, in keeping with the business acumen he had always possessed. I relaxed even more.

"They're asking for almost five and one half times the amount of the increased line," I said. "This seems excessive to me because the acquiring company has a seven-year history of significant profitability."

"You're right, that's excessive," he said. "Don't worry. The bank will ultimately back off, if it's really serious about financing the transaction."

This conversation was a breath of fresh air. I was now convinced that my father had not lost his cognitive abilities. Getting rid of Grace will be a cinch, I thought. All I had to do was show Dad the evidence, and Grace would be history.

Nonetheless, I was still concerned about my dad's appearance. K.C.'s description had not prepared me for the person I was now seeing with my own eyes. Same old voice, smile and easy manner, but, God, he looked awful. I was reluctant to comment on his appearance for fear of angering him and starting the important conversation to come on the wrong foot. So I decided to try what I thought was a neutral question.

"Dad, why are all of those pills on the floor in the bathroom?"

"Oh, sometimes they fall out of my hand, which trembles a lot lately," Dad said. "I have trouble bending over to pick them up, so I just wait for Grace to clean them up."

This seemed like a reasonable response, although I still was not pleased by what I had heard. I pushed a little further. "Dad, I'm concerned about how many pills are on the floor. Are you taking your medicine?"

"Oh, yes, Son," he assured me. "Every morning I take all of my medicine, just like the doctor ordered. The doctor says I'm doing great, Ed."

"But Dad, who makes sure that you take what you're supposed to?"

I could tell that he was starting to get defensive. In a tone of voice that said "back off," Dad said, "Ed, let's not talk about my medicine. I take what my doctors prescribe. Grace makes sure that I follow the doctors' orders. And my doctors all say I'm in good health for my age. Now, let's talk about something else."

Dad had never had trouble communicating his feelings. In fact, he was a little quick to anger in his later years. He was an independent person who obviously did not want his kids nosing around in his private life. Knowing this, I decided it really wasn't important to determine whether Grace was properly monitoring Dad's meds. My goal was simply to get rid of her and get my father some reliable caregivers. The ammunition was tucked away in my briefcase, but I didn't want to fire the bullets until K.C. arrived. I could hardly wait to make my case; I was looking forward to exposing Grace's treachery. However, while waiting for K.C., the last thing I wanted to do was to light Dad's short fuse about some pills on the floor, so I backed off. Way, way off.

I dropped my probing about Dad's meds, and we had a nice, neutral conversation about K.C.'s children. The talk meandered to the weather in California versus Maryland and on to the NBA playoffs. While we were debating the prospects of the Chicago Bulls, I heard a car in the driveway, and I knew K.C. had arrived. I don't know if it showed on my face, but my heart was starting to pound. In just a few minutes it would be "show time," and I needed to get mentally focused.

K.C. was through the door without delay, and I could see she hadn't changed since I had seen her the previous year. For as long as I could remember, K.C. had always looked liked she had stepped out of a fashion magazine. No matter what she wore, she looked perfect. Every hair in place, petite and trim and always dressed in an attractive outfit. This evening was no different; she looked great.

K.C. was also one of the most bubbly people I knew, and truly a good person. She was always around to help our father when Mom was sick. Then, after Mom died, K.C. was constantly "on the job," looking out for Dad. It was extremely painful for K.C. when her marriage of fourteen years broke up in 1985. She was never one to hold a grudge, however, and she worked hard to maintain a good relationship with her ex-husband. When she walked into the family room it was as if she brought the sun with her. I could see the glow of happiness and love on Dad's face when he saw his little bird.

After kisses and hugs all around and some small talk about the family, we all sat down in the family room, and I got down to business. I pulled my chair directly in front of Dad so that we were almost knee to knee, looked him in the eye and delivered the message I had been rehearsing on the airplane. "K.C. and I are greatly concerned about your welfare," I began. "We want you to stop using Grace because she has been taking advantage of you." So far, so good. Dad was at least listening. "I want to ask a few questions, and I do not want you to fly off the handle and get mad," I continued. "Then, I want to show you something that will make your blood boil. I've flown three thousand miles to be with you because K.C. and I love you, and we have some real concerns about your welfare." Then I asked him to make two promises: "Will you promise not to get mad? And will you promise to answer a few questions?"

My hope that Dad would be receptive disintegrated quickly. He immediately became defensive, already not liking the subject of the conversation. I could almost see the grey hairs rising up on his neck as he looked from me to K.C. and back to me.

"What concerns? What is this about? Grace is a wonderful person. She's been my savior since Sue died. You know she has been with the family forever. She is wonderful to me." Dad was getting worked up. I knew that he was capable of getting so angry that he would lose his ability to listen to reason. But I had to keep going.

In a lower tone of voice, while I continued looking him straight in the eye, I asked him again if he would answer a few questions without getting mad. I repeated that I loved him, but I needed some important questions answered. Would he cooperate? Dad said he would, but his voice betrayed his reluctance to discuss matters pertaining to Grace. Nevertheless, I pressed on with my first question.

"Dad," I began, "I understand that you have been paying money to a church. What is this church, and why are you paying money to it?"

I could almost see the wheels in his mind turning as he debated whether to abide by his promise and answer my questions. With an air of indifference, Dad explained that Grace's son was the minister of a recently formed church south of San Diego. "The church is poor," he said, "because it has only a few members, most of whom are unemployed." He told us that Grace, a religious and God-fearing Christian, had taken him to the church on several Sundays. Sometimes he was recognized by the minister (her son), who asked the parishioners to pray for Dad's salvation from his sins. At the end of the service, Dad would give a donation to the church, which was "just a few dollars."

A few dollars! I wondered if Dad had any idea that the amount he had given to the church totaled several thousand dollars. I resisted the temptation to ask him why he had given any money to a church, given the fact that he was Jewish. Instead, I asked him why one of the larger checks had the notation "fashion show" on the memo line, and another said "musical instruments."

Dad's answer was straightforward, albeit irritating for me to hear. "The church had a fashion show as a fund-raiser, which I went to with Grace. Her daughter was the fashion designer. After the fashions were modeled, some by Grace herself, I decided to buy them all for Grace." Again, he indicated that the money he spent for the clothes was "only a few dollars." I was furious, realizing now that Grace was apparently the appointed fund-raiser for the church, and Dad was the fund.

The musical instruments purchase was yet another stunning story involving the poor fledgling church. It seemed the church was in need of some musical instruments for an ensemble it hoped to organize. During one prayer session (with Dad probably sitting front-row center) the minister offered up prayers for a savior to help them with funds for this most important purchase. In my imagination I could see the minister with his hands stretched up toward the heavens, calling on the great creator for help while looking directly at Dad with a loving smile. Of course his prayers were answered on the spot by their patron saint on earth, Ben Carnot, who funded the musical instruments. Dad explained that "it was only a few dollars."

Was Dad so sick that he couldn't see what was happening? "How many dollars?" I asked. I just couldn't resist asking this question, even though I knew I was treading on thin ice.

"I don't remember the exact amount," Dad claimed.

I knew the number, however, which was far from a few dollars. On the basis of the checks I saw, Dad's charitable contributions, along with the money he was giving Grace, could have funded the musical instrument needs and new uniforms for the entire Ohio State marching band.

I could see in Dad's eyes that he was confused and getting more angry by the second with my prying questions. As our eyes locked, I knew he was rapidly losing his attention to anger, so I decided it was time to present my evidence. "How often do you pay Grace?" I asked.

Dad fought the question. "Ed, I don't want to talk about this any more."

"Dad, you promised to cooperate," I reminded him.

Reluctantly, Dad indicated that he paid Grace "once a week." He didn't know the day he paid her; it was up to Grace to remind him when her check was due because he couldn't remember things as well as he had in the past. He did remember that she was paid $400 per week.

Dad was getting angry. His volatile personality was taking over, and the love in the air was dissipating quickly. "What's this all about? I told you, Grace is an honorable, highly educated person from a wonderful family." He went on, "Ed, stop this. I don't want to talk about Grace any more."

It was time to cut to the chase. "I have something to show you, Dad." I reached for my briefcase to pull out the photocopies of his checks for the last year, when the phone rang.

Dad's easy chair was always strategically placed in arm's reach of the telephone, which was sitting on the corner of a nearby desk; however, when I had moved my chair in front of his in order to talk to him face-to-face, I ended up closer to the telephone than he was. I stared at the ringing phone in irritation and realized that my heart was racing from the stress of just getting some background facts about Grace from my dad. Now here I was, about to present the compelling evidence that would bring an end to this nightmare, and I was being interrupted by someone who could not have picked a worse time to call. The phone rang a second time. I looked at my father, and I picked up the receiver.

"Hello, Carnot residence."

"Hello, this is Grace."

Are you kidding me? This is a bad dream! She was supposed to be in China! I was so taken by surprise, given the heat of the moment, that I said the first thing that popped into my mind. "I thought you were in China." Grace was effervescent on the other end of the phone. She said she had cut her trip short because she was not having a good time: she was back from China and wanted to talk to Dad to see how he was doing. She was going on about how much she missed Dad, and while she was rambling on, I cut her off in mid-sentence.

I had regained my composure, calmed down, and after taking a deep breath I delivered the message I had been looking forward to since my sister first told me about Grace's abuse of dad. "Grace, you are never to call this number again. You are not to come by the house ever again. You are not to have any contact with my father."

I couldn't tell if she was shocked or had already prepared for the worst. But her response was easily anticipated under the circumstances. She said, "Why? What are you talking about?"

I didn't miss a beat. In a calm and even tone I said, "Grace, you know why," and I hung up the telephone, slamming it into its cradle.

Back from China. I didn't believe her for a moment. I knew you couldn't just change your plans in China, a communist country, and return to the States as easily as you hop onto a commuter plane from New York to Boston. I was no expert, but I assumed it was equally, if not more, difficult to change airline reservations in China as in the third world countries I had visited. There is a lot of paperwork; sometimes a visit to an embassy is required along with a substantial penalty for a new ticket. I realized that Grace had never gone to China. She was probably just taking some time off from bleeding the walking wounded.

Grace obviously knew something was afoot when Dad told her son Thomas that his services were not needed because I was coming to visit. She must have decided to call to test the waters. I knew when I hung up that Grace clearly understood the reason for her abrupt termination, but I could only imagine the conversation that was going on in her house right then. I would have loved to be a fly on the wall when she delivered the message to her children. I wondered if she was saying, "The jig is up, we need to get packing," or "Can you believe that SOB Ed? Where does he come off telling me that I can't take care of Ben? I have only acted in his best interest, haven't I? All of the good years I have given to Ben, and Ed has the nerve to tell me that I'm fired. I'll talk to Ben and get this straightened out." Impossible to know what she was thinking and saying, but I had a feeling that I would find out in the future.

My daydreams were cut short, however, because Dad exploded in anger. World War III was now underway. "How could you do that to Grace?" he yelled. "She is such a fine person!" Dad was hot, hotter then I had ever seen him. Reaching for the telephone he said, "Let me call her back and apologize. Ed, what right do you have to come into this house and fire Grace? This is my house. Where do you come off—?"

I was physically and emotionally shocked, as if an actual explosion had gone off in the room, and I responded reflexively, reacting without even thinking about what I was doing. I physically restrained Dad from picking up the telephone receiver by putting my hands down hard on his hand, and then I grabbed the entire telephone from under his hand. Dad stood up to reach for the phone, but I was already on my feet, with the phone in my hands, holding it away from him. Dad took wobbly steps toward me, trying to get more leverage to grab the phone, but I kept backing away from him. At the same time, I was watching Dad, hoping and praying that he would not fall while trying to get the phone from me. He was so unstable that he ultimately planted his right hand on the desk for support and stayed there, not wishing to test his legs further.

I was feeling out of control myself. Never in my life had I physically interfered with my father. The mere act of holding my father's hand down on the receiver and then grabbing the telephone was a show of force that I never would have thought I was capable of. "You do not hit your sister," I had been taught. No one ever had to tell me that you also do not hit your parent; I knew better. Yet here I had as good as hit my father. I had pushed his hand down on top of the phone so he couldn't pick it up, and then I had pulled the phone away from his grasp. I couldn't believe what I had done. All the confidence I had maintained until Grace's call was now gone. Tears were beginning to well in my eyes as I was flooded with emotions. I barely got the words out that I needed to say. "Dad, you have to look at this. Grace has been stealing money from you," I said softly, hoping to calm everyone down, including myself.

By this time, K.C., too, was up and out of her chair, by our father's side with her hands gently on his shoulders. She helped him back into his chair, telling him it would be best if he sat and listened to what I had to say. I think both Dad and I were grateful for her calming presence and her ability to help cool somewhat the highly charged emotions in the room. Dad didn't resist K.C.'s efforts. As he sat, even though he was breathing heavily, he delivered some not-so-nice opinions about my intrusion into his life, which I ignored. He had a right to be mad about my firing Grace, because he had not seen the evidence in my briefcase.

I sat down as well and reached for my briefcase. Once I had it on my lap, I released the two brass latches, opened the lid and reached inside, pulling out a sheaf of papers that were secured by a large paper clip. While fumbling with my briefcase, I could almost feel Dad's eyes boring through me. When I looked up, I saw a face that was contorted with rage. Dad was still breathing deeply, trying to get himself under control. I took a few deep breaths myself to regain my composure. Then, in a soft monotone voice, I explained that K.C. had gotten photocopies of all of Dad's checks for the last year, and that the checks told a vivid story of rampant financial abuse by Grace.

First, I showed my father the charts I had prepared using the information from the copies of his canceled checks. They clearly proved that Grace, who should have been paid about $21,000 per year, had received more than three times that amount during the past year, and it looked like she was on track to do the same for this year. Then I gave Dad the photocopies of the checks.

My hopes began to rise somewhat because Dad seemed interested in what I was saying. He had calmed down a bit, although he was still breathing heavily. My charts were quite detailed, showing for each check the check number, the date written, the payee and the amount, partly because I knew Dad appreciated scrupulous attention to detail, but mainly because I didn't want him to have any doubt about the accuracy of the tally and the extent of Grace's malfeasance. I wanted to drive home the point of how Grace had consistently fleeced him over time.

I was starting to feel better and more confident as I continued with my presentation. By this time Dad also appeared to have cooled down to almost normal, so it was easier to talk to him even though I was still shaking from our altercation. I explained how all of the information on the charts had been cross-referenced to the front and back photocopies of the checks, so Dad could easily confirm their accuracy and see Grace's endorsement on each check.

I waited a moment or two for this information to sink in, and then I reminded Dad that Grace was supposed to get paid once a week. I pointed out that, according to the charts, on many occasions Dad had signed two paychecks per week; unbelievably, he frequently had signed three and sometimes even four.

I wanted my father also to realize how he had been abused by the church. I went over with him a similar presentation of the checks made out to the church, a sum that was anything but a "small amount of money." I didn't even get into the religion issue. The facts were compelling enough without the garnish.

The hook had been well set, I thought. Now it was time to sit back and see if the presentation had sunk in. There was no doubt that I had Dad's attention. I could see that he was carefully looking at his signature on each check, spending time with each sheet of paper. It appeared that after checking Grace's endorsement, Dad was verifying the charts' accuracy, comparing the check number, amount and date to the copies of the checks. As each moment passed, I was more confident that a guilty verdict was assured. Grace was about to get her comeuppance.

I glanced at K.C. who gave me a furtive "thumbs up," a smile, and a slight nod of her head. I was feeling so good that I sort of wished Grace could be there to face the public humiliation of Dad telling her to get out of his life forever. No, better this way, gone and forgotten forever. I indulged in other delicious thoughts. Maybe Dad would call the police. I pictured the police taking her away in silver bracelets. It would be a beautiful sight for my sister and me. I was feeling so good that I allowed a slight grin of satisfaction to spread on my face. While waiting for Dad's edict, I even started thinking about changing my airline reservations to go back home earlier then I had planned.

I was confident that in a few more minutes, after he had fully digested the evidence I had prepared, Dad would look up from the papers and say to both of us, "Thank you for looking out for me," which was all we needed. I was prepared to respond, "It's okay, Dad, we love you." Then, maybe I could bring out the guardianship papers. At that point it should be easy to get Dad to sign, so that a train wreck like Grace could never happen to him again. I was itching to get ready with the guardianship papers, but I squelched the impulse, waiting until my father gave me the opening I was expecting, probably within the next few seconds.

After what seemed like hours, but was probably only minutes, Dad looked up and started to talk.

My heart was pounding. I realized I was so anxious to hear what my father had to say that I had inched forward on my chair until I was sitting on its edge. What I heard from my father would be indelibly inscribed in my mind.

"There must be some mistake. I will talk to Grace. I will take care of this." That was it. Dad stopped talking and looked from K.C. to me and back to K.C. Only silence followed.

A wave of heat spread over me, beginning in my face and then moving down my body to my toes. I felt as if I had just stepped into an oven. I could not believe what I had just heard. "What did you say?" I stammered. "Mistake, how could there be some mistake?" Yelling now, and having really lost my temper, I continued. "You have the evidence in spades. She is raping you and you can't say anything more than 'I will take care of it.'?"

K.C. was less loquacious, but just as forceful. "Dad, she is not good for you. Grace did good work for you in the past; she took care of Mom and Sue. We know that she took good care of you. But no longer. She has changed. She has been taking advantage of you. You should be grateful that we figured this all out before it was too late."

No further response from Dad. He had rendered his judgment and there was not going to be an appeal. Not tonight at least. Here was the person I had always admired for his sharp mind and strong ethical fiber who for some reason could not confront the truth. "Dad, she has been stealing from you, probably for years," I added in a loud voice. "What do you mean, 'there must be some mistake?' She's a thief!"

Dad was unshaken in his judgment. Sitting in his chair, he came to Grace's defense: "She is a fine person. There has to be an explanation. I will take care of this when I see her." Then, looking at me, he continued in a stern voice. "Ed, this is none of your business."

"Dad, what do you mean it's none of my business? This is robbery, larceny, and who knows what else. Not only is it my business, it's the business of the District Attorney."

"Ed, I don't want you getting involved," Dad said. "When I see Grace, I will discuss this with her. I am sure there is a plausible explanation. I don't want to discuss this anymore."

Frustrated and seeing that the conversation was going nowhere, I told my father, "Grace is not coming back. If she does, I will go the District Attorney's office myself and swear out a criminal complaint against her." I really didn't know what one did at the DA's office to get the process rolling, or what specific crimes had been committed, but I felt it was essential to sound like I was serious about taking all steps necessary to separate the two of them permanently. The message, not the factual content, was most important.

Dad was extremely agitated as K.C. and I went on about Grace's abuse of him. "Ed," he said, as he leaned forward and pointed his finger not two inches from my face, "Don't you tell me how to run my life. Grace is a good person; she has taken good care of me for many years." There was more from my dad, but I had tuned him out. He was going on and on, repeating the same thoughts using slightly different words. This situation was much more serious than I had anticipated. I had been confident that as soon as I presented the evidence of Grace's abuses to my dad, she would be out of the picture, gone and forgotten. However, I was hearing from Dad that Grace was the only person he wanted to care for him, despite some "irregularities," which Dad was sure would be explained when he spoke with her.

I was speechless. Grace had become the most important person in Dad's life. Even more important than his daughter and his son.

The talking and yelling went on for what seemed like hours. K.C. tried again to reason with Dad about Grace, covering the same ground as I had and adding some observations of her own about how inadequate Grace's care had become. She told him that he did not look well nourished; she emphasized her concern that he was not taking his medicine; and, of course, she repeated that Grace had been grossly overpaid. "These checks speak volumes, Dad. You cannot simply ignore them. They are not an isolated instance of a mistake, but a repeated pattern of abuse of you by Grace."

But Dad would hear nothing of these arguments, rejecting them with his comment that Grace was taking good care of him and repeating that K.C. "should mind her own business."

It became clear that nothing was going to be resolved that night. Inwardly, Dad was the proverbial brick wall. He would not yield. Given the hour and the fact that all that could be said had been said, it was time to give up for the evening and go to bed. Dad was already making some not-so-subtle comments about being tired, which were designed to break up the "party." I looked at my dad, and he seemed to have aged even more in the last few hours. He looked like he had been beaten down. His shoulders were sagging, his eyes watery, and his face drawn, but his resolve and commitment to Grace were like iron.

I picked up on Dad's theme, saying that I was tired myself, having traveled three thousand miles that day. Getting some much-needed shut-eye sounded appealing. I could only hope that after a good night's rest, Dad would acknowledge Grace's abuses and agree that she was bad for him. Not a realistic thought, I knew, but a hope. I was entitled to have hope.

Long-Distance Caregiving: What You Can Do

For many years, my version of long-distance caregiving was limited to an annual visit to San Diego and weekly telephone calls to my father. When I learned how Grace was taking advantage of Dad, I quickly discovered what can and cannot be accomplished when you don't live in the same city as your parent. I was lucky; I had a sister who was living in San Diego when my father's situation began to spiral out of control. But countless others are not so fortunate. You might be surprised to learn that of the estimated 30 million caregivers in the United States, 7 million of them are caring for someone older than 55 who lives at least an hour away (Seff, 2002).

Measures can be taken to help you be an effective caregiver for an aging parent, whether you live thirty or three thousand miles away. Remember, the last thing you want is the type of confrontation I had with my dad. However, with some forethought, you can take steps that will not only protect your loved one but will also give you peace of mind. There are three stages to plan for, each of which is absolutely essential:

1. Advance planning
2. Ongoing caregiving
3. Acute or emergency measures

Of course, you will need to adapt the following suggestions to your own circumstances, but by employing as many of them as possible, you can create a blueprint for successful long-distance caregiving.

ADVANCE PLANNING

The goal of advance planning is to develop a comprehensive plan of care for your parent or parents while they can actively participate in the planning process. Much of your success will depend on how much planning you do with your parents at a time in their lives when they are able to recognize and appreciate the need to plan for their future care. You alone, however, know your parents and probably have a reasonably good idea of how much of your involvement they will tolerate. Still, if you plan a family meeting before your parents' needs become acute, you can discuss their wishes and concerns, express your own concerns and agree upon the best steps to take, which, in the end, will make everyone feel more comfortable.

The Family Meeting

Plan a meeting that will include you, your parents, your siblings and anyone else who is likely to be closely involved in their current or future caregiving. Arrange a time when all parties who live out of town can be present. It's important that, before the meeting, everyone involved has a clear understanding of the current situation and the options under consideration for the future.

The best scenario is to have this meeting while both of your parents are still living. Then, when only one parent remains, if dissent over a care plan arises, it can be helpful to remind that parent that the steps you are taking are part of a plan that both parents devised earlier. But even if only one of your parents is still living, a meeting of this type can be equally effective and, in some cases, even more important.

As a prelude to the meeting, set your parents' fears to rest about why such a meeting is necessary. Tell your parents that it is important that their wishes be known ahead of time, so the family can provide them with the care they desire if the time comes when they can't make their own decisions. Reassure your parents that you are not trying to worm your way into their private affairs or wrest control of their assets from them. Explain often that your sole purpose for suggesting a family meeting is to avoid having to make decisions for them in the future that they would not approve. The only way to accomplish these goals is to address certain issues ahead of time, no matter how uncomfortable such a discussion might be for all involved.

A family meeting of this nature is bound to be emotional, which can steer you off track in a hurry. Don't rely on your memory to cover every item you believe is important. Write your priorities down and circulate your ideas to the family members before the meeting, so there will no surprises about the topics for discussion. Also, ask your family members for suggestions of other issues to be added to the agenda.

It's important to avoid having anyone feel left out of the agenda-planning process. Your goal is for everyone involved to feel well informed about the purpose of the meeting. The best way to achieve this goal is to distribute, well before the meeting, a "final" agenda that includes suggested topics you have received from everyone who will attend.

During the meeting, follow the agenda, recording what is said so there will be no misunderstandings later. Although each family's needs and desires are unique, the following is a list of the most important subjects that should be discussed *and settled.*

•**Residence.** Are your parents adamant about remaining in the family home until death? Do they envision an eventual move to a senior community that provides assisted living? How do your parents feel about nursing homes? These are critical issues to decide early, because they affect nearly every other care decision down the line.

•**Legal Issues.** This would be an ideal time to discuss a general durable power of attorney or a revocable trust. At a minimum, suggest a dual-signatory checking account. (The advantages and disadvantages of general durable powers of attorney and revocable trusts are explained in chapter 1.) A dual-signatory checking account requires that both your parent and whoever is appointed as the second signer must sign all checks. If the second signer is you or a sibling, this provides an added layer of protection against inappropriate expenditures. The disadvantage of this arrangement is that it is changeable at the will of your parent. You will recall that my dad closed his checking account with K.C. as the co-signatory and opened instead a more traditional account requiring only his signature.

Even if your parents aren't immediately ready to act on any of these ideas, you will have at least paved the way for a subsequent discussion. As part of this meeting or in anticipation of it, I strongly suggest that you ask your parents' permission to contact their attorney to ask him or her to discuss with them the legal issues outlined in chapters 1 and 5. A benefit of this approach is that you will get the name of your parents' attorney if you don't have it, and, more important, the attorney will strongly endorse the recommendations you are reading about in this book.

You should ask the attorney to speak with your parents about these legal issues before the family meeting, and try to get a resolution ahead of time so you do not have to spend time on these matters during the meeting. You also might consider asking your parents' attorney to attend the family meeting in order to have an independent third party present whose opinion your parents respect.

•**Finances/Insurance.** A more delicate conversation, but an important one, concerns whether your parents have the financial resources and/or insurance to cover health problems and caregiving needs that might occur. If you have not done so by now, you should find out the location of your parents' assets (bank accounts, real property, stock accounts, etc.), and, if they seem receptive, perhaps even the size of their estate. Get the name of your parents' accountant, who will be invaluable if you have to locate your parents' assets. My father began discussing these subjects with me when I started college. Whenever I returned to San Diego, he would sit me down in his office and tell me how his records were kept, where his assets were located, and who to contact should the need arise.

I know, however, that many of my clients are extremely reluctant to discuss such financial issues with their children. Their reluctance is based on a fear that if the children learn about the size of their estate, they will be less willing to work hard to make their own way in the world. Instead, they will look to their parents for support. I respect this position. If your parents fall into this category, ask them to provide information about their assets to someone who is not a family member, perhaps their accountant or lawyer, just in case you have to step in and take control if one or both of your parents become incapacitated.

I also suggest that you review with your parents all insurance policies. Depending on their health, it might be advisable to suggest securing a healthcare policy that would be a supplement to Medicare. You might also discuss long-term healthcare insurance plans. Insurance options are discussed in detail in chapter 6.

•**Power of Attorney for Healthcare, Living Will.** Both of these critically important legal documents are explained in chapter 5. Make sure they are on your agenda because they present the best opportunities for your parents to be specific about their feelings concerning extraordinary life-sustaining measures and to what extent they will be administered should the need arise. Better yet, I again suggest that your parents' attorney help resolve these issues before the family meeting.

•**Caregivers.** A recent AARP survey indicates that approximately 89 percent of those surveyed want to stay in their current residence for as long as possible (Bayer, 2000). If your parents have expressed a desire to remain at home, you will need to have a discussion about employing a continuum of caregiving services, ranging from light housekeeping and meal preparation to nursing care, as your parents' needs increase. If you or your siblings live in the same city as your parents, you should agree on what your and their involvement in caregiving should be. Selecting a caregiver is one of the most critical and difficult decisions to be made. See chapter 8 for guidance to help you with the selection process.

These are the primary issues to include on your agenda for the family meeting. I'm sure you will think of others that are specific to your family's circumstances. Before, during, and after your family meeting, be sure to stress to your parents that you are acting solely out of love and a desire to provide them the best possible care and protection-all in accordance with their wishes.

In a perfect world, you would get through this agenda with time to spare for a family dinner. Unfortunately, this is not a perfect world, and the issues being discussed are weighty. The process will be slowed down by each family member weighing in with an option. Don't worry.

If decisions are not reached on all critical issues, and it would be difficult to reconvene a family meeting within the next few weeks, appoint one member of the family to resolve the remaining issues. This selected family member must be willing to shoulder the additional responsibility of acting as a liaison to the others and keeping everyone apprised of the decisions made in their absence. Under these circumstances, it is best to establish at the meeting an outside date for the resolution of issues with the family liaison or through another family meeting. Without a sunset date for these issues, they will hang around forever.

Gathering a family together is a special occasion that should not be squandered. Try to plan a family dinner for after the meeting. It will give everyone a chance to relax after a conversation that is sure to take an emotional toll. No one wants to admit that a loved one, especially a parent, is facing the many problems associated with old age. So take advantage of your time together to give everyone a chance to share the love of family.

Above all, don't try to plan for every eventuality for the rest of your parents' lives. It is impossible to foresee everything that could happen up until the end. Treat advanced planning as an evolving process. I like to suggest planning for five years out. Three years thereafter, get the family together again and plan for another five years. This way you don't have to look too far over the horizon, and you will always have a current roster of your parents' wishes. As long as your parents are competent, it is of the utmost importance to get their opinion on these critical issues so that when they start to slip, everyone agrees on how to take care of them because it was fully discussed when your parents could express their desires. Finally, to avoid problems in the future about what was decided at the family meeting, each person who attended should receive a copy of a memo summarizing the decisions that were made.

ONGOING CAREGIVING

You've taken every preventive measure you can think of, and you've completed all your advance planning. As a long-distance caregiver, though, what do you watch for as time goes by? One of the problems with long-distance caregiving is that often caregivers and care receivers will differ in their perceptions, especially when only one parent is alive. At times it may seem that your parent refuses to admit a problem, and, at other times, even a small difficulty can be exaggerated. How you respond can vary, too. Some caregivers are filled with anxiety, imagining the worst and overreacting to insignificant problems (Heath, 1993).

On the Telephone

Frequent telephone conversations with your parent can provide many clues to how things are really going. As with my calls to my dad, I knew what to expect from him when we spoke each week. When the tone of the conversation changed and his responses were dramatically different, it was a clear signal that something was wrong. Often your parent will be reluctant to admit to a problem, but if you start with gentle questioning about things in general, then move on to more specific conversation about health issues or other potential problems, you might get some clues. It's helpful, too, for both of you, if you plan to speak on the telephone at prearranged times.

In Person

Visiting your parent in person is your best opportunity to assess the current situation. Ideally you should schedule regular visits, but if this is not possible, enlist the aid of a sibling or other family member, a church or temple member, or a friend who lives in the same city as your parent to perform regular checks. The following are some potential trouble spots that you or someone else should be looking for:

•**Medications.** Ensure that your parent's caregiver (and your parent, if possible) understands which medications are to be taken, at what times, and the proper dosage of each. Make a chart to hang in a convenient spot with spaces for checkmarks for the caregiver to record each medication as it is taken.

•**Physical Appearance.** Much can be learned by simply observing your parent's appearance. Is your parent's clothing clean? Do the socks match? How does the clothing fit? Does your parent look well-groomed, have good color, and appear physically sound? Has there been a significant weight loss or gain? Observe your parent's behavior, too, for indications of lessened cognitive ability. Look for signs of confusion or loss of ability to perform simple tasks.

•**Condition of the Home.** Is your parent's once-tidy home showing signs of neglect? Is there food in the refrigerator? Is any of it spoiled? Is dirty laundry piling up? Are there pills on the bathroom floor? Be alert for signs that your parent may be unable to properly care for the home or perform such tasks as grocery shopping. Also, assess the home for safety hazards such as frayed electrical cords, loose carpeting or rugs, broken windows, or insect infestations. These are signs that your parent may need more professional care at home.

•**Mail.** Look for piles of unopened mail. This could be a sign that bills are not being paid and that your parent is losing the ability to handle day-to-day finances.

Ideally, you should try to schedule doctors' appointments for your parent while you are visiting for two important reasons:

1. You can learn a lot by accompanying your parent to the doctor: information that can reassure you that all is well, or information that tells you it's time to make some adjustments in your parent's care plan.
2. The doctor will feel comfortable talking to you on the telephone. If the doctor understands the close relationship you have with your parent, he or she may be less inclined to adhere rigidly to the laws pertaining to patient confidentiality discussed in chapter 5.

Even though you are far away, you can accumulate some tools to ease your anxiety and to help you in case an emergency arises.

•Keep a phone book from your parent's city at home with you.

•Have your parent's doctors' names and phone numbers handy.

•Make a list of friends, neighbors, clergy, and others (and their telephone numbers) who are in regular contact with your parent.

•Familiarize yourself with what local agencies can offer in the way of support, such as meal delivery, social opportunities, and transportation.

•Write down where your parent's important documents are located.

•Keep a list of the name and recommended dosage of the medications your parent is taking so that if necessary you can ask specific questions about each one.

ACUTE OR EMERGENCY MEASURES

By the time I realized there was a problem with my father's caregiving, it had already reached the emergency stage. Although I was able to accomplish a small measure of advance planning by having Dad give me power of attorney, I simply wasn't prepared for how badly his situation had deteriorated. Thus, K.C. and I had to take immediate, emergency steps to try to protect him.

If you're living far away and you get a phone call that sets off alarm bells, you must be prepared to make some quick decisions. However, before you jump on the first plane headed for your parent's city, perform a brief assessment of the situation.

•Call your local contacts (doctors, siblings, friends, helpers) to get feedback as to the severity of your parent's situation.

•Try to put the current situation in the context of your parent's normal reactions. As I noted earlier, some parents overreact, some underreact. How does your parent tend to evaluate problems?

•Assess your own reactions, as well. Do you have a tendency to overreact to what could be a small problem? If so, then it's even more important for you to gather information from others before you race to your parent's side.

•Ask yourself how you and your parent will probably feel if you don't go, or if you delay your trip.

Some situations, of course, will be immediately identifiable as bona fide emergencies, such as an accident, other medical crisis, or a caregiving emergency like my father's. In that case, the decision is clear. It's time to get to your parent as quickly as possible. If a medical emergency is at hand, the doctors will need someone who is empowered to make decisions for your parent, and, if you've been successful in your advance planning, you will have the necessary documents (for example, Power of Attorney for Health Care and Living Will) with you to affirm your decision-making authority. Emergencies are much easier to cope with if you don't have to waste time wrangling with legalities.

No matter what your parent's emergency situation might be, the fact is that you can best handle it if you are there in person. Decisions will need to be made, and it's hard to think clearly and make good choices when you're far away. Also, once there, you will have allies in those who are on-site to help oversee your parent's care. Chances are you will be faced with some tough decisions. Having someone else to share the responsibility can greatly ease your burden.

Don't be surprised if, in spite of your best intentions and efforts, you meet resistance from your parent when trying to plan for caregiving eventualities. Remember, this represents a significant role reversal between parent and child, one that might easily be resented. Try to keep your manner gentle and your plans as non-invasive as possible without sacrificing your parent's well-being. You are navigating uncharted waters, and the key to success is to be both vigilant and flexible.

CHAPTER 3

An Uneasy Truce

K.C. left after hugging both Dad and me. As Dad escorted her to the front door, we made tentative plans to get together in the morning. Dad waited for K.C. to get into her car safely before he turned off the outside light and locked the door. When he came back to the family room where I was still standing, I gave him a hug and a kiss on the cheek. Dad reciprocated, but without much enthusiasm. This was a clear sign to leave further discussion of the "Grace issue" until tomorrow. I fervently hoped that the gravity of what Grace had done would sink in overnight, and then maybe Dad would appreciate our efforts to protect him.

We said goodnight, and Dad left the family room for his bedroom, obviously distraught, upset, and maybe a bit disoriented. Remembering that my suitcase was still in the trunk of the rental car, I unlocked the front door, turned on the outside light and went out into the cool air. After retrieving my bag, I lingered for a moment before going in, savoring the peace. It was a welcome respite from the volatile few hours I had just experienced. I went back inside and secured the house for the evening.

During my mom's illness, Dad had moved out of the master bedroom and into K.C.'s old bedroom, which was at the other end of the hall from the master bedroom, so that he could sleep without being disturbed by the constant noise of Mom's caregivers helping her throughout the night. Now Grace had taken over the master bedroom, with its king-size bed, walk-in closets, private bath and sitting area, which was where I was bunking during my visit. I made my way to the master bedroom, suitcase in hand, and as I unpacked, I took in my surroundings.

The master bedroom was now decorated in "early Grace." She had obviously moved in, bag and baggage. I saw many framed pictures decorating two end tables and a large double dresser. One picture was of a man in clerical garb; I presumed he was the minister of the church Dad had been so generously supporting. Grace was in several of the photos along with young men and women, who I assumed were her grown children. The instant I saw her, I remembered her: a little overweight, sweet smile on her face, hair tastefully styled. I couldn't help remarking to myself that she had a beautiful family. It was still hard to accept that Grace was capable of such heartless exploitation of my father.

A couple of other items caught my attention, included a treadmill and a sewing machine on a stand. Both looked brand-spanking new.

I looked in the closets for no particular reason except that I was being nosy and didn't want to turn in yet. The room had two large closets that were packed with clothes on hangers. Not the clothes that had belonged to my mom or Sue, which I knew had been given to Goodwill after their deaths. These were nice-looking clothes, brightly colored suits and dresses. I couldn't tell if the garments were all new or just well cared for.

Complementing the clothes were dozens of pairs of shoes on the floor of the closets. Dress shoes, primarily, but also several pairs of casual shoes and sandals. From where I stood, these shoes looked new, with no scuffs or scratches that I could see. I refrained from looking in the many dresser drawers, which I assumed were equally well stuffed. I had seen enough. I knew that Dad had probably paid for everything in the closets if not the entire room. It did not take a genius to realize that there was a lot of Dad's money in these "gifts."

I was getting a headache. For one thing, I was flat-out tired; for another, there was a strong smell of perfume in the room. I had noticed the scent when I first walked in, but now it was starting to bother me. The smell hung in the air like a vapor. I went into the bathroom to find some aspirin, and I saw that Grace had taken over in there, too. Exotic lotions, soaps, and shampoos were spread out all over the counter. I looked in the medicine cabinet and all of the drawers, but I couldn't find anything resembling an aspirin.

I decided to check with Dad. Maybe he keeps the aspirin in his bathroom, I thought. I walked down the hall to Dad's bedroom, but I actually had another motive. The aspirin was not as important as my plan to kiss Dad goodnight one more time and reassure him that I was just trying to do what was best for him because I loved him. As I neared the closed door of Dad's bedroom, I could hear his voice. It sounded like he was talking on the telephone. Before knocking, I paused to listen. I immediately felt guilty for eavesdropping on my father and invading his privacy. It surprised me that I would stoop so low as to listen to my father's private conversation.

It was obvious that Dad was talking on the telephone to Grace. I heard him promising her that "Ed will be gone in a few days and things will be okay." Hearing this made my heart hurt even more. Before our confrontation, I had been confident, almost cocky, in my belief that when Dad saw the evidence, Grace would be out of a job. Instead, he was making plans to welcome her back into his home. Even in my exhausted state, I finally understood that the chances for a speedy resolution of the Grace issue were evaporating. I didn't even bother to knock on his door. I was so upset that I forgot about the aspirin and my headache. I turned around and went down the hall to my bedroom and went to bed. I just wanted to sleep. I pulled the blanket up hoping that maybe when I woke, this nightmare would be over.

My head hit the pillow and I was out like a light. Shortly, when I was somewhere between the twilight zone and deep sleep, I became aware that someone was in the bedroom. I woke with a start. My father was standing in the doorway. The bedroom was pitch black except for a small ray of light coming from the nightlight in the hall, which helped Dad find the bathroom.

"Dad what you are you doing?" I asked as I lifted my head off the pillow and struggled to get into a sitting position. Dad was obviously agitated; I could tell even in the dim light. His voice was low and sounded almost fearful, and he appeared to be holding onto the door frame for balance.

"Ed, I just wanted to find out when you are leaving."

"Why?" I asked.

"I just wanted to find out when you are leaving," Dad repeated.

"Dad, I'll leave when all is well. Now please go to bed, I'm tired."

"Okay, I just wanted to know when you are leaving," he said again.

"I told you, Dad. Now, please go to bed," I said as I laid my head back down on the pillow.

That was the conversation; nothing more was said. After a few seconds, Dad turned around in the dim light and left the room, and I listened as he shuffled down the hall. I rolled over to glance at the clock on the nightstand. One-fifteen in the morning. I was absolutely exhausted. It was 4:15 A.M. on the East Coast, where I lived.

Sleep came immediately, but soon I became aware of someone in the room again. I awoke with a start, and there was Dad in the doorway.

"Dad, what are you doing?" I asked for the second time.

"Ed, I just wanted to know when you are leaving."

Now I was getting angry. Exhaustion and sleep deprivation were taking their toll and my voice did not hide my feelings.

"Dad, I *told you* that I will leave when we get everything resolved."

"When will that be?"

"Dad, please go to sleep. I will take care of everything. I love you. Now please go to sleep."

"Okay, I just wanted to know when you were leaving."

Dad acted as though he didn't remember our previous conversation about my departure date. He must have been so upset or stressed that he had blocked the conversation from his mind.

Again, I heard Dad amble down the hall. I thought I heard him close his bedroom door, although I couldn't be sure. I looked at the clock again and was stunned to see that only forty-five minutes had passed since our first fitful discussion.

I laid my head back down on the pillow and was asleep in an instant, only to be startled awake again by my dad lurking in the doorway to the bedroom. We had yet another conversation that was the same as the previous two. What was even stranger was Dad's reaction to my answer about when I'd be leaving. It was as though he was hearing it for the first time; he acted as if he had never questioned me about my departure date, even though by now we'd had the same conversation three times in the last few hours.

Sleep was out of the question now. I was having trouble compre-hending that my father didn't understand what he was doing. He was so distressed about Grace's termination that he wasn't functioning ration-ally. As I tossed and turned in bed, trying to get some sleep, my mind wouldn't shut down. I kept thinking about K.C.'s and my unsuccessful conversation with Dad earlier in the evening, and then the three bizarre nighttime visits. I realized that I was probably more confused than Dad. Things just didn't make sense. Dad wasn't angry at Grace for bilking him, but he was upset that I was hanging around, preventing him from seeing her. What a mess, I thought. I told myself that things always looked bleakest in the wee hours of the morning. Maybe so, but the events of the day had left no doubt in my mind that Dad was no longer the father I had known. He was different. A lot different.

I woke up at 4:15 A.M. Pacific time, 7:15 A.M. eastern time, the time I normally get up. At first I was disoriented and not sure where I was, a condition that lasted only a few seconds before I remembered all too clearly. I looked at the clock and realized I must have slept some, although I didn't want to calculate how long for fear of learning how lit-tle shut-eye I had actually gotten. I lay in bed thinking about the previ-ous night's events, and I even questioned whether the three middle-of-the-night encounters had really happened. I knew they had, but I want-ed to believe otherwise. Maybe today would be better, I thought, although I wasn't optimistic.

I used the phone in the bedroom to call my office voice mail and then called my wife to fill her in on all that had happened. It was nice hearing her voice and words of support. After I finished my calls, I lay back in bed, closed my eyes and tried to get some more sleep, which proved to be impossible. My mind knew it was time to get up even though my body screamed out for rest. By 6:30 A.M. I heard my father moving around.

As long as Dad was up, I figured I should get up also. I showered, dressed and joined him in the family room, where he was sitting in his chair, reading the newspaper and listening to a morning talk show on television. Dad looked up with a smile and asked me how I had slept. I told him that I was still tired from the trip. I asked how he had slept, waiting to see if he would mention anything about the late-night visits to my room. Curiously, Dad said only that he had slept well.

Despite my inner turmoil, I put on a happy face and suggested that we go out for breakfast. Looking at my father in the natural light of the morning sun, I realized again that he really was a shadow of his former self. In addition to not taking his medicine, as confirmed by the pharmacy of drugs on the bathroom floor, I was convinced Dad was malnourished. Dad proposed a local Mexican restaurant he said he frequented with Grace. I didn't respond, but I'm sure my face gave away my feelings about hearing "her" name first thing in the morning. Ignoring the Grace reference, I suggested that I call K.C. to see if she wanted to join us. Dad thought this was a nice idea and followed up with some complimentary comments about K.C., how she was always on the go with her children, what a good mother she was, and how she was always willing to take him whenever he needed a ride.

I was beginning to realize that my father had become so complicated that I could no longer predict his reactions. How could someone who so obviously loved his daughter, as evidenced by his continual praise of her, sit by when Grace had pushed her? None of this made sense to me.

Also, I couldn't tell whether Dad was making a sincere effort to be agreeable after the previous night's events or if he had indeed forgotten what happened. Chances were he was trying to be agreeable, maybe to get me out of his hair quickly. It really didn't matter to me what his motive was right then. I was looking forward to having breakfast with my dad and K.C.

K.C. answered the phone on the second ring. She said she was up, although I doubted her. I heard the hesitation in her voice when she answered the phone, like she was trying to wake up as opposed to being awake. I knew that she wouldn't want to make me feel guilty for waking her. I extended the invitation for her to join us for breakfast, but she declined and suggested that I take Dad to breakfast and spend some time with him, which was fine with me. We agreed on a time to meet at the house.

Before hanging up, K.C. told me that she had called Dad's doctor, Dr. French, last night after the blow-up. She told Dr. French about Dad's abnormal reaction to the information we had provided about Grace and how agitated he seemed. I was surprised that K.C. had been able to get through to the doctor so late. Apparently, Dr. French had been Dad's doctor for many years, and he had given K.C. his home telephone number for emergencies. Dr. French was also concerned about Dad after hearing K.C.'s report. He told her he was going to be at the hospital all the next day, doing rounds and paperwork, and he had asked K.C. to bring Dad there for a check-up. I hung up the phone, grateful for the foresight she had shown by calling Dr. French. I wished I could have told K.C. about Dad's visits last night and his telephone call to Grace, but with Dad in easy earshot I decided to wait for a better, more private, opportunity to share this information.

"Well, Dad, breakfast is going to be a guy's outing. K.C. will catch up with us later."

Dad made some effort at humor when he said, "It's her loss." I readily agreed, and we smiled at each other as if we were two college kids, off to play a prank. I felt immeasurably better seeing my dad smile and hearing him crack a joke.

We left the house, deciding that I would drive Dad's black Cadillac while he gave directions. For as long as I could remember, Dad had always had a black Cadillac, which, according to him, is "the finest car on the road." We engaged in some small talk on the way to the restaurant, but I desperately needed some coffee to kick-start my batteries. After a short drive, we arrived at the restaurant in Ocean Beach and were greeted by the hostess, who obviously knew Dad. My guts did a belly flop when she asked, "Where is Grace? I hope she's not sick, is she?" Dad explained that Grace was in China. Now I wasn't sure if he even remembered last night's telephone conversation when Grace announced that she was "back" from China.

The restaurant had a Mexican décor *á la* 1950s, and I vaguely remembered it from my younger days. Juke box in the corner, which now played CDs instead of 45s, a few hanging piñatas, a bunch of "XX" beer signs, and framed posters from the late 1960s announcing bullfights in Tijuana, Mexico. The facilities were sparse: a long counter for service and an assortment of heavy, dark-stained wooden chairs grouped around six or seven stainless steel tables with gray laminated tops.

We settled in at one of the tables, and the waitress brought coffee for Dad the way he liked it, steaming hot in a mug; I got mine in a cup. It didn't matter to me what the coffee was in as long as it was hot and strong. Dad and I looked at the menu for a few minutes. I realized food was not a high priority for me right then, but I figured I should eat something to give me strength. It was going to be a long day, and I was hoping to accomplish a lot.

The restaurant offered a good assortment of Mexican dishes that under normal circumstances would interest me, even for breakfast. Chiles rellenos, cheese enchiladas, and shredded beef tacos were my favorites, and they were sadly lacking in Maryland. Ignoring the Mexican delicacies, Dad ordered a combination plate of two scrambled eggs, toast, refried beans, and bacon. My appetite was nonexistent, so I ordered the same. It seemed simpler to follow Dad's lead, for some reason. As soon as our order had been taken and the hostess (now the waitress) had disappeared, our eyes met and Dad wasted no time.

"So, when are you leaving?"

He caught me off guard. I still wasn't sure if Dad remembered last night's three conversations on this subject in the wee hours. Maybe he was hoping for a different answer than he had gotten last night, or maybe he believed he was asking the question for the first time. I hadn't a clue. So I brushed off the question and came back with one for him.

"Dad, what are you going to do about Grace?"

Dad sought refuge in the same nonresponsive rhetoric of the night before.

"I will discuss the checks with Grace. I am sure there is an explanation for the checks. Grace is a good person, Ed. She wouldn't hurt me." He continued to offer up this defense, which he obviously believed, but it made no sense to me. I wondered if the subject of the checks had even come up during his phone call to Grace the previous night. But I wasn't about to raise the subject of his late-night telephone conversation with her. This was out of the question because it would require an admission that I had violated his privacy by eavesdropping outside his bedroom door. Instead, I kept my mouth shut and listened.

"Ed, Grace is from a good family. I don't want to do anything to hurt her." Then, after taking a breath, "Ed, when are you going home?" My father was making no effort to disguise his feelings on the issue of Grace and my continued presence in San Diego.

I could not believe my ears. My head was now pounding with a reprise of my headache from the night before. I could hardly contain my anger. If Grace had been there at that moment, I think I could have killed her, I was that angry. Grace and her son had bilked Dad out of thousands of dollars, and Dad was concerned only about not hurting her. How could he not realize that Grace was taking him to the cleaners? This was insane!

If Grace had been delivering the care Dad needed, then I might have had some appreciation of Dad's concern for her welfare. I knew, however, that at the same time Grace was picking Dad's pockets, she was abusing his trust in her, as evidenced by his physical condition and the pills I had seen scattered on the floor of Dad's bathroom.

I tried another tack. "Dad, the only way to avoid hurting Grace is never to see her again. If she comes around again, I will call the District Attorney and swear out a criminal warrant." As soon as the words were out of my mouth, I realized this was not the right thing to say. The morning wasn't even an hour old, and already we were at odds.

Dad was starting to steam again. "Ed, this has nothing to do with you. Don't get involved in my life. Stay out of this." Then he repeated, "I don't want you to hurt Grace."

I didn't want Dad to get so mad that he wouldn't eat, although it was clear from the tone of his voice and his body language that he was pretty upset already. I decided to hold my tongue. "Fine, Dad, let's talk about it later." I could barely disguise the disgust in my voice. We both stopped talking and suddenly became interested in looking at the pictures on the walls, the menu, playing with the sugar packets, doing anything as long as our eyes didn't meet and we didn't have to talk.

This certainly was not like the many happy breakfasts I'd had with my dad when I was a child. This was more like a face-off between matador and bull in a very small ring. Maybe the bullfighting posters on the wall were symbolic of my situation with my father. Usually, the end of a bullfight comes when the matador is victorious and the bull dies. I shuddered inwardly at the image. How will this confrontation with Dad end? I wondered. Would we be friends again, or would one of us trample the other? Which of us was the matador and which the bull?

The food came and I ate, but I didn't taste what was passing from my fork to my mouth. I couldn't understand how my father could be so irrational when it came to Grace. I looked over at Dad and noticed he had just sort of pushed his food around his plate with his fork. He had eaten maybe half a slice of toast when the waitress came by to warm up our coffee, and he asked her for the check and a doggie bag.

"Dad, you haven't even touched your food. Please eat something."

"I know, Ed, I just don't eat much."

"Could you try to eat something?"

"Ed, I'm not hungry."

"Dad, you look terrible. How about trying?" He replied by saying he wanted to go home. That was it. I knew that Dad was not going to eat any more. The check and doggie bag were delivered to our table, and over my dad's objections, I paid the bill. As we were leaving, the waitress reminded Dad to "Say hello to Grace for me."

Dad said, "You can count on it."

I shuddered again as we walked back to the car.

Instead of going straight home, I suggested we take a ride around the city. San Diego has many beautiful sights; there are jewels to be seen everywhere. Plus, it was still early and I wanted my dad to get out and feel the sun on his face. Actually, I was hoping that he might wake up from the fog he was in and come out from under the spell of Grace. Maybe a little California sunshine would help.

Dad agreed to a ride. We first drove to Mission Bay, where hundreds of beautiful boats are docked. From Mission Bay we made our way to the San Diego harbor, where the big Navy ships are anchored. As a kid, I had toured the warships with my dad on visiting days. In those days, the Navy would have an open house on a ship almost every weekend. Dad loved machinery, and during our tour of the Navy ships, he would tell me about the working of the ship's boilers, generating equipment, gun batteries and things as simple as the winch that pulled up the anchor.

We left the harbor area and worked our way to Shelter Island, a man-made island where several restaurants, yacht brokerages, harbors, and the Kona Kai Country Club are located. In my younger days, the family had kept a membership in the Kona Kai Club, which was a nice place to mingle with the movers and shakers of San Diego. As we passed the Kona Kai, Dad spoke of the wonderful times at the club with the family. My memory was different, however. I had spent many summers with my mom, my sister, my aunt, and her children at the club, which was not more than fifteen minutes from the house. We would swim, sail small boats, eat a lot, and socialize with other club members and their guests. I did not remember my dad being there with us.

Dad had worked hard during the years that Mom, K.C., and I were enjoying the good life at the club. He believed that with hard work you could overcome any obstacle. Dad often told me that when he and my grandfather, whom everyone called Poppy, purchased their laundry business in La Jolla, residents weren't receptive to members of the Jewish faith buying a business in their community. Prior to the completion of the sale, the city fathers had approached the seller of the business and suggested that he not sell to my father and grandfather because they were Jewish. The seller told the city fathers that if they were so concerned, they should buy the business themselves. After the sale, Dad and Poppy worked hard to make the business successful. Together with about 150 employees, they took the business to ever-increasing revenues and bottom-line profits. Poppy worked in the plant as the eyes and ears of the owners. Dad was the outside salesperson and also the chief mechanic. He knew how every piece of machinery operated, even better than the two engineers they employed.

He was a stickler for preventive maintenance, which meant that on Saturday afternoon, after the business shut down for the rest of the week until Monday, Dad and a select few employees would repair, replace, and clean the equipment. If this could not be accomplished by the end of Saturday, a crew came in on Sunday to complete the work. So Dad worked long hours and often seven days a week.

Usually, Dad left the house by seven in the morning and didn't return until five-thirty or six in the evening. So, as kids growing up, K.C. and I usually did not see our dad during the day or much on the weekends. I couldn't conjure up memories of my father spending many happy days with the family at the club. It didn't matter, though, because my dad seemed to be enjoying his memories of family outings to the Kona Kai. I was just glad that we were talking and having a good time together.

As we completed our circle of the island, Dad said he wanted to go home because he was tired, so we headed back to the house. The drive home from Shelter Island took all of ten minutes, and the rest of a long and undoubtedly tumultuous day loomed ahead of us.

Dementia and the Elderly: What You Can Do

Years ago, when an older person showed signs of forgetfulness or exhibited odd behavior, we would nod knowingly and say "senile." Many of us assumed that senility was just part of getting old. But it has been determined that senility, now called dementia, is not part of the normal aging process. The most extreme form of dementia is Alzheimer's disease. We'll discuss Alzheimer's in greater detail later in this chapter, but it's important for you to know that if you notice changes in your parent's cognitive ability or behavior, it doesn't necessarily mean Alzheimer's disease is the culprit. Mild forms of dementia do not always progress into Alzheimer's disease. Even if cognitive or behavioral changes are significant, there are many possible causes that merit investigation before deciding that your parent has fallen victim to Alzheimer's disease.

In hindsight, I realize that my father was showing signs of mild dementia and depression (which is discussed in chapter 9). For example, when Dad repeatedly woke me during the night to ask when I was going home, without remembering that he had already asked me several times, he was exhibiting signs of short-term memory loss. Also, when he tried to liquidate his portfolio, he was obviously showing poor judgment, another sign of dementia.

It's hard for us to admit that our parents are changing, and I think it's even harder to be objective about seeing the changes for what they really are. We have a tendency to think that inappropriate behavior can be controlled, regardless of what might be the underlying cause. This was clearly a problem for me. I was unwilling to accept that my father was incapable of understanding how Grace had been abusing him.

Not all caregivers who abuse the elderly have coal for hearts. Sometimes, when caregivers abuse the elderly, it can be a result of frustration and a lack of understanding of dementia and its effects. They mistakenly believe that if the older person only tried harder, the behavior problems would disappear. The caregiver's frustration escalates into punishing behavior. Obviously, if your parent suffers from any form of dementia, it's critical to educate whoever is in charge of caregiving about both the causes and effects of dementia. (Techniques for selecting educated caregivers are discussed in chapter 8.)

My hope is that once you understand more about dementia, you'll be able to develop the objectivity you'll need to help your parent get the best and most appropriate care and treatment.

DEMENTIA

Dementia is a disorder of the brain that may or may not be progressive. Some causes of dementia are treatable, including fever, dehydration, malnutrition, thyroid disorders, minor head injury, or adverse reaction to medications. If you or a caregiver notices signs of dementia in your parent, the first step is to have a physician eliminate any of these potential causes.

The following is a list of ten warning signs to watch for that might suggest dementia in your parent:

1. **Short-term memory loss.** We all forget things. Even as young adults we can misplace our car keys or forget a frequently dialed telephone number. What distinguishes this type of memory loss from one caused by dementia is that eventually we will remember the forgotten information. People with dementia will not. For example, your parent might ask you the same question, over and

over, forgetting both your answer and the fact that the question has already been asked.

2. **Difficulty with familiar tasks.** A client of mine used to knit beautiful afghans. As dementia set in, she forgot how to perform this skill she had known since she had been a young woman. Has your parent forgotten how to cook? Have your father's wood-working tools become a mystery to him? Does your mother begin a task only to be unable to finish it? Be alert for signals that everyday tasks may now be exceeding your parent's ability to perform them.

3. **Difficulty with language.** Everyone struggles for a lost word occasionally. People with dementia, however, frequently forget simple words or use the wrong words to try to convey what they mean. This creates enormous frustration because they lose the ability to make themselves understood; consequently, their wants and needs go unfulfilled.

4. **Disorientation.** Has your parent gotten lost while driving to a familiar destination or been unable to find the way home? Often, people with dementia can get lost even while walking in their own neighborhood or on their own street. Time disorientation is common, too. Does your parent awaken in the middle of the night and start preparing for the day as if it were morning?

5. **Poor judgment.** Has your parent started making unwise decisions? Is your mother giving away family heirlooms to strangers? Does your father go for a walk and leave the front door wide open? These are signs that judgment is becoming impaired.

6. **Inability to think abstractly.** You and I might have trouble setting an electronic clock. People with dementia might be unable to grasp the concept of numbers and how they represent time.

7. **Misplacing things.** Has your parent put something in an inappropriate place, such as ice cream in a cupboard instead of the freezer? I have a client who misplaces her underwear and then accuses her housekeeper of stealing it. Another client has called the police on several occasions to report her jewelry stolen only to find out later that she has placed the jewelry in an inappropriate location. Often, people with dementia misplace an item and then are unable to find it later.

8. **Mood swings.** Changes in mood are normal for everyone, but people with dementia have unexpected, radical mood swings, going from a normal state to rage and then dissolving in tears in an instant.

9. **Personality changes.** Does your parent not seem like the same person he or she once was? Does your parent seem fearful, suspicious, or easy to anger? Significant personality changes can be a sign of dementia.

10. **Loss of initiative.** People with dementia can lose interest in the world around them. Is your parent refusing to leave the house? Is your parent no longer interested in friends or activities that were once important and enjoyable?

I believe now that my father exhibited at least five of these ten signs of dementia. As his symptoms were progressing, I could not accept that he might be suffering from dementia and needed help. Don't make the same mistake. If any of these signs describe your parent, and the symptoms seem to be affecting your parent's quality of life or safety, a visit to the doctor is in order. Doctors can diagnose dementia and its probable cause through a series of physical exams and tests. Don't accept signs of dementia as a normal by-product of growing older. There might be a possibility for treatment and elimination of the problem.

ALZHEIMER'S DISEASE

Now that Alzheimer's disease has become so prevalent and widely recognized, many people with aging parents are watching carefully for signs of mental deterioration that might indicate the beginnings of this devastating disease. The warning signs for Alzheimer's are by and large the same as for other forms of dementia. Alzheimer's, however, is categorized by three distinct stages.

Stage 1. At first, your parent may experience forgetfulness, poor insight, difficulty with calculation, repetition of questions, and a minor degree of disorientation (Bell, 1996). This stage of Alzheimer's usually lasts from two to four years, sometimes longer. Stage 1 patients usually still enjoy life, but they may experience frustration with how their symptoms interfere with their daily activities. As a result, they may become moody or emotional.

Stage 2. As the disease progresses, memory worsens, words are used more and more inappropriately and some basic self-care skills are lost. Loved ones may confuse night and day, and fail to recognize family and friends (Bell, 1996). During this second, moderate stage of Alzheimer's, patients require close supervision because they also tend to get lost easily, even in familiar places. Home care may become necessary at this stage, which is the longest phase, usually lasting from two to ten years.

Stage 3. In the final stage, the family member must be fed, becomes incontinent, bedridden, uncomprehending and mute (Bell, 1996). This most severe stage of Alzheimer's usually lasts from one to three years. Patients require 24-hour care and supervision, and they typically suffer from hallucinations and delusions. Friends and family members usually are no longer recognizable, and patients are unable to care for themselves.

Approximately 4 million Americans have Alzheimer's disease, and researchers predict that 14 million will be afflicted by 2050. The reason for the upward spiral in numbers of cases is simply because we are living longer. Of those who reach the age of 85, nearly half have or will develop Alzheimer's disease (Alzheimer's Assoc., 2002). Unfortunately, once Alzheimer's strikes, little can be done to remit its course, although researchers are working hard to develop drugs to treat the disease.

Should your parent's diagnosis be progressive dementia, even Alzheimer's disease, there are things you or your parent's caregiver can do to make life easier. However, you needn't wait for a diagnosis. To the extent that you can implement the suggestions below, go ahead. Then, as your parent declines, preparations will already be in place to make his or her life easier.

Remember, once dementia is diagnosed, your loved one is excused 100 percent of the time (Driscoll, 1994). This must be your mantra. Memory loss is a disability. People with dementia can't remember, and they can't remember that they can't remember. It may be difficult to accept that your parent has changed mentally but, in the long run, it will be easier for everyone if you can accept that your parent has a physical disability rather than a behavior problem.

If you are not the primary person responsible for your parent's care, spend some time instructing the caregiver to take the following measures.

•Be a good listener. As communication skills decline, pay attention to body language and encourage use of gestures, signs, and pictures.

•Modify the home environment gradually as needed, and simplify daily routines. For example, if you need to "parent proof" the house for safety reasons, do one room at a time so that your parent doesn't have to adjust to an entire house full of changes all at once. Routines should be kept simple; for example, breakfast-bath-dress-walk, etc., in that order, every day.

•Ask "yes" and "no" questions and allow plenty of time for comprehension.

•Keep directions simple, and give just one step at a time.

•Repeat instructions in exactly the same way.

•Use labels with words or pictures on drawers and shelves to identify contents.

•Lay out clothes in the order they are to be put on.

•Plan failure-free activities, such as reminiscing with family photo albums or listening to favorite music.

•If a confrontation begins, avoid it by leaving the room.

•Be patient, cheerful, gracious, considerate, and reassuring.

•Expect the unexpected.

(Adapted from the *San Diego Eldercare Directory,* 2002)

Remember, it is counterproductive to try, on your own, to sort out the probable causes of your parent's behavior and decide what the best course of action might be. Enlist the aid of others—friends, other family members, caregivers—who are familiar with your parent. Get their insight, combine it with your own, and seek help from professionals.

Your parent deserves the best quality of life possible. Don't allow dementia to rob your parent of that quality when it's very possible that treatment is available.

If the diagnosis is Alzheimer's disease or another form of progressive dementia, remember that your parent will still be able to enjoy life for quite a few years. And there are many agencies and support groups that can offer help and ideas for both parent and caregiver. Take advantage of these wonderful groups. Their knowledge and experience can truly help make a difficult time much easier for you and your loved one. A good resource to help you find the support you need is the Alzheimer's Association, a national organization that provides education and support for people diagnosed with the condition, their families and caregivers. The Alzheimer's Association can be reached at www.alz.org, or at (800) 272-3900.

CHAPTER 4

Police to the Rescue

*H*ome again. We settled into the family room with Dad in his usual chair next to the telephone. We were talking about baseball and how the San Diego Padres might fare this season, when K.C. arrived with another woman in tow. I could tell Dad was genuinely happy to see K.C. He got up, giving her his usual Cheshire cat grin and a big hug. Dad seemed pleased to have his family together once again. I too gave K.C. a hug and kiss. We all seated ourselves in the family room, then looked at each other in silence.

Either my imagination was taking the lead, or tension was already starting to build. Dad was staring at the woman K.C. had brought with her, and I realized that the next few minutes would dictate whether he would still be happy to have his children there with him.

K.C. broke the silence. "Dad, I'd like you to meet Jane Buchanan, your new caregiver." Fresh from the agency, Jane was a well-groomed, middle-aged woman.

Jane seemed personable, saying with a smile, "Ben, I have heard nice things about you. I'm looking forward to working for you."

At first, Dad seemed taken by surprise. I wasn't sure if he had heard Jane. He certainly didn't acknowledge either her introduction or her words, which, as a gentleman, he would have done under normal circumstances. Instead, he brought up Grace. "Ed, I have a caregiver. Grace is only on vacation. I don't need another caregiver."

I didn't understand why his objection was directed at me because, in this case, the messenger was K.C. Not that it really mattered, because we were a team, but it was beginning to sink in that I was going to play the role of the heavy in this drama, whether I wanted to or not. "Dad, I told you. Grace is not coming back. Also, she is not in China. She never went there. China is just another one of Grace's lies."

Dad's eyes narrowed and his face contorted. He was instantly angry. I don't think I would have been surprised to see steam coming out of his ears. He yelled, "I want her out of the house!" He was pointing at Jane, but staring directly at me. Then, in a cooler voice, Dad said, "Ma'am, this has nothing to do with you. I am sure you are a nice lady. But would you please leave?" No one moved. Jane, K.C., and I were speechless and immobile in our chairs.

I had never heard my father yell so loudly, but I knew I couldn't back down. I calmly explained that if Dad did not want to give Jane a chance, K.C. could arrange for another caregiver, but "Grace is not coming back, never, never again."

Dad would hear nothing of this. He became more assertive. He got up, pointed his finger at Jane again and said, "I want her out of this house! I want her out of this house now!"

"No, Dad," I said in a calm voice. "She stays or we get someone new. It doesn't matter to us. As I said before, Grace is not coming back."

There didn't seem to be any way to make Dad understand that the past was gone, and his children were trying to help him move in a better direction with the rest of his life. Clearly he didn't want his kids inter- fering, and he did not want our help. "Ed, where do you come off telling me who I can see? I don't need you to run my life. I have done well enough without you. Now, get her out of here. Ed, if you don't get her out of this house, I'm going to call the police."

Although shocked, I maintained a calm and even voice, saying "Suit yourself, Dad. Jane is not leaving until you at least talk to her. If you don't like her, then we will find another caregiver. I hate to repeat myself, but Grace is not coming back. Never. Now, get with the pro- gram. I suggest that K.C. and I leave the room and you two talk to each other. What do you say?"

"I say you are full of s--t, Ed. I want *you* out of my house, also. Now get out."

"I'm staying, Dad. K.C.'s staying, and Jane is staying until you talk to her."

"Ed, if she does not get out of the house, I swear, I will call the police."

"Do what you have to do, Dad."

I was stupid to challenge my father to call the police, but I was revert- ing to my training as a litigator: Never budge. Never give in unless absolutely necessary. Make the other side blink first. My acute lack of sleep was undoubtedly fueling my anger, too. However, I still could not understand Dad's blind devotion to Grace in the wake of overwhelming evidence that she was a thief. I wanted Dad to understand, once and for all, that Grace was not coming back, and he had better get used to the idea that another caregiver was going to take her place.

Much to my surprise, Dad picked up the gauntlet. He called the police. I watched him as he dialed 911.

A police cruiser pulling up to a house in this quiet neighborhood was an unusual occurrence. Disturbance calls were out of step with Point Loma's middle-class, suburban lifestyle. But having heard my dad report a dispute to the 911 operator, I knew that it would not be long before the police arrived.

While waiting for the police, we sat and stared at each other in silence—a reprise of what had happened at breakfast when Grace's name had come up. K.C. tried to break the ice when she told Dad that she had spoken with Dr. French, who wanted to see him today for an exam. Instead of diverting his anger, K.C. succeeded only in increasing the tension. Dad tersely replied, "I don't need any exam. I'm not going to the doctor's today. Now would you please get this lady out of my house?"

K.C. said, "Dad, we have to work something out with a new caregiver. Would you at least speak to Jane? I think you will find that she is a nice person who wants to take care of you. I really believe you will like her if you give her a chance. Please talk to her."

In response to K.C.'s plea, Dad shook his head violently from side to side. Not only did he not want to talk to Jane, now he wouldn't even speak to K.C. I looked at the walls, glanced at my dad, Jane, K.C., and then at the garden outside. I was getting good at this silence game, having learned the rules earlier at breakfast.

After a few minutes, I walked to the living room window, which offered an unobstructed view of the street to the corner, three houses down. Soon I saw a black-and-white police car pull up and park at the foot of the driveway. Without waiting for the police officer to come to the front door, I left the house to greet him as he was getting out of his car.

Officer Martinez was a nice-looking man, about six feet tall with a medium frame. From the look of the ribbons on his chest and the signs of age on his face, he was obviously a veteran of many years of service to the community. His very appearance commanded respect. I stuck out my hand to greet Officer Martinez and introduce myself, but he was not particularly interested in shaking hands. Blunt and to the point, he asked, "Who is in the house and what is the problem?"

I explained that my father was extremely angry about a new caregiver that my sister had brought to the house to take care of him, and he wanted her to leave. I gave the officer some background information about how Grace had embezzled a lot of money from Dad. Officer Martinez asked, "Would your father press charges against Grace?"

"Probably not," I said. "In fact, he wants Grace back as his caregiver." Officer Martinez shook his head in a way that indicated that he understood what was going on.

I also told Officer Martinez that we were trying to get Dad to Mission Ridge Hospital for an appointment with his doctor. I asked the officer if he could transport Dad to Mission Ridge, but he told me that he could only take him to the hospital if he "was a harm to himself or a harm to others." There it was again. That simple phrase that was proving to be such a huge obstacle in our attempts to help Dad.

Still, I had to try. I told Officer Martinez that Dad was a harm to himself because in the last year he had paid Grace almost three times her salary, and just a few days earlier he had tried to liquidate all of his assets. Dad's plan was to give away all of his money to someone, probably Grace, so he was obviously a harm to himself.

"Unfortunately, that doesn't count," responded Officer Martinez. He went on to tell me what I already knew: that "harm to self" means physical harm. "What you have described is financial harm. Your dad can give away everything he owns. As long as he is somewhat competent, there is nothing I can do." Officer Martinez suggested that we go into the house and talk things over with Dad.

I had no idea what Officer Martinez intended to do when he spoke with my father. Although the officer did not know it, Dad was a person who respected the law and law enforcement officers. Dad believed that a police officer's job was extremely difficult and that officers were constantly putting their lives on the line for a mostly ungrateful public. He had often told me that he felt police officers were not appreciated for the wonderful work they do.

We walked together up the porch steps and into the house, and Officer Martinez took over immediately. K.C. and Jane were still sitting in chairs against one wall of the family room, and Dad was still in his favorite chair. It was clear as we entered the room that there had not been a lot of conversation after I left to meet the police officer. The tension showed on everyone's face. No one in the room had ever had dealings of this sort with the police, and we had no idea what to do or what to expect.

As soon as Officer Martinez walked into the family room, Dad sat up straight in his chair. The officer walked across the room and selected a chair, which he pulled up next to Dad. Taking a seat he asked, "Ben, what is the problem?"

Dad was obviously nervous and upset. His body was shaking perceptibly, probably because the rush of adrenaline from his earlier explosion was over. He was now tired and spent. In a soft, somewhat shaky voice, he told Officer Martinez, "I want that lady"—pointing to Jane—"out of this house. This is my house and I want her out." He then repeated himself in a quivering voice. "This is my house and I want her out." Silence followed his demands.

I broke the silence. I wasn't sure if it was relevant to Dad's demands or not, but I turned to the officer and explained that what my father had said was not exactly true. "The house is actually owned by my sister and me. We inherited one half of the house when our mother died and our dad"—nodding at my father—"gifted to us the other half."

Officer Martinez turned his head back toward Dad and asked, "Ben, is this true? Do they own the house?"

Dad sort of let his head hang down, exhaled a deep breath he apparently had been holding, and said in little more then a whisper, "Yes, it is their house."

Speaking directly to Dad, Officer Martinez asked, "If I get everyone out of the house, will you go to your doctor with your son?"

Dad thought about this for a few seconds, and a grin painted his face as he lifted his head like the emperor who has prevailed in battle. With the assurance of an aristocrat he said, "Yes. Yes, that would be fine with me."

Officer Martinez got up from his chair, still looking at Dad, and took a short step toward him, saying, "I don't want any misunderstandings, Ben. If I get everyone out of the house, you have agreed to go to the doctor with your son. Do we have a deal?"

Dad said, "Yes."

Officer Martinez then offered his right hand to Dad and said, "Shake on it." While the other three in the room watched in amazement, the two of them sealed the deal with a hearty handshake.

The policeman pointed his finger in the direction of K.C., Jane, and me, and said in a booming and commanding voice, "I want all of you out of this house, now!"

I was amazed. Officer Martinez seemed to me to be a genius in the psychology of the elderly. In a painless manner, he had resolved Dad's emergency call to his satisfaction, and, at the same time, he was helping me get Dad to his doctor's appointment.

Officer Martinez's order reminded me of an incident involving a favorite client who called to tell me that a SWAT team of heavily armed customs inspectors were executing a search warrant at his engine-repair facility. The inspectors wanted my client and all of the employees to move to the lunchroom until they could be interviewed and the items in the search warrant seized. The client was calling me for advice, describing the heavily armed SWAT officers on the roof and surrounding the building, as well as those inside, herding people at gunpoint from their offices throughout the building into the lunchroom. My advice was simple and direct: "Listen to the man with the gun."

With that advice in mind, when Officer Martinez told us to get out of the house, pronto, I stood up, and so did my sister and Jane. We walked to the front door, with Jane in the lead. Behind us, Dad followed with Officer Martinez. As we were exiting the house, Officer Martinez stopped on the porch by the front door, while we continued walking single file from the porch to the driveway. I stopped and turned to look at Officer Martinez, who pointed his finger at me and motioned with his hand to indicate that he wanted me to join him on the porch for a private conversation.

I retraced my steps, and when I got within comfortable speaking distance, Officer Martinez told me that before he had pulled up to the house, another police officer had radioed him about a van parked on the side of the road, about two blocks from the house. The occupants were just sitting in the van, and they looked suspicious. When the second police officer stopped to ask them about their business in the neighborhood, they indicated that they were going to 1649 Turn View Drive to visit with the owner of the house, whom they identified as a close friend. The other officer had heard the radio call to Officer Martinez dispatching him to 1649 Turn View Drive, and he asked Officer Martinez to find out whether the occupants of the van would be welcome at the Turn View address.

The people in the van were identified as Grace and some of her family members. Officer Martinez had told the other police officer to stay with the van until he could establish what was happening at the house. Once he had sized up the situation, he asked that K.C. not go to the hospital with Dad and me, because he wanted to supervise Grace removing her personal effects from the house. He needed K.C. to ensure that only Grace's property left the house.

Upon hearing this information, I surmised that Grace and her children had planned to visit my dad, but after driving by the house and seeing K.C.'s car as well as a car they did not recognize in the driveway (my rental car), they didn't want to make an appearance while Dad had company. So they were probably just waiting for us to leave when the police car pulled up next to their van.

I could not thank Officer Martinez enough. At last, someone was willing to help. I knew he could have decided not to get involved as soon as he determined that this was a civil controversy. The jurisdiction of the police is limited to criminal matters, and once Officer Martinez had confirmed that Dad would not testify against Grace, there was no criminal matter for him to address. Thus, he could have simply left us to our own devices. Instead, he was one of those rare public servants who was willing to take the extra steps to help. Officer Martinez was a godsend to our family.

I left Office Martinez on the porch and walked to Dad's car where he was waiting by the front passenger door. I unlocked the door and held it open for Dad to get in. While he was getting into the car, I whispered to my sister, who was standing near the right rear passenger door, "Don't get into the car. Stay here for a minute." K.C. nodded silently, indicating that she understood. I quickly walked to the driver's side of the car, opened the door and slid in behind the steering wheel, closing the door and starting the engine in one motion. After making sure that Dad had his seatbelt fastened, I got out of the car, telling Dad that I would just be a minute, I had something to tell K.C.

Not wanting to leave Dad unattended in the car for very long, I gave K.C. the basics of what Officer Martinez had told me and suggested she get the details from him. I returned once more to the porch so I could shake Officer Martinez's hand and thank him again for his help. He modestly replied, "Just doing my job." Officer Martinez accompanied me back to the car, and through the open window patted Dad on the shoulder and told him to take care of himself. Dad beamed at the officer's concern, and he also thanked him for his help.

I pulled away from the curb in a bit of a daze. Events were unfolding so rapidly, I was having trouble trying to sort them all out: Dad's angry outburst at the new caregiver, his calling the police, Grace and her family lying in wait, the coincidence of the call to the police precipitating the roadside investigation of Grace and her family, and the expert engineering of the situation by Officer Martinez. I'd had enough surprises for one day, but I suspected more might be on the horizon.

Working with Officials: What You Can Do

Had I let my imagination run wild, I probably could have predicted many different scenarios that might have resulted from my father's situation. Never in a million years, however, could I have imagined that the police would become involved. Although it was an unsettling experience, I was grateful for the professionalism and the expertise displayed by Officer Martinez. He single-handedly defused a volatile situation and helped me get my father to the doctor, an outcome I don't think I could have achieved on my own.

HOW THE POLICE CAN HELP

If you or your loved one resorts to calling the police, your situation has already spiraled out of control. It is only natural to want to avoid police involvement (and I will give you some direction in that regard later in this chapter), but if the unimaginable should become reality, there are things the police can do to help. When Officer Martinez arrived at my father's house, his first priority was to make sure no crime was in progress and no one was threatened with physical danger. Once he determined that everyone was safe, his work was done. He rightfully could have removed himself from the situation and referred us to a social services agency.

Officer Martinez (like most police officers) was well-schooled in how to defuse domestic disputes. In a matter of minutes he was able to resolve our immediate trouble to the satisfaction of everyone involved. Moreover, he seemed familiar with incidences of unscrupulous caregivers, and he was willing to go beyond his basic duty to make sure Grace cleared out of my father's house. I must stress, though, that this was voluntary on the officer's part. It is unrealistic to assume that a police officer will be your safety net. Had Officer Martinez been less caring, or had a police emergency arisen elsewhere, he would have been gone, and we would have been back where we started.

Your city's police force does care about your elderly loved ones. Check with your local police station to find out what programs are offered. In San Diego, for example, the police and the sheriff's departments jointly offer a program called You Are Not Alone. If an elderly person is enrolled in the program, a member of the Retired Senior Volunteer Patrol (RSVP) will drop by on a regular basis for a visit, just to make sure everything is okay. The RSVP volunteers are also trained in helping the elderly; however, unlike the police, they have plenty of time to spend with your parent, just talking if necessary.

Most police departments (usually in conjunction with the District Attorney's Office) are a treasure trove of information on how to protect the elderly, and are an especially good source of tips for home safety. The following are some suggestions provided by the elder abuse unit of the San Diego D.A.'s Office:

•Lock your doors and windows.

•Identify who comes to the door before you open it. A peephole in the door is preferable, but a sliding chain on the door works well, too. Ask strangers for identification.

•Make a list of your valuables (jewelry, antiques) and take photographs of the items. Keep the photos in a secure place such as a safe deposit box.

•Keep your checkbook and additional checks in a safe place.

•Do not keep large amounts of cash at home.

Discuss these safety measures with your parent and with your parent's caregiver. You might be surprised at how often an elderly person becomes a crime victim simply because a door or window was left unlocked.

Your local District Attorney's Office will have information about current con-artist schemes targeting the elderly. This type of information is usually available on your local District Attorney's web site. The scams vary, but listed below are some of the more common ones that seem to pop up on a regular basis:

- **Bogus Charities.** The elderly person is approached either at the door or by telephone with a request to donate to a legitimate-sounding charity. Be very wary of such calls. Many so-called charities are bogus, and the money is diverted directly into the pockets of the crooks.

- **Home Improvement Scams.** These are among the most common abuses of the elderly. The elderly person is approached, normally by at least two individuals posing as contractors. The unsuspecting victim is persuaded that a roof, driveway, or other part of the home needs immediate repairs. The contractors quote a high fee for the work, and after obtaining a substantial up-front deposit, disappear. Even in those instances when the work is actually done, it is usually shoddy and almost worthless.

  Warn your parent to be wary of contractors who use high-pressure sales techniques such as "This is a one-time, limited offer." Another common tactic is to say that the work on the house will be used for promotional purposes with neighbors; thus, a "special, reduced price" is being offered. However, if the offer is not immediately accepted, it will be given to someone else in the neighborhood, and your parent will have to pay a higher price.

Should your parent fall victim to such a scheme, remember, in every state the law says that contracts for home improvements must contain a three-day right of rescission (a cooling-off period). This means that if your parent cancels the contract within seventy-two hours, the entire deposit must be refunded, and there will be no obligation under the contract. This law will not help your parent with the stranger who runs off with a deposit, but it does help with other contracts that are signed at the house. Also, encourage your parent to call the Better Business Bureau (BBB) about any home-improvement contractor, or, better yet, make the call yourself. The BBB is a great source of information about contractor complaints.

- **Thefts from Within the Home.** The elderly person is approached at the door by at least two individuals who use a ruse to enter the house. Such ruses include requests to use the bathroom, permission to use the telephone to call 911 to report an accident that happened down the street, or something as innocent-sounding as asking for a glass of water. Once inside, one of the individuals will keep the elderly person occupied, while the other individual rummages through personal belongings, stealing cash and jewelry.

- **Bank Investigator Scheme.** The elderly person is contacted by telephone or outside the bank by a stranger who flashes an official-looking badge and identifies himself as a member of law enforcement. The stranger asks for help in catching a dishonest bank employee. The elderly person is persuaded to go inside the bank to a particular teller window and withdraw a large sum of cash, and then meet the "official" outside. Once the cash is handed over, the stranger gives a bogus receipt for the cash and a phone number to call him at the police station about the status of the investigation. Then he disappears with the money.

•**Sweepstakes Scam.** A telephone caller explains that the elderly person has won a substantial prize, but to collect that prize, he or she must first send a money order for up to $4,000 by overnight mail.

(Provided in part by the San Diego County District Attorney's Office)

DISTRICT ATTORNEY

The District Attorney's Office exists for the purpose of prosecuting criminals. As the cases of elder-abuse increase, many D.A.'s are creating special elder-abuse teams or units to specifically address crimes against the elderly. The D.A.'s office usually works hand-in-hand with the police to disseminate information to the public to help ensure elder safety. In many cities, elder-abuse crimes carry penalties similar to those for hate crimes. Awareness of crimes against the elderly is increasing, and most district attorneys are working hard to find ways to protect our older loved ones.

Elder abuse crimes fall into four main categories:

1. **Physical abuse,** including assaults, batteries, sexual assaults, false imprisonment and endangerment.
2. **Physical neglect by a caregiver,** including withholding medical services or hygiene that exposes the elderly person to the risk of serious harm.
3. **Mental abuse,** including making threats or the infliction of emotional harm.
4. **Financial abuse,** including theft of personal items such as cash, investments, real property and jewelry.

(Provided by the San Diego District Attorney's Office)

Although district attorneys have become quite aggressive in prosecuting cases of elder abuse, financial abuse remains the crime that is most difficult to pursue if the victim is unwilling to press charges. This, of course, was the case with my father. I would have immediately gone to the D.A. myself had I not been told repeatedly that unless my father was willing to go after Grace, she could not be prosecuted. This is a loophole in the law that I hope will be remedied one day. As long as this loophole exists, you must be ever vigilant in protecting your parent from financial exploitation.

Some states are enacting new statutes to help elderly victims recoup their losses from fraud or financial abuse. These new laws provide civil remedies (in the form of lawsuits) and allow for criminal prosecution for financial exploitation. This is a step in the right direction; however, the victim still must overcome the reluctance to take action against the abuser. Without a cooperative victim, there can be no legal action. Also, even if legal action is taken, built-in problems still hamper the odds of success:

•Difficulty of proving the case

•Cost for the lawyer

•Slim possibility of actually collecting damages or recouping exploited money from the perpetrator

•Slow pace of the judicial system

•Lack of knowledge about elder abuse among lawyers, prosecutors, law enforcement officers and judges.

(Stiegel, 2000)

The good news is that legislators are becoming more aware of the challenges faced by victims of elder abuse and are working to change policy and practices. As a result, many more cases of elder abuse are showing up in the courts. In California, for example, the Elder and Dependent Adult Civil Protection Act authorizes the award of attorney's fees for elder-abuse cases, and sometimes even punitive damages. The act also allows a lawsuit to survive the victim, which means the heirs can continue the law-suit if the victim dies. In Illinois, victims of financial abuse can now col-lect triple damages in addition to attorney's fees and court costs. Maine's recent statute addresses the improper transfer of real estate, personal property or money between an elderly person and a caregiver. Such trans-fers are automatically voided unless the elderly person was represented by independent counsel specifically for that transaction.

As you can see, new ground is constantly being broken in the cause to protect our elderly citizens. Still, these are baby steps, and it will take time to write and enact laws that truly offer the best protection. You'll find my thoughts on how the laws should be changed at the end of the book.

AGENCIES

When you sense that your parent's situation is becoming troublesome, you can take steps before it degenerates into emergency status and you feel the need to involve the police or the District Attorney. Nearly every community has some form of Adult Protective Services Agency, whose purpose is to offer links to supportive services for the elderly.

Staff members at Adult Protective Services are specially trained in issues affecting the elderly. Most offer services such as the following:

•Abuse investigation

•In-home assessment

•Mediation

•Plan-development for stability

•Referral to community services

Many people are unaware of the myriad support systems available for the elderly. These support systems are particularly helpful for children who don't live in the same city as their parent in that they provide several layers of protection. When you know that someone is delivering meals, stopping by for a visit, or overseeing case management for your parent, if anything is amiss, you'll find out quickly.

If your parent doesn't require 24-hour caregiving, it might be well worth the effort to arrange for as many of these services as seem appropriate. In my father's case, he had a single caregiver who was responsible for nearly every facet of his life. Hindsight proved that, in our case, this was a recipe for disaster. Had there been a steady parade of specially trained people delivering meals and checking on him, he wouldn't have been as susceptible to being conned.

Another benefit of having these trained professionals in constant contact with seniors is that they encourage them to get involved in their community to whatever extent they are able. They know of volunteer and social opportunities and can lead your parents to something that might help rekindle their enthusiasm for life.

Finding the right fit of options and services for your parent will take some research on your part. I can't overemphasize, though, just how valuable these services can be in becoming part of the network of people and programs that have the common goal of ensuring your parent's welfare.

CHAPTER 5

Involuntarily Committed

*D*riving to the hospital, I realized I had much to be grateful for. First, that K.C. had managed to get an appointment with Dad's doctor on such short notice, and second, that Officer Martinez had persuaded Dad to let me take him to the hospital. I was further grateful that after all the excitement and trauma of the previous hour or so, the drive to the hospital was blessedly uneventful. Dad even attempted some conversation, commenting on how nice Officer Martinez had been and noting how hard it is to be a police officer, even in a low-crime area like Point Loma.

I agreed with everything Dad said, while inside I was saying a silent prayer of thanks for Officer Martinez. I was glad to learn, too, that Dad liked Dr. French. "Dr. French is a fine doctor, Ed. He cared for your mother, you know, and Sue was his patient, too." I resisted the urge to ask whether Grace had used the services of the good doctor, as well.

Mission Ridge Hospital is a relatively small facility about a twenty-five-minute drive from the house, flanked by medical offices, a pharmacy, and a collection of fast-food restaurants. I parked Dad's car and he got out unassisted. Together we walked toward the emergency room, where K.C. had told me I should have Dr. French paged. We learned from the receptionist that Dr. French was running late and had not yet arrived. But he had already ordered some blood work and other tests in anticipation of Dad's arrival. So Dad followed an orderly to begin his tests, while I settled into the waiting area.

I took in my surroundings, noting that this seemed to be an unusually quiet emergency room, not that I was an authority on emergency rooms. It didn't seem to be the hub of activity I always saw on *ER,* the television show I watched religiously. The waiting area had just a few chairs and only two other occupants. Piped-in elevator music was mostly drowned out by the television, which was tuned to a game show that no one seemed to be watching. I glanced briefly at the selection of worn magazines and realized I was too tired to make the effort to read. The long trip to California and lack of sleep were catching up with me. So I sat quietly in my chair against the wall, closed my eyes and tried to gather my thoughts. It took a huge force of will even to think.

The more I thought about all that had happened, the less I could see a clear way out of this mess. Given the events of the last twenty-four hours, I knew Dad would never agree to appoint me or even K.C. his guardian, at least until the "Grace issue" was resolved. Since the lawyer I had consulted had offered no alternatives, I was down to no real options. What had appeared to be the easy task of getting rid of Grace now seemed next to impossible. This realization didn't mean that I was going to give up. Too much was at stake for my father.

My one ray of hope right now was a man I had never met, Dr. French. Maybe he could help. I believed that all Dad needed was to get his meds regulated and start eating three squares a day. Then, he would be back to his old self and realize that Grace should get the boot. It was obvious that the caregiver K.C. had selected was not going to work out. Although Jane had seemed eager to please, Dad responded to her as if he had grabbed a live wire. Maybe a different caregiver was the solution. I made a mental note to talk to my sister about this possibility, and maybe I could discuss it with Dr. French, too. I was still mulling over our dismal predicament when the orderly came out.

I was stunned by the size of the guy. As he approached me, I was engulfed by his shadow. I was about to ask him why he wasn't playing for the NFL, but he stopped me cold with this statement: "Your father asked me to tell you that he wants to go home." These were not the words I wanted to hear. Right now the hospital was a sanctuary for Dad; indeed, it was the only sanctuary I could think of at the moment.

"What does the doctor say?" I asked.

"He hasn't arrived at the hospital yet."

I thought for a minute and then said, "Please tell my father that he should not leave until the doctor has seen him." At this point I believed my father would be more willing to listen to the orderly than to me. "Tell him that Dr. French will be here in a few minutes, and he left specific instructions that he wanted to see my father. If you could, please make it seem important that he stay for a little bit longer. My father is sick, and I think it's imperative that he wait for Dr. French." I felt uncomfortable confiding to a stranger that my father was sick. It wasn't my nature to share problems with anyone outside my family. But I knew I needed some help from someone, and the orderly seemed willing to help me. He nodded his approval and disappeared behind the door to deliver the message.

Within minutes, a middle-aged man emerged from inside the emergency room and approached me. I breathed a sigh of relief when Dr.

French introduced himself. As we shook hands I told Dr. French how genuinely happy I was to see him. Dr. French thanked me and said that Dad had always said the nicest things about my family and me. I was gratified to learn that Dr. French knew Dad well enough to be familiar with his family members.

Dr. French wasted no time in giving me an overview of Dad's health status. He told me my father had been his patient for many years, and he saw Dad regularly because of his various ailments. My father had a mild heart problem. He also had high blood pressure, which was under control, and age-onset diabetes, which was controllable as long as Dad took his medicine. Dr. French mentioned a few other ailments, as well, but in the blur of confusion and fatigue, I didn't catch everything he said.

Dr. French was a talker. He asked about K.C. and then about Grace. Rather than enlighten him about Grace's recent entry into the ranks of the unemployed, I simply said that she was recovering from her trip to China. Even in my tired state I could hardly deliver the message with a straight face. Dr. French didn't seem surprised to hear that Grace was in China. He asked me to "give her my best," a request that forced me to bite my tongue in restraint. I had no intention of giving Grace's anyone's best unless she was inside a jail cell.

Instead, I began to give Dr. French some background information. I was telling him about the pills covering the bathroom floor, and my father's lack of appetite and mental acuity when, out of the blue, the floodgates opened. I gave Dr. French the entire picture, sparing nothing. I told him how Grace had duped Dad into signing paychecks several times a week. I added in the unusual contributions to the church and Dad's irrational instructions to the stockbroker to liquidate his portfolio. By the time I got to Dad's unwillingness to confront the reality of how much Grace had exploited him, I could see that I had Dr. French's rapt attention.

Dr. French needed to know everything, I reasoned, so that he would admit Dad to the hospital to get his meds regulated and some decent food in him. Dr. French indicated that now he was also extremely concerned about Dad. But even though he acknowledged the highly unusual conduct from the patient he had known so long, his next statement was not encouraging: "Regulation of medication and nutrition does not qualify as medical necessity." Therefore, Dr. French could not admit Dad to the hospital. Needless to say, I was not happy to hear this news.

Approaching desperation, I asked Dr. French about an admission for observation or any other way to get him in. I was hoping Dr. French would appreciate the severity of the situation and come up with a creative way to get my dad into the hospital for the care I truly believed he needed. I wanted my father to be in the best possible environment so he could get healthy again. I was praying that a day or two in Mission Ridge would be the magic bullet to get Dad back on track.

Dr. French said that an involuntary admission for psychiatric evaluation was possible only if Dad was a "harm to himself or a harm to others." So, once again, I smacked right into that bureaucratic roadblock. I explained to Dr. French that Dad was obviously a harm to himself because he had ordered his stockbroker to liquidate all of his worldly assets. Predictably, Dr. French said, "Ed, unfortunately, this is not enough. Harm to self means physical harm. I am sorry, but as a lawyer you surely understand that your dad can be admitted only if he is a harm to his person or his conduct puts someone else at risk of harm." Trapped by the truth, I had to acknowledge that I understood.

Dr. French excused himself, saying it was time for him to see Dad, and disappeared through the door where the orderly had gone. I was drifting off to sleep, thinking about my conversation with Dr. French, when

I heard the door open once more. I looked up to see the orderly, Dr. French, and Dad heading toward me. Dad had the lead, and stopping not more than three feet in front of me said in a stern voice, with his hand outstretched and almost touching my nose, "Give me the keys to the car, Ed, I want to go home!"

I knew that Dad was probably as frustrated as I, but for different reasons. He wanted only to get back to the environment that was his comfort zone: home, with Grace taking care of him. I wanted only for my father to get the treatment I believed he needed, but the system was working against me. The two stubborn bulls were at it again.

Looking at Dr. French, I asked if Dad was being discharged. Dr. French indicated that he had concluded his physical examination and everything was fine. However, he wanted us to wait in the ER a bit longer, until the lab results came back. I cringed when I heard Dr. Fench's message. "Your father has insisted on leaving, and I don't have the legal authority to detain him." I knew Dad had heard what Dr. French said, so I said, "Dad, let's wait a little bit longer for your lab work, and then we can go home."

Dad was not to be deterred. He looked straight into my eyes and with barely concealed anger said, "Ed, give me the keys to the car, I want to go home. *Now!"*

He yelled "Now" so loudly that the others seated in the waiting room looked away in obvious discomfort at witnessing our dispute. My own temper was starting to flare, and I was in no mood for a discussion. *"Dad, we are* waiting for your labs. *We are not* going home until your lab work comes back."

With fury in his eyes, Dad lunged at me and grabbed me around the throat. "Ed, I want the keys. Give them to me." Nothing could have prepared me for this. Something obviously broke inside Dad, and he could no longer take the pressure of the last twenty-four hours. Still, I never would have predicted that he would attack me physically. Swimming through layers of shock, I finally perceived that the orderly was now holding my father's arms behind his back, and Dr. French was telling me that he was committing Dad involuntarily for observation.

I was in a daze. It had happened so quickly and I was so stunned that I honestly did not really remember the sequence of events between the time I saw my father lunging at me and his being restrained by the orderly. My father hadn't hurt me, so I was somewhat surprised to hear that Dr. French had decided to admit Dad. This was music to my ears, naturally, but I was confused about what had changed the doctor's mind. While collecting my thoughts, I noticed that my father was breathing rapidly and deeply, as if he had just finished running up several flights of stairs and was trying to catch his breath. He wasn't resisting the orderly, who was still holding his arms behind his back.

When I could think rationally again, I asked Dr. French why he was admitting my father now, when just a few minutes earlier he had led me to believe that an admission was impossible. "What about the harm to self or harm to others test?"

He told me that when Dad lunged at me, he had said, "I'm going to kill you if you don't give me the keys."

I knew my father didn't mean it literally, and I marveled at the irony. Dad's efforts to liquidate everything he owned and give away all of his assets—probably to Grace—did not qualify as harm to self, but an excited utterance of an exhausted, malnourished, frustrated, and probably confused person met the other part of the test. Dad was now considered a harm to others.

I was not going to argue with Dr. French's "sound" medical judgment. My goal was accomplished, even though in a backhanded way. Dad was going to get much-needed medical attention from trained professionals and three square meals a day, no matter how it had been accomplished.

Dad was escorted back though the door of the ER. I knew that my father was out of it and truly needed the rest and observation he was about to get. I thanked Dr. French for his help and left Mission Ridge feeling optimistic that Dad was on the road to recovery. For the first time since the confrontation with Dad, I felt good.

I felt a brief pang of conscience about feeling good that I was leaving my father in the hospital, but I knew deep down that this was best for Dad and that I *should* feel good that he was getting the care he needed. An added benefit to Dad's hospitalization was that Grace would not have access to him, so he could begin the healing process. I realized that, for Dad, losing Grace was akin to the death of a loved one. But I also knew that time softens the wounds of permanent separation. Dad's wound needed to heal, and this was just day one of their permanent separation.

I returned to the house, where K.C. was waiting. When she saw that Dad was not with me, she immediately expressed concern, but I told her all was well and that I'd fill her in as soon as she told me what had happened in my absence. K.C. jumped right into an amazing story of how Grace, dressed in her Sunday best, along with her two sons and her daughter, took all of her worldly possessions out of the house in an assembly line, under the watchful eye of Officer Martinez and another police officer. K.C. was positively effusive with joy when she described how Officer Martinez stood by the front door with Grace's sons, while the other officer posted himself in the master bedroom with Grace. The procedure Officer Martinez put into effect was simple and efficient. K.C. escorted one of Grace's sons from the front door to the master bedroom where Grace would identify her property in front of the other officer. The son would pick up the item, and K.C. would escort the son to the front door, where he would exit the house and go to the van where Grace's daughter was doing the packing. This process was repeated over and over. K.C. described all of the designer purses, dresses, shoes, and expensive hats that Grace had accumulated, which she said were new or nearly so. K.C. would know. She was the fashion expert of the family.

There was no question in K.C.'s mind about who had paid for Grace's clothing. K. C. told me that Grace was from a poor family. Obviously, she had hit the mother lode with Dad.

K.C. said it took a couple of hours for Grace and her kids to remove her possessions. When all was done, Officer Martinez had gone out to the loaded van and had a talk with its occupants. When he returned, he told K.C. that he had told them they were not to return to the area, and there would be consequences if they didn't heed his directions. The van pulled out and left; shortly thereafter, "Saint" Officer Martinez and his fellow officer left, as well.

I then shared with K.C. the unbelievable events I had experienced with Dad, relating how Dr. French would not admit Dad because he was not a harm to himself or others until he had made a grab for me out of sheer frustration and threatened to kill me.

Our mutual debriefings ended with the setting sun and we realized that food was in order—in fact, necessary. Neither of us had eaten anything since the morning. We decided on a local Italian place, a short drive away. I was tired, yet somewhat energized by the recent positive turn of events.

Our conversation over pepperoni pizza and root beer was warm and hopeful. We discussed our children and mutual friends. I filled K.C. in on my wife and kids in much the same way as I had my father the evening before. In turn, K.C. brought me up to date on her kids. Most of all, we talked about growing up.

We were never close as children. In fact, we fought like cats and dogs during our formative years. Despite our rocky childhood relationship, most of our conversation that evening focused on wonderful memories of family activities. We talked about how our parents took us out to the finest restaurants the area had to offer so that we would know our way around menus comfortably. We were always encouraged to taste before eliminating a dish from our "interested" list. K.C. and I reminisced about the trips our family had taken, the many get-togethers with our grandparents who lived around the corner when we were growing up, the contribution of our parents to civic activities, and a host of other pleasant memories.

We could relive the past for only so long, though, before the conversation inevitably returned to our father, what had happened to him and what the future possibly held. I was convinced that after Dad was stabilized in the hospital, if we could secure reliable care providers, all would be well. K.C. was not so sure that adequate caregivers were the solution. She believed it might be better to get him the type of care he needed in a facility geared for older people. As an option, K.C. mentioned that she had been doing some research into nursing homes, and she had found an assisted-living facility nearby that she wanted us to visit.

The mere mention of the words "nursing home" made my head throb. We both knew that for Dad the idea of going to a nursing home was worse than a death sentence. The laundry business he had owned with our grandfather really took off with the introduction of linen supply. Dad was one of the first to come up with the idea of buying the linen and then renting it to the customer for a fee. The profit margins were astonishing. After three washings, the cost of the linen was recovered, and thereafter each washing was handsomely profitable. Dad brought in so much linen-supply business that eventually the laundry was operating two, sometimes three, shifts a day. The principal source of the linen supply business was nursing homes.

At that time, in the late 1950s, nursing homes were virtually unregulated and the place of last resort for leaving a loved one. People talked about nursing homes in the same hushed whispers they might talk about a married person having an affair.

Dad saw the nursing-home business from the worst possible vantage point. The linens coming into the laundry were always soaked in urine and spotted heavily with feces, which meant that the residents were lying in their own waste for who knew how long. The halls of the nursing homes were dark and dank, and the residents were often strapped in chairs, wearing food-stained night clothes. Paint was frequently peeling from the walls, and food that looked barely edible was served to the inmates/residents. This is what Dad saw when he visited the nursing homes on his sales calls, and it had a profound effect on him.

Both K.C. and I recalled vividly the many conversations at the dinner table where Dad would describe, in more detail than we wanted to hear, what he had seen that day while visiting nursing homes. An integral part of those graphic descriptions of the horrors Dad saw was his statement that "I wouldn't put my worst enemy in a nursing home." From the time we were young children he had made us promise never to put him into a nursing home. This was a commitment that we had affirmed to our father not once, but many, many times.

We had seen firsthand Dad's opposition to a nursing home as an option for our mother. He believed that a nursing home was not a place for his beloved wife under any circumstances. It was not an easy task for Dad and, in fact, it was physically burdensome to keep caregivers in the house twenty-four hours a day for the better part of twenty years to care for Mom. He would tell us individually and jointly that Mom would never be put into a nursing home as long as he was alive. She was his special person who deserved much better then the deplorable conditions a nursing home had to offer at that time.

So, when K.C. mentioned the idea of an assisted living facility, we both knew we were treading on dangerous ground. Even our idle conversation on the subject sent a shiver up my spine, as if Dad could hear our blasphemous words from the hospital almost fifteen miles away. I knew if we tried to put Dad into a nursing home against his wishes, it would be an unparalleled assault on his psyche. But I trusted K.C.'s judgment, so in spite of the obvious problems with our father's opinion of nursing homes, I agreed to visit the place she had found.

Dinner wound down and exhaustion took over. I paid the bill and drove back to the house looking forward to a good night's sleep—finally. I stopped the car on the street to let K.C. out, said goodnight and waited for her to get into her car and drive off toward her home. Once she was gone, I parked the car in the garage, hit the automatic door switch and heard the garage door close with a thud behind me as I entered the pitch black house.

It was almost eerie, standing in the family room, reliving the events of the day. I saw the ghost of Officer Martinez pointing his finger at all of us while telling everyone to leave the house. I smiled to myself thinking how resourceful he had been to get Dad out of the house easily so that he could be taken to see Dr. French. I pictured in my mind the assembly line of Grace's children removing her possessions from the house under the watchful eyes of two of San Diego's finest. Again, I expressed silent thanks for the delivery of those two officers. Finally, I considered the positive implications of my father's permanent separation from Grace. I was confident that with the stabilization of Dad's meds combined with a nourishing diet, he would once again think clearly and would want to have nothing to do with the person who had exploited him for almost all he was worth.

I realized I was well past gone. Exhaustion was an understatement for my current condition. I immediately made my way to the bedroom, where I fell on the bed and was asleep in seconds. Sometime during the night, I woke long enough to take off my clothes and put on a nightshirt.

Making the System Work for You: What You Can Do

Sadly, cases of elder abuse are becoming more common. Fortunately, our legal system is recognizing the increased incidence of elder abuse. Existing laws are being tightened up and new laws are being enacted to help protect our loved ones. Many states, for example, have instituted mandatory reporting requirements if elder abuse is observed by employees of health facilities, law enforcement officials, or health and social service workers.

As I noted in chapter 4, elder abuse crimes generally fall into four main categories:

1. Physical abuse
2. Physical neglect
3. Mental abuse
4. Financial abuse

Abuse that can be substantiated under any of these categories is a prosecutable crime. The first two categories, physical abuse or neglect, are usually easy to observe and document, simply because the evidence is visible. Bruises and broken bones cannot be ignored, nor can the signs of physical deterioration because of neglect.

Financial abuse presents unique problems when, as with my father, the victim refuses to admit a crime has taken place. My father refused to acknowledge that he had been victimized by Grace, and without his corroboration, the legal system was powerless to help him. Even when my sister and I had proof that Grace was fleecing my dad, the legal standard of "harm to self or to others" proved to be an almost insurmountable obstacle in our attempts to help him.

The law has not yet adapted enough to help elderly people who have formed such a strong psychological bond to their caregiver that they will deny abuse out of fear of abandonment. This was clearly the case with my father. He had the cognitive wherewithal to realize that Grace had cheated him, but he couldn't contemplate being left alone, without her. As a virtual shut-in, my father's only remaining friend was Grace, whom he was unwilling to lose, regardless of the price. His unwillingness to acknowledge her scheme or to press charges threw everyone involved into a legal limbo. We had the facts, we knew a crime had been committed, but we were powerless in the eyes of our legal system.

Until the laws change to allow adult children the latitude to help their parents when they are truly in need, we must adopt the Boy Scout's motto: Be prepared.

In chapter 1, I talked about various powers of attorney and revocable trusts that can be set up to help you and your parents prepare for healthcare issues and other decisions relating to their well-being. Then, in chapter 2, I gave you ideas for advance planning to try to anticipate as many eventualities as possible. There are other tools that can be immensely helpful to you and your parents, particularly with regard to healthcare issues. One is a power of attorney for healthcare, which usually is drawn up in conjunction with a living will. Each is useful in its own way.

POWER OF ATTORNEY FOR HEALTHCARE

A power of attorney for healthcare is somewhat different from a general durable power of attorney in that it allows the person designated as attorney-in-fact to make only healthcare decisions for the principal—not financial or legal decisions. This document can be crafted to your parent's individual needs, but it typically includes a provision that healthcare decisions are to be made by the attorney-in-fact only after consultation with the principal (your parent) in an attempt to determine the principal's preferences, even if he or she can communicate by only rudimentary means, such as a blink of an eye or a hand squeeze to indicate yes or no.

Further, the power of attorney for healthcare covers decisions about healthcare circumstances, such as those listed below:

•Use of experimental procedures

•Access to medical records

•Hospice care

•Change of physicians

The benefit of the power of attorney for healthcare is that obstacles are eliminated before they arise. Under the law, doctors are not required and are sometimes prohibited from discussing the medical condition or the course of treatment for your parent with anyone other than the patient. I have seen cases in which the doctor followed these rules to the letter, to the great consternation of the adult child who wanted only to help with the parent's care. In one case, a middle-aged woman was in a coma, survived only by her adult son. The doctor would not discuss his patient's condition with the son. A power of attorney for healthcare grants consent ahead of time; thus, doctors are relieved of the legal responsibility to withhold your parent's medical information from you.

Most spouses will grant a power of attorney for healthcare to each other. After one of your parents is deceased, it is imperative that the surviving parent sign a power of attorney for healthcare appointing one or more of the adult children to make healthcare decisions for that parent. Alternatively, when your parents prepare an initial power of attorney for healthcare, they can designate their adult child as a secondary agent to fill the role should one of them die or become incapacitated.

You can see from the above partial list of issues covered in the power of attorney for healthcare that we are talking about a comprehensive document designed to allow the attorney-in-fact to make major health-care decisions for the parent. Even though the attorney-in-fact is required to ascertain the parent's opinion on a specific medical question at the time it is being considered, the attorney-in-fact still has the authority to make the ultimate decision, using his or her best judgment of what the parent would want absent the present condition.

Sometimes this creates a moral dilemma for the attorney-in-fact. For example, should you authorize an experimental procedure that might relieve pain and suffering even though the procedure will shorten your parent's life? Or should you let your parent continue to live in pain and let nature take its course? There may be no right answer at such a critical time; however, if you had previously discussed with your parent the issue of the use of experimental procedures versus a shortened life, possibly without pain, you would have a strong compass heading to follow.

The only shortcoming a power of attorney for healthcare has is that, like other powers of attorney, it can be revoked. This is not likely to happen, however. In my more than thirty years of legal practice, I have yet to see a power of attorney for healthcare revoked.

LIVING WILL

A living will differs from a power of attorney for healthcare in that in a living will, your parent makes clear his or her wishes about the use or continued use of extraordinary life-support procedures. As you know, medical science has progressed so that it can sometimes artificially prolong life indefinitely. The most basic form of a living will allows your parent to decide ahead of time whether or not to be kept alive by machines. The beauty of this document is that it takes out of the children's hands the decision about whether to use or continue using such extraordinary healthcare measures.

In all states, the law on living wills is tied to the same basic medical test: Is death imminent and will it occur whether or not life-sustaining procedures are used? If it is determined that this is indeed the case, then through a living will your parent can express a desire that life-sustaining procedures not be used and only medication to relieve pain and suffering be administered. The decision to use or not use life-sustaining procedures is made only by your parent's doctor using this standard. The child is not required to make this decision.

I strongly recommend that a safeguard be built into the living will in states that allow only one doctor to make the ultimate decision. That safeguard would require the unanimous opinion of two doctors—your parent's treating physician and an independent doctor who has examined your parent—that the use or continued use of extraordinary life-support procedures would serve no useful purpose. In my experience, this additional language has alleviated the fear that the doctor may be temped to "pull the plug" too quickly.

Furthermore, you needn't fear that a living will compels the doctor to discontinue life support without consulting family members. Even though not required to do so by law, in my experience, the doctor will always talk with the family members first. However, the living will is a wonderful way for the parent to relieve the child from the difficulty of making the ultimate decision. Some years ago, I was in the intensive care unit waiting room with a client whose father was hanging onto life by a thread. The doctor came out and said, "Harry has no brain waves. Do you want us to use 'heroic measures'?"

My client said, "My father has executed a living will," which she had with her and gave to the doctor. The doctor indicated that he understood and would follow Harry's desires. While a tragic moment indeed, it struck me how wonderful it was that my client did not have to make the decision about whether her father should be allowed to die naturally or kept alive by machines.

Although a living will does not necessarily have to spell out your parent's wishes about every life-sustaining measure, it can specifically address those that your parent may feel strongly about, such as ventilators, artificial feeding, or resuscitation. Many parents have strong opinions about the right to die with dignity. The living will is the instrument by which they can make sure their wishes are respected and carried out.

GUARDIANSHIP/CONSERVATORSHIP

In chapter 1, I talked briefly about guardianship (or conservatorship—in some jurisdictions, the terms are interchangeable). In fact, I had drawn up guardianship papers before I came to San Diego with the hope that my father would sign them and appoint me his guardian. Had I been appointed guardian for Dad, I would have "stood in my dad's shoes" with complete authority to make all decisions for him.

A guardianship is the next step up from the revocable trust I discussed in chapter 1—and it's a big step. If a guardianship is secured, *all* formal control by your parent over his or her personal affairs is relinquished. As ominous and shocking as this may sound to you, it is your very best tool to prevent financial exploitation and abuse by a caregiver, mainly because a guardianship is difficult to revoke.

Guardianships are either voluntary or involuntary; the authority each grants is the same. Your parent can voluntarily appoint you as guardian. Obviously, this requires a great deal of trust between parent and child, because your parent is essentially allowing you (or whoever is appointed guardian) to have complete control and decision-making power over everything. If your parent voluntarily agrees to appoint you alone as guardian (or in combination with other siblings), your worries are over. You would have complete control over your parent's personal, legal and financial affairs.

The major problem with voluntary guardianships, which my clients will rarely state in front of their children, is the parent's fear that if a child is appointed as guardian, the child will become stingy with the parent's care because the child is in a conflicted position. Obviously, the less the child spends on the parent, the more the child stands to inherit. Personally, I don't always buy into this fear. However, to alleviate this concern, I suggest the parent appoint a trusted independent person as guardian, such as the family accountant or attorney or a good friend, thereby taking the child entirely out of the process. Another alternative is to appoint the child and the independent person as co-guardians, with the independent person making all financial decisions, and the child being responsible for all other decisions pertaining to the parent.

The second principal concern about a guardianship that I hear often from my clients is much more difficult to overcome. Some parents are concerned that they are losing their dignity by giving up complete control over their property. In many families, control of the purse strings guarantees love, affection and attention from the children, as crass as this may seem. The best way a child can respond to this fear is with honesty and love, telling the parent that he or she has done well, accomplished a lot and has much to be proud of, but now some help is needed. I also suggest that the family attorney be asked to discuss with the parent privately the advantages of voluntary guardianship.

This is a tough situation for all. If your parent is reluctant or unwilling to consent to a voluntary guardianship, you still can employ some of the other measures I've discussed, such as a general durable power of attorney. Once your parent has had more time to think about a voluntary guardianship, you might be able to revisit the subject in the future.

Should you and your parent agree on a voluntary guardianship, it must be filed with the court, so you probably would require the assistance of an attorney. As guardian, you would be legally obliged to act in the best interests of your parent. Further, the court will supervise the relationship to assure proper treatment of your parent. Obtaining a voluntary guardianship is a best-case scenario, but it is a step that many parents are unwilling to take, until it is too late. Often, by the time the children realize the parent has reached a point where guardianship is desirable—or necessary—the parent is in no frame of mind to grant it. Then the children must wrestle with the difficult decision of petitioning the court for an involuntary guardianship.

If you are considering seeking an involuntary guardianship, the following information will help guide you.

1. An involuntary guardianship can be ordered by the court after a hearing in which the parent, the person asking to be the parent's guardian and two expert witnesses testify. The expert witnesses are usually two psychiatrists, one for the parent, who will testify that the parent is competent, and one for the adult children, who will testify

that the parent is incompetent. This is the proverbial battle of the experts with the judge having to decide which expert to believe.

2. If the testimony convinces the judge that the person is incompetent, the judge issues an order appointing another person, usually a family member, as guardian, which means that person now has complete control over the incompetent person's affairs.

3. The judge usually requires that the guardian submit an accounting of the income and expenses and the current value of the estate at least once a year. This allows the judge to monitor the guardian's activities.

4. The judge also usually requires that the guardian post a bond. The bond is an insurance policy protecting the estate from the guardian taking or using assets in a manner not in the best interest of the incompetent parent. The cost of the bond is paid for by the estate, and it is expensive.

5. The appointment of the guardian can be revoked only by a judge, which would require another hearing and the judge's determination that the incompetent person has regained competence.

Involuntary guardianships are much trickier than voluntary guardianships; I compare them to high-stakes poker. A fine line often exists between competency and incompetency. My father was a good example of someone straddling that line. He seemed rational most of the time and was still capable of thinking for himself and making some decisions. But he was beginning to show signs of mild dementia, he obviously wasn't making good financial decisions—given his call to his stockbroker—and he was apparently incapable of seeing how Grace was taking advantage of him. Despite these facts, had I pursued involuntary guardianship on the basis of the information I had at that time, I doubt if I would have been successful.

The odds of securing an involuntary guardianship when the parent is at least partially competent are practically nil. However, the risk of destroying your relationship with your parent is 100 percent. No parent would welcome being yanked into court to be accused of being incompetent by his or her child. Should you decide to pursue involuntary guardianship, you must be prepared for the worst, whether you succeed or not.

In most jurisdictions in the United States, the "harm to self or harm to others" standard is practically impossible to overcome if the parent is even marginally competent. Remember, the only reason my father was admitted to the hospital was because he lost his temper and physically attacked me. Thus he was deemed capable of causing harm to others.

Also, keep in mind that an involuntary guardianship procedure is costly. You will need a lawyer to represent yourself (or the person seeking to be named guardian). You will also need to hire a lawyer to represent your parent. Usually the two psychiatrists will have to evaluate your parent and attend the hearing to testify to the competency of your parent. When you start calculating the costs for two lawyers and two doctors, you can see that involuntary guardianship is an expensive proposition.

I hope you never have to face the prospect of securing an involuntary guardianship for your parent. You can greatly reduce the chances of such a scenario if you work with your parent (or parents) while they are still of sound mind and capable of making good decisions.

RELATIONSHIPS

I would like to suggest another powerful advance-planning tool that you can use to avoid problems before they begin. If you are able, develop relationships with those who have financial connections with your parent. This measure can go a long way in protecting your parent.

K.C.'s good relationship with the branch manager of Dad's bank was invaluable to us in determining just how far Grace had already gone in siphoning his funds. Without the branch manager's help, we would have been left in the dark. As incidents of financial abuse of elders are increasing, banks are beginning to realize that they have a responsibility to be an active partner in the protection of our aged citizens. Many banks sponsor special training for their employees to learn how to spot account abnormalities that might signal a scam or potential financial abuse. In some cases the government is stepping in. In California, for example, the state legislature has established a pilot training program for bank employees to learn the many ways seniors can fall victim to financial abuse. Likewise, many District Attorney's offices and Aging and Independence agencies are offering free training to bank employees about what to do if they suspect elder abuse. Such programs are still in their infancy, though, and you would be well advised to find out if your parent's bank has taken any measures to institute policies and programs designed to protect their elderly customers. However, even if your parent's bank is on the cutting edge of elder protection, don't let your guard down. Act on the suggestions below to avoid problems before they occur.

1. Make an appointment with the bank manager or customer service representative of your parent's bank. Explain that your parent, while still relatively independent, might be susceptible to a scam or other financial abuse, and you are hopeful that you can count on the bank's cooperation in protecting your parent. Ask if the bank has any procedures in place to flag an elderly person's account for the purpose of spotting abnormal activity. Also ask if the bank's tellers have had any special training to be alert for possible victims of financial abuse. Ideally, you would arrange for the bank to contact you immediately if they notice unusual activity.

A popular scam targeting elderly people involves a so-called Canadian lottery. An official-looking letter notifying recipients that they are "winners" is followed up by a telephone call from a sweet-sounding woman who persuades victims to send in a "processing fee," usually several thousand dollars, in order to claim their prize. One elderly woman withdrew a large sum from her bank account twice in the same week, and the bank never questioned her. An alert, trained teller would have noticed the large withdrawals and gently questioned the woman. Granted, bank employees are sensitive about invading the privacy of their customers and alienating them. But, in this day and age, it is incumbent upon banks to lend a hand in protecting our elder population.

2. If you are a signatory on your parent's account, request that a copy of the monthly statement and canceled checks be mailed to you. The duplication will likely incur an additional fee, but the peace of mind it provides is worth it. When you receive the statement, be sure to take the time to review it for anything that appears out of the ordinary.

3. Talk with your parent about keeping only a small amount of money in the checking account, enough to cover one month's expenses. Then, arrange to replenish this account each month with a regular, automatic transfer from a savings or money-market account.

4. Insist that your parent's checking account **not** have overdraft protection. Often, people will have several accounts within the same financial institution: checking, savings, money market, etc. If your parent writes a check on a checking account with overdraft protection, it would be honored even if the account did not have sufficient funds. Many banks will simply transfer funds from another account to cover checking account overdrafts. But if your

parent's account is flagged for no overdraft protection, an unusually large check would not clear even though your parent signed the check. A bounced-check charge is easier to swallow than the possible loss of thousands of dollars.

Make a list of everyone with whom your parent has financial dealings. Try to meet with all of them, either in person or by telephone, to enlist their support in watching out for your parent. You will undoubtedly have to dispel some suspicion that you are meddling in your parent's affairs or trying to get control of the finances. You should be able to reassure these professionals that you are simply trying to take the necessary steps to protect your parent without sacrificing his or her independence. All you're really asking is to be notified of anything unusual or unexpected, such as a closed account or, as was the case with my father, an attempt to liquidate investments. Include the following financial representatives on your contact list:

- •Bankers

- •Tax Accountants

- •Financial Planners

- •Stockbrokers

- •Insurance Agents

Everything I have suggested to you so far—power of attorney, revocable trust, power of attorney for healthcare, living will, voluntary guardianship, even developing relationships with your parent's financial contacts—has been recommended so your parent can continue making many independent decisions. Each tool has a specific purpose, and each is beneficial to both you and your parent. The effort you expend on persuading your parent to take advantage of these tools will pay off in a large way should your parent ever lose decision-making ability. The biggest benefit is shared by both you and your parent: peace of mind.

CHAPTER 6

Dad's Doctor: Advocate or Adversary?

*M*orning came and I awakened to the sounds of birds singing outside. My first thought was that the situation with Dad was going to improve today. Still lying in bed, I looked around the bedroom, noticing how bare it now seemed without Grace's pictures and personal items. The emptiness was gratifying. I hoped it would be just as easy to rid Dad of Grace as it had been to rid this room of her possessions.

I called K.C. to check in, and we agreed to meet mid-morning. We planned to first go see our father, and then if we had time, to visit the assisted-living facility K.C wanted to check out.

As I still had some time before meeting K.C., I moved to the family room to sit and reflect. Given Dad's attachment to Grace, I knew that he needed friends and a social outlet. Could the facility K.C. mentioned last night satisfy this need? It was obvious that caregivers could not.

Dad needed to be with people his own age. Maybe the assisted-living facility was the solution. I promised myself to keep an open mind about the upcoming visit.

My reverie was interrupted by the ringing telephone. On the other end was Dr. Weaver, the psychiatrist Dr. French had asked to evaluate Dad at the hospital. He had "good news." My father had told him everything, and Dr. Weaver had concluded that Dad was "fit as a fiddle and ready to go home."

More then a little shocked by this broadside, I asked Dr. Weaver, "What did Dad tell you about the reason he was in the hospital?"

"Ben told me that he got into an altercation with his brother in the elevator by the hospital waiting room about the keys to his car. It was a massive misunderstanding. He was terribly embarrassed and all was forgiven."

I took a few deep breaths, and told Dr. Weaver, "Ben's brother died in 1945. His altercation was with me, his son, and it took place in the hospital's Emergency Room. Evidently my father is so confused that he doesn't know who he was fighting with or where the fight took place."

After a moment of silence, Dr. Weaver suggested that under the circumstances, more tests and observation in the hospital were warranted. What a relief!

I asked Dr. Weaver about visiting Dad. Dr. Weaver told me that there were no set visiting hours for the lockdown unit. Upon hearing those two words, my stomach did a flip-flop. "What is the lockdown unit?" I asked.

Dr. Weaver said, "I thought you knew that your father had been put in a secure ward because he was a harm to others."

"Is my father in a padded cell?"

"No, not at all. He is sharing a room with another patient. In fact, Ben is currently a member of the 'normal population.' He has access to all services on the ward; however, he cannot leave the ward." Dr. Weaver continued in a rapid-fire voice, obviously trying to ease my shock on hearing that Dad was in a locked-down part of the hospital. "You're probably wondering what normal population means. It means that we do not believe there is a substantial risk that Ben will harm himself or others in the ward, as long as he takes his medicine. We are keeping him under close observation, and we continually assess his condition."

Dr. Weaver further explained that "Ben does not have contact with anyone in restraints or anyone who is assigned a 'special room,'" which was something of a relief to hear, even though I wasn't entirely certain what a special room meant. Dr. Weaver told me that everyone in the lockdown unit had or was suspected of having a psychiatric condition whereby they were at least potentially a harm to themselves or a harm to others. "So fights can break out among the patients, which is why they are monitored so closely. It is sort of a trade-off. It is important for the patients to socialize with others, but the hospital staff must be prepared to act quickly to prevent the patients from getting involved in fights. The patients who become combative are weeded out to special rooms."

I was not comforted by Dr. Weaver's words. From his description, Dad could be in great danger. I knew that Dad presented no harm to himself or to anyone else, despite what Dr. French had concluded the day before. Even though I didn't like the description of where my father was being kept for treatment and observation, rather than cause a problem where there might not be a problem, I chose to thank Dr. Weaver for his call and indicated that my sister and I would be visiting our father in about an hour. Dr. Weaver requested that we meet him as soon as we arrived at the hospital, before we visited with Dad. He asked that we page him. I got the impression that Dr. Weaver was trying to prolong the conversation with unnecessary verbiage to make up for his incorrect diagnosis of my father.

I hung up the phone feeling less sure about the direction of Dad's care. How could a trained psychiatrist be so easily persuaded by Dad that the incident that resulted in his hospitalization was only an aberrational mishap that had occurred between him and his brother? Why hadn't the doctor sought confirmation of the information Dad provided before rendering his diagnosis that my father was fine? Why the rush to judgment? This man was a trained professional. Was he perhaps just having a bad diagnostic day, or was there reason to be concerned about his competence? What should I do?

I concluded that I would be in a better position to evaluate what was happening to my father and the competence of Dr. Weaver once K.C. and I saw Dad in the lockdown unit. I left the house and drove to K.C.'s house, which was only a few miles up a two-lane road toward the lighthouse that used to mark the entrance to San Diego Harbor.

I pulled up in front of her house and honked a few times. K.C. came out, smartly dressed and with her usual smile, got into the car and gave me a kiss on the cheek. While driving to the hospital, I told her about my unsettling conversation with Dr. Weaver. K.C. shared my anxiety. Dr. Weaver's decision to discharge Dad was formed on only a thinly constructed story that could easily have been refuted had the doctor made the effort to verify the facts he heard. We decided that for now the best plan was to watch Dr. Weaver closely and speak with Dr. French if we had more concerns. We also talked about visiting the assisted-living facility after seeing Dad. K.C. told me that the home was flexible about a meeting and tour, so we had no need to rush.

I turned into the hospital's drive, but this time I parked in the visitor's lot instead of the emergency room lot I had used the day before. K.C. and I made our way through the large double doors that marked the entrance to the hospital. In the middle of the room was a semi-circular desk, where two women were seated under a large "Information" sign hanging from the ceiling. One of the women was wearing a volunteer badge, and after a search on her computer, she found the information that would lead us to Dad's room. Maybe it was my imagination, but I was convinced the volunteer had a different look on her face after reading on the computer screen that Dad was in the lockdown unit. Or maybe I was just feeling uncomfortable and embarrassed because my father was confined to the psychiatric ward.

After a few wrong turns, we finally arrived at a wing without any signage to identify it. However, we saw two nurses seated at a desk blocking the entrance to the hallway. Repeating the routine from the information desk, one of the nurses punched in Dad's name and date of birth and told us that there was an order that Dr. Weaver was to be notified when we arrived. She abruptly got up from her chair, stepped out from behind the desk, and asked us to follow her. The nurse escorted us past the desk and down the hallway to a closed door, telling us to wait by the door while she notified Dr. Weaver that we had arrived.

The door where we were left to wait was solid metal with a small glass window. K.C. and I did the normal thing: We looked through the glass to see whatever we could see. Beyond the door was a continuation of the hallway where we were standing. From our vantage point we could see doors evenly spaced down each side of the hall. Probably the doorways to rooms, I thought. What stood out most clearly was a group of patients, all dressed in identical light blue hospital gowns and matching hospital-issued slippers, shuffling up and down the hall in an elongated circle, one person walking behind the other. Each "inmate" moved single file down the hall to the door at the end, made two left turns, then continued back up the length of the hall toward us. I estimated that maybe fifteen people were silently doing the shuffle. Their movement was strange. No one was stepping or walking with a natural stride. They all appeared to be sliding their feet along the floor in a uniform manner.

It was impossible to guess how long this follow-the-leader routine had been going on. I reminded myself that these people were sick. Dr. Weaver had told me that everyone in the unit was in some way a danger to himself or to others. As far as I could tell, no one looked sick, but the subtleties of mental illness were obviously outside my expertise. I thought perhaps the shuffling was some sort of treatment, even though it looked like little more than a way to kill time or a way to get rid of pent-up energy by getting the body moving.

I saw hard-looking men with tattoos and beards who looked like they were on a day pass from the local Hell's Angels chapter. Others looked emaciated and worn by time, people who probably had spent years on the streets. Then there were those who looked utterly ordinary, and among that group was Dad.

K.C. and I both gasped as we saw him. Dad was doing the shuffle with everyone else. He looked dazed and disoriented. I was again shocked by how thin he was. At that moment the realization hit me hard. There was my dad, in the lockdown unit, and he was very sick. My heart ached at seeing him under these circumstances. It took all my effort to maintain my composure. This was quite a shock from the fantasy I had been living since yesterday, when I truly believed that all would be well with Dad in a few days.

Dad did not see us looking through the window as he walked by the door. In fact, no one in the line acknowledged the two faces staring in from the other side of the small window. After Dad shuffled by us several times without showing any signs of recognition, we concluded that we must be looking through a one-way window, otherwise Dad would be looking right at us each time he approached the door. This would also explain why no one else acknowledged our presence. K.C. and I stood in silence, watching our dad and the others, until the sound of footsteps coming from behind us forced us to tear our eyes away.

We turned to see a man approaching in a white coat with "Bernard Weaver, M.D., Division of Psychiatry," embroidered in red on his pocket. We shook hands over introductions; then, Dr. Weaver reached into his pocket and took out a key connected to a flexible, coiled cord and asked us to follow him. He inserted his key into the lock in the door with the window, turned it and pulled opened the door, ushering us into the hallway. Once inside, he relocked the door behind us.

Having crossed the threshold, I concluded that we too were now captives of the lockdown unit. Noise that had been inaudible on the other side of the door was now easily heard. Far down the hall, I heard the drone of a television set. Before following Dr. Weaver down the hallway, I turned around and looked back at the window in the door to confirm that it was one-way glass, as we had suspected. We were wrong; the small window was crystal-clear glass from this side, as well. So why didn't Dad acknowledge us? Each time he approached and passed the glass in front of K.C. and me, we had made a stronger effort to get his attention. We smiled. We waved. We had even knocked on the glass to get his attention. Nothing worked. He never acknowledged his children on the other side of the glass as he approached and passed by the door. I made a mental note to ask Dr. Weaver about Dad's strange behavior.

Our presence had a surprising effect on the conga line. Instead of walking to the door we had just come through before turning and shuffling back, it was as if the door had been moved five feet down the hall. Each patient simply made an earlier turn, without missing a step. When Dad came to the head of the line, before he turned he smiled at us. He didn't stop to talk, but kept moving with the group, as if some unwritten protocol dictated that one doesn't break up the flow of the line, even

if visitors have arrived. I was at a loss to understand how Dad had fall-
en in step with the rules of the line in the short time he had been there.
But at least he had recognized us. This was something. I had many
questions for Dr. Weaver and I hoped he would be able to answer
them.

Dr. Weaver took us about halfway down the hall, stopping in front of
a door with a sign that read "Small Conference Room." Using the same
key he had used to let us into the unit, he unlocked the door and ush-
ered us in. The room was dominated by a brown, circular conference
table the size of a small kitchen table, with six matching chairs placed
around it. Off to the side was a small table that held a telephone, which
was resting atop a worn copy of a telephone book.

I didn't like the room at all. It made me feel like I was in a box. Interior
offices with no windows, such as this one, had always made me feel
slightly claustrophobic. I squelched my discomfort and sat with K.C. on
one side of the table, facing Dr. Weaver, who had positioned himself
directly opposite us. Dr. Weaver had a kind face. I was eager to hear what
he had to say.

"The results of your father's blood work have come in. He is severely out of balance chemically. I have visited with Ben on the unit, and
I've consulted with Doctor French, who also examined your dad earlier
this morning."

The fact that Dr. Weaver had conferred with Dr. French made me feel
better about his professionalism.

"Doctor French would be happy to discuss your father's health with
you if you would call him," Dr. Weaver said. "It is our opinion that Ben
is suffering from some mild dementia in addition to his other ailments,
such as his diabetes, heart issues, and fluid in his lungs. Furthermore,
his esophagus is not directing all his food to his stomach; some food is
going to his lungs. Also, he complains of constant pain in his feet." To

temper Dad's agitation, Dr. Weaver told us he had given him some medication to "take the edge off." K.C. didn't seemed surprised by the laundry list of Dad's health issues, probably because she had accompanied him to the doctor on many occasions and was more in tune with his condition. I, however, was shaken by the extent of Dad's ailments, many of which I had apparently missed when Dr. French and I had spoken in the Emergency Room.

Dr. Weaver explained that once Dad's blood chemistry was stabilized, he would be as okay as possible, given his other ailments. Dr. Weaver emphasized that unless Dad took his medications as prescribed and ate a balanced diet, he could easily have another episode that could be more severe and perhaps life-threatening.

I wondered what Dr. Weaver meant by "episode." Was he talking about my dad allowing his care provider to fleece him and still caring for her more than he cared for his children? Was he talking about Dad trying to liquidate his assets? Or was he talking about him being easily agitated? I left these questions unasked, because I knew what Dr. Weaver's answer would be. Something about medicine being an imprecise science, and that the best way try to prevent Dad's out-of-character conduct was to keep him on his meds, keep him well fed, and keep an eye on him all the time. An admirable goal, I silently conceded, but what were the realities? Keeping Dad on his meds and keeping him fed might be possible, but keeping an eye on him all the time was going to be tough. Dad was not one to take direction from others when he had his mind set. So, when it came to Grace, I was no longer sure we could keep the two of them apart.

Dr. Weaver was still speaking, but a lot of it was medical mumbo-jumbo that didn't exactly stick. However, we nodded our heads when Dr. Weaver paused, indicating that we understood. Without question, we understood the importance of Dad taking his meds and eating well.

K.C. and I made it clear to Dr. Weaver that we cared about our father and wanted to do everything possible to ensure his speedy recovery. Dr. Weaver seemed to understand.

Still, he had bad news for us. "In order for your dad to stay in the hospital, he has to be a harm to himself or to others." He and Dr. French "had concluded that Ben no longer met this criterion; therefore, he should be discharged immediately."

My stomach tensed up into a knot. "Are you serious?" I asked Dr. Weaver, looking him straight in the eyes. And then counting on my fingers for emphasis, I presented my argument for Dad remaining in the hospital:

"One, he attacked me in this very hospital yesterday, in the presence of Doctor French and an orderly. Two, he threatened to kill me if I didn't turn over the car keys. Three, he told you he had a fight in the hospital with his brother, which was impossible because Dad's brother died fifty years ago. Four, during the last year he has signed checks to his caregiver for nearly $100,000, when she should have received less than thirty thousand, and, five, he called his stockbroker just a few days ago, instructed him to liquidate all of his assets and issue a check payable to cash. And you say he should not be hospitalized! And you say he is not a harm to himself?" I was boiling mad by the time I reached the end of my litany of episodes.

Dr. Weaver didn't seem shocked by my outburst. He was a professional, used to dealing with anger. He started out by replying that it was best not to kill the messenger. "Everybody has your dad's best interest in mind. Unfortunately, there are legal constraints that govern what we can do. The incidents with the checks and the stockbroker do not count as harm to self or harm to others. I truly regret this, but I don't make the rules."

I knew that Dr. Weaver was right, but I was still unwilling to accept that giving up all of your worldly possessions and becoming a pauper or a ward of the state did not qualify as harm to self. How could the law I loved so much let me down when it came to my father? I knew if an attorney recommended that his client give his family members all of his assets in order to qualify for Medicaid assistance, the attorney would be committing a federal crime. Yet, Dr. Weaver, Officer Martinez, and my attorney friend were all telling me that if an eighty-two-year-old man suffering from mild dementia "voluntarily" gives away his worldly possessions and thereby becomes a ward of the state, well, that's okay. No harm, no foul.

What a screwed-up legal system, I thought. It just did not make sense that there was no remedy in the law to protect an elderly person from himself, and yet allow the person to manage his financial affairs with dignity. I held my tongue on the issue, though, because Dr. Weaver was the decision maker here, and I had to keep him on our side. He was acting within certain legal constraints when it came to keeping a patient in the hospital. It was my job to get him to test the outer boundaries of those constraints and find a way to keep my father from being discharged immediately.

While not calm, at least I wasn't steaming while I listened to Dr. Weaver's attempt to explain the other issues I had raised, my father's attack on me and his misstatement of why he had been hospitalized. Dr. Weaver was convinced that these were isolated incidents caused by his unregulated meds and the shock of Grace's dismissal. It was too early in Dad's treatment for Dr. Weaver to comment conclusively on Dad's feelings toward Grace.

"It could be that your father is under her influence, or perhaps he has fallen in love with her to the point that he cares more for her than for his children." Dr. Weaver speculated "It was possible Ben may have wanted to show his love for her by giving her a lot of money." He didn't know for sure. The answers to these "difficult and admittedly troubling" questions would have to be resolved through counseling sessions, which he was recommending.

What a crock, I thought. The idea that Dad loved Grace was inconceivable to me. I was not going to debate with the doctor our relative worth as Dad's children vis-à-vis Grace. Even though I was angry with Dr. Weaver for even raising this possibility, I had to stay focused and not let my welling anger get the best of me.

"Is there any way that Dad could stay a bit longer to get the medical attention we feel he needs?" K.C. asked. I echoed my sister's question and added my concern that Dad would not be properly cared for if he went home, because we had not yet selected a new care provider for him. I felt it was essential to interview the care providers offered by the agency before letting them attend to our dad. We desperately needed some time to get caregivers lined up. I pointed out too that Dad had not acknowledged us when we were standing behind the door, looking through the glass, and he only barely acknowledged us with a smile when we were inside the unit. I questioned whether under these circumstances Dad was ready to go home.

Dr. Weaver explained that Dad's minimal recognition of us was probably the work of the sedative he had prescribed, which should be wearing off because he had received the dose the night before. So Dad's conduct inside the unit was not justification for a continued stay. As for the other issues we had raised, while Dr. Weaver was sympathetic to our problems with getting healthcare providers lined up, our issue did not constitute medical necessity, which was the hurdle that had to be met to warrant a longer stay. Dr. Weaver ended by saying, "My medical opinion is that the only way Ben can continue his stay in the hospital is under a voluntary admission."

Eureka! A ray of hope. So there was a way for Dad to stay. Dr. Weaver said that Dad would have to sign a form, voluntarily admitting himself for observation. In other words, he would have to check into the hospital the same way he would a hotel. Dr. Weaver further indicated that Dad's insurance probably would not pay for the stay. I quickly volunteered that if the insurance company did not pay the bill, I would guarantee payment. Then I looked at K.C., who was looking at me. I knew we were both thinking the same thing. We had our work cut out for us to get Dad to admit himself into the hospital.

Our business concluded, Dr. Weaver offered to get the necessary forms for Dad's signature and then bring our father into the conference room so we could spend some time together.

The minute Dr. Weaver was out the door, we started talking. "Can you believe this guy? What an idiot!" I said.

K.C. was equally vocal. "How much longer did he intend to keep us in misery about his decision to discharge Dad before telling us about the voluntary admission option? Is he some sort of sadist?"

We were both also offended by Dr. Weaver's suggestion that Dad might have loved Grace more than us, his own children. The idea that Dad could care romantically for Grace at all was simply off our radar scope. Dr. Weaver was rapidly becoming one of our least favorite persons.

We were just as outraged at an antiquated legal system that offered us no help. But our resolve was firm. Even if the system was so stacked against us, we would beat the system. The two of us were standing shoulder to shoulder on a mission to save our father from himself. An unexpected benefit of our miserable situation was that it was bringing K.C. and me closer with each passing moment. We were united in achieving our objective, and nothing was going to get in our way. Our first order of business was to get our father to sign the voluntary admission form. I said a silent prayer for help.

Dr. Weaver's return, a few minutes later, was signaled by the sound of the door lock retracting. He came into the conference room holding a one-page form, which he handed to me. It was titled Consent for Voluntary Admission. Dr. Weaver's explanation of the intricacies of the one-page form was short and to the point. "If Ben signs on this line"— pointing to the bottom of the page—"we can keep him in the hospital for a few days. If he signs, he must do so in the presence of a witness who must sign on the other line and date the form. Neither of you can act as a witness to your dad's signature." That task was reserved for a non-family member. Dr. Weaver suggested that we use the nurse as a witness. "If you need a witness, call the nurse's station at extension 333. Do you understand?"

K.C. and I said "Yes" at the same time. Dr. Weaver told us that he was going to bring Dad to the conference room, and then he would be making rounds. If we wanted to talk to him further, we should ask the nurse to have him paged. We all shook hands and K.C. and I politely thanked Dr. Weaver for his help.

Again, Dr. Weaver disappeared out the door, this time to get our father. There wasn't much time for conversation, because in a matter of seconds, it seemed, we again heard the door lock shift to the open position. Dr. Weaver walked into the room, followed by our dad.

We simultaneously stood up from the table to greet him. Having seen him before through the glass in the door and again while we were standing in the hallway with Dr. Weaver, I wasn't as surprised by his appearance as I might otherwise have been. I did notice, however, that Dad had not shaved. I don't think I had ever seen my dad with a day's worth of stubble on his face. I assumed he hadn't shaved because the hospital didn't want him to have a potentially dangerous weapon like a razor.

It was hard to tell who was happier to see the other. Dad gave each of us a warm hug and a smooch on the cheek. We reciprocated with hugs and kisses of our own. As Dr. Weaver excused himself to go see other patients, we sat down around the conference table, thanking the doctor for his time and promising to get in touch with him if we felt another meeting was necessary.

We were brimming with questions, which Dad fielded without any problem. He said that he was "feeling fine." He was rooming with another man whom he described as "a large drink of water with a full beard who had a mishap on his motorcycle." From what we could discern, his biker roommate, under the influence of something undoubtedly illegal, had been stopped by the police. After a knock-down brawl with the local constabulary, he had been brought to the lockdown unit for observation. Dad said his roommate kept him up all night, moaning about his many injuries and recovering from the ill effects of his recent high. Dad thought his roommate was a fine person. They were getting along like two old friends. This was typical of Dad. He always had a place in his heart for the underdog and always saw the best in his fellow man, regardless of his station.

While feigning interest in the roommate's medical problems and Dad's prognosis for the unfortunate fellow's recovery, we were understandably more interested in how our father was doing. Dad said again he was "fine." He was eating and taking his medicine. For entertainment, he could go to a communal dayroom and participate in exercise classes or watch television. The other entertainment option, walking up and down the hall, Dad did not mention.

Dad made one statement that made me laugh. "Ed, you should see the security around here. It is unbelievable. The locks and back-up systems would make this place harder to break out of than a jail." I had to smile because it reminded me of my father of old, who had known the inner workings of all the machinery in the laundry and the Navy ships we visited, which gave me hope that perhaps Dad could be on the road to recovery. His comment about security sent me a message that some of Dad's old interests were being stimulated in this seemingly sterile environment.

He told us that he didn't need anything, but that he would like his slippers from home, some personal items, and maybe some magazines. It appeared that Dad was somewhat resigned to staying in the hospital for a while, even though he did ask several times when he was going home. Taking advantage of the opening, we explained that Dr. French and Dr. Weaver wanted him to stay just a few more days, but he had to sign "this paper for insurance purposes," a white lie, but it seemed justified under the circumstances. Dad said he was willing to stay a bit longer if that was what the doctors recommended, but not more then a day, because he wanted to get home.

I took a deep breath and handed Dad the form, along with a pen, and watched as he signed the paper. Hoping against hope that he wouldn't read the title of the form, I gently told Dad that he needed to add the date next to his name. Without hesitation, he dated the form and handed it back to me.

We knew that Dr. Weaver had asked that Dad sign in front of a witness, but this was a golden opportunity that we couldn't pass up. I would explain to Dr. Weaver later why the nurse was not called in as a witness. I was fairly certain that Dad would acknowledge his signature to the nurse or Dr. Weaver, if necessary.

K.C. and I both breathed an audible sigh of relief now that we had accomplished our immediate goal. K.C. asked whether Dad wanted her to bring any candy or sweets to eat. He must not have heard the question, or maybe he was ignoring it, because in response, Dad asked, "How is Grace?" Not a good question from my point of view. I did not want to cause another war like the one that had happened at the house after I first arrived in San Diego, so I ignored Dad's question and responded with one of my own.

"Dad, can you tell me about why you called Arthur and asked him to liquidate your portfolio?" Since my dad seemed lucid, at least temporarily, and was obviously interested in talking, I decided to risk asking him about the call. This mystery was something I had been unable to address two nights before, when Dad flew off the handle after I had discharged Grace. I hoped the fact that my father was in the hospital would restrain his tendency to get angry, and maybe we would hear the real reason for the call. I desperately wanted to understand better what was going on in his life.

Dad seemed almost eager to talk to us. He couldn't get his story out fast enough, and it finally sounded like we were getting closer to the truth.

"Grace wanted me to help her son's church pay for the land for a new building and some of the construction expenses. Her goal was strictly charitable," he emphasized. "Grace suggested that the stockbroker have the check made out to cash to make it easier to deposit into the church's building fund." Dad believed that if he did not accede to Grace, she would get upset and he would lose her. "I didn't want to lose Grace, so I agreed to help the church out." Surprisingly, this made perfect sense to Dad because Grace had promised to take care of him for the rest of his life if he would do this "one small thing" for the church.

Even though I had been certain Grace was involved in whatever scheme was cooking, hearing it confirmed nauseated me and made me angry—extremely angry. I heard what Dad was saying about her love of the church, but I knew in my heart the "gift" was not for the purpose Grace had told my father. I believed that Grace was going to the well one final time, for the big payoff.

For some reason, Grace was not content with her salary increase to $100,000 per year. Maybe she was growing tired of being Dad's caregiver,

I speculated, so she had threatened to leave Dad unless his entire life savings were paid to the church. Judging from all the new clothes I had seen in the bedroom she used to occupy, it was obvious that she was enjoying *la dolce vita*. I doubted that any part of the six-figure check she was anticipating from the sale of Dad's stocks would find its way to the church. With Dad drained of all of his money, I was sure that he would never see Grace again.

The seeming insanity of my father being duped into agreeing to sell all of his assets because of his obviously strong feelings for a high-priced caregiver was impossible for me to understand. It just did not make sense, even in the context of Dad's being in love with Grace. Grace was not the sort who would turn heads. She was not a trophy girlfriend, not even a tarnished, shopworn trophy. What was going on? My father was too smart for this. That is, he always had been, but obviously was not now. I was convinced, more then ever, that my father must never, ever see Grace again. This was Day Two of my father's formal separation from Grace, and, if I had any influence, the separation would be permanent.

The strain of the day and the evening before, as well as the new meds, were obviously starting to take a toll on Dad. I realized I had been so engaged in hearing Dad's explanation of what had transpired with Grace, the church, and Dad's stockbroker that I failed to appreciate how exhausted he looked. Spending the night in a strange environment and probably not being able to sleep because of his biker-buddy roommate had also taken a toll. Dad needed to get some rest. He was yawning continually and his eyelids were at half mast. The pause in our conversation was conveniently interrupted by the click of the lock retracting, the door opening and Dr. Weaver's return, signifying that our visit was over.

Dr. Weaver announced that he "wanted to see how things were going." I told him that we were having a good discussion, but my father looked tired, and I thought maybe he should get some rest. Dad readily agreed.

Dad got up and gave us each a hug. As he was walking out the door, held open by Dr. Weaver, he turned to us and said, "Ed, promise me that you will do nothing to hurt Grace. She is a good person and she comes from a good family."

I looked at my father, a broken man whom I loved dearly. Not wanting to show the intense anger I was still feeling, I swallowed hard and said, "I promise."

If put to a test, I honestly wasn't sure what I was willing to promise at that moment. My list of reasons to be angry with Grace was growing longer. My feelings of animosity toward her were so strong that it was hard to even say her name without it sounding like a curse word. But I had made a promise to my dad. Given our history, I knew promises were to be taken seriously.

When I was quite young, maybe eight years old, I was showering with my dad in the stall shower in the master bathroom. This was always fun for me because the shower had two heads, one at a normal height and the other midway between the upper shower head and the floor. We played a game. Dad got the taller showerhead because he was bigger. I got my own showerhead to control at kids' level. Each of us would soap down and then rinse off under our showerhead. Dad would shampoo his hair and then do mine, being careful not to get the shampoo into my eyes. After we were both fully lathered, we would rinse under our showerheads again. Finally, it was my job to turn off both showerheads.

On this particular evening, when the two of us exited the shower and reached for the towels lying on the counter, Dad looked down into the shower and saw a wad of gum on the drain. "Whose gum is that?" he asked, looking at me. It was pretty obvious whose gum it was because Dad didn't chew gum. And since I chewed gum all the time, I was the only logical candidate to claim its ownership.

"I don't know," I responded. Obviously, the story of George Washington and the chopped-down cherry tree had not made an indelible impression on me. This temporary lapse in my moral education was about to be corrected. Following an intense discussion, which was more like an interrogation, I 'fessed up, with tears in my eyes. "Yes, it is my gum."

What followed was not pretty. Dad made it clear to me that I was not to lie to my parents. The punishment was swift and sure. Dad smacked me hard, several times, grabbing my arm so I could not get away, leaving red welts on my behind. With each slap, Dad yelled, "You don't lie to your parents. Do you understand?" I understood. The message was painfully loud and clear.

I had not forgotten this incident, forty years earlier. From that time forward, being honest with my father was a priority. Not that I was a saint, but whenever I did lie, even those little white ones like the one to my father to get him to sign the voluntary admission form, I felt guilty because I would recall my ethics lesson in my parents' bathroom. So I was really conflicted about my promise not to hurt Grace. Should I act on my legal training and go after Grace with a vengeance, both civilly and criminally, or should I honor the promise made to my father? This was not a question I was prepared to answer just yet. But it was an issue I knew I would have to confront eventually.

Dad left and we remained seated at the conference room table. The door was ajar, and I heard Dr. Weaver directing Dad to the dayroom, telling him to "Wait for me there." Dr. Weaver then came back into the room. I explained that Dad had signed the form. Dr. Weaver made no mention of his instruction that Dad should sign in front of a nurse. Looking at the document, he said "Good," and then indicated that Dad could stay for a few days more.

I reiterated my concern that my father was fixated on Grace for reasons that made no sense to me. Dr. Weaver said that this was something that he hoped would resolve over time, "if it really is a problem for your Dad." The slow burn inside was starting again, but I didn't want to get into it with Dr. Weaver. Again, Dr. Weaver had raised the possibility that Grace could be more important to Dad than his children were. Instead of challenging Dr. Weaver, K.C. and I thanked him for his help and said goodbye.

While walking to the car, I told K.C. that for me the jury was still out on Dr. Weaver. "But for now he's the only game in town for us. We can replace him later. I believe the best plan for the short term is to stay on his good side in the event we need his help." K.C. agreed and gave me a squeeze around the waist, which said it all. We were a good team, brother and sister united in our desire to help our dad.

Assessing Your Parent's Insurance: What You Can Do

In chapter 2 I emphasized the importance of discussing insurance with your parent or parents while planning for future needs. With healthcare and prescription drug costs spiraling into the stratosphere, careful insurance planning becomes even more critical in your overall plan. Prescription drug costs alone are increasing at a rate of 15 percent annually for elderly people (Oluwasanmi, 2002). Social Security's Medicare plan no longer offers the comforting safety net it once did. Even though this government healthcare plan is better than nothing, additional or supplemental insurance policies can markedly decrease your parents' fear of financial catastrophe as their needs increase.

Obviously, insurance cannot take care of every possibility. But with careful evaluation of your parent's financial status and medical conditions, you can formulate a plan that should give you both increased peace of mind. Let's look at all the options. My hope is that you will find the right combination of plans to finance your parent's needs and avoid stress and possible impoverishment as aging progresses.

MEDICARE

Medicare is a health insurance program, funded by payroll tax deductions, for people 65 years of age and older. It is administered by the federal government, and always seems to be in crisis because of budget deficits and increasing healthcare costs. Almost every year it seems that benefits are reduced and premiums are increased. Still, it is the primary healthcare plan for millions of elderly Americans, and it is a godsend to those who have no other insurance. Medicare is composed of two parts:

Part A

Medicare Part A coverage helps pay for care in hospitals as an inpatient, for skilled nursing facilities, hospice, and some home healthcare. Most people do not have to pay premiums for Part A coverage. If your parent or your parent's spouse paid Medicare taxes through payroll deductions, there is no cost for Part A coverage. If your parent or your parent's spouse did not pay Medicare taxes, Part A coverage can be purchased. The Social Security Office can be called toll-free at (800) 772-1213 for information on purchasing Part A.

Part B

Part B helps pay for doctors' services, outpatient hospital care, and other medical services such as physical therapy and some home health-care. Part B coverage requires a monthly premium, which was around $60 per month in 2003. Part B coverage is optional, and if your parent chooses to have it, the premium will be deducted from monthly Social Security payments.

Medicare coverage has become an essential financial tool for American elders. It does have some drawbacks, however, which should be a catalyst for conversation with your parent about additional coverage. For example, the program does not pay for extended nursing-home stays, assisted living facilities, home healthcare, or the vast majority of prescription drugs. Medicare will cover a maximum of one hundred days in a nursing home, and sometimes the coverage is a little as twenty days.

Additionally, people with basic Medicare coverage are having a more difficult time finding doctors who will treat them. Because of diminishing reimbursement rates, many doctors are electing to no longer treat Medicare patients, which reduces the choice of doctors and increases waiting time for appointments. These factors should motivate you and your parent to consider the option of supplemental coverage.

MEDIGAP POLICIES

Medigap, or supplemental, insurance policies are offered by companies in every state. Medigap policies are traditional, fee-for-service programs that have to meet the federally mandated criteria listed below:

1. **Hospital coinsurance.** Medicare pays for the first 60 days of hospitalization (less the initial deductible). Medigap plans pick up after the first 60 days and pay a set amount for days 61-90 and an increased

amount for days 91-150. The amounts change from year to year, but in 2003 the rate was $210 for days 61-90, and $420 for days 91-150. Once Medicare's days 1-60 coverage and Medigap's days 61-150 coverage are used up, Medigap provides for an additional 365 hospital days over your parent's lifetime. These 365 days are called "lifetime reserve days" and are a benefit that can be used only one time; they are not renewable from year to year. These 365 days don't all have to be used at once and can be spread out over many years.

2. **Part B services.** Medicare pays 80 percent of medical services and 50 percent of mental health services. Medigap covers the remaining 20 percent for medical services and 50 percent for mental health services.

Some of the benefits of Medigap supplemental coverage include the following:

1. Your parent can see any doctor, anywhere in the country.
2. Specialists are easily accessible, without primary doctor referral and without large out-of-pocket expenses.
3. Premium costs vary depending on the policy, but copays and deductibles are usually covered, so costs are predictable.

As with basic Medicare coverage, very few Medigap policies offer prescription drug coverage. However, the savings in healthcare costs afforded by a supplemental policy can help make up for the out-of-pocket expense for medications.

MEDICARE HMOs

Many elderly people have elected to enroll in a Medicare Health Maintenance Organization (HMO) such as Kaiser, Secure Horizons, or Blue Cross, to name a few. Medicare HMOs have contracted with the federal government to provide health benefits to persons eligible for Medicare who choose an HMO over Medicare's traditional fee-for-service program. A Medicare HMO is a recommended way for your parent to maximize healthcare coverage while minimizing out-of-pocket expenses. Medicare HMOs follow the same model as traditional HMOs and are actively involved in the planning and delivery of healthcare services. Like other plans, Medicare HMOs have benefits and drawbacks.

Benefits

1. **Cost.** The primary benefit of a Medicare HMO is cost. Such programs typically have low premiums and co-pays, which can be a great help if your parent has limited income.
2. **Prescription drugs.** Some Medicare HMOs offer prescription drug coverage, but the coverage is usually limited to drugs on their approved lists, and they tend to favor generic over brand-name drugs. Because of the huge increases in drug costs, the Medicare HMO program can be an attractive option for those who require a wide array of prescription medications.

Drawbacks

1. **Choice of doctors.** If your parent enrolls in a Medicare HMO, choice of doctors is usually limited to those in the HMO's network.
2. **Specialists.** Seeing a specialist almost always requires a referral from the primary care doctor.
3. **Coverage away from home.** Healthcare services are usually limited to the HMO's service area. If your parent has chronic health

problems but still travels frequently, this would be a major consideration in deciding whether a Medicare HMO is a good option.

Although the Medicare HMO program seems to have more drawbacks than other plans, the drawbacks are relatively minor. If your parent has been in an HMO previously, the necessity of working within the system will seem like second nature rather than an obstacle to good healthcare.

MEDICARE PPOs

A test program in twenty-three states began in 2003 to offer Medicare Preferred Provider Organization (PPO) coverage. The main difference between Medicare HMOs and PPOs is in access to specific doctors and specialists. The Medicare PPO has a network of doctors, but your parent would be able to see any doctor outside the network (for a higher cost). Also, unlike an HMO, your parent would not need a referral from a primary care doctor to see a specialist. Some PPOs offer prescription drug coverage, but like most HMOs, the coverage is limited to drugs on their approved lists. The major drawback to the PPO plan is cost. Premiums and co-pays are usually higher than with an HMO.

MEDICAID

Medicaid is a program that is jointly funded by the federal and state governments to provide healthcare services to low-income people. Many people, even those who have been self-sufficient their entire lives, are unprepared for the financial devastation that a serious or long-term illness can wreak. It's comforting to know that Medicaid exists as the ultimate back-up plan should all other options be exhausted.

Although the federal government has established broad national guidelines for Medicaid, each state is responsible for the governance of its own program.

1. Each state sets its own eligibility standards
2. Each state determines the type, amount, duration, and scope of services.
3. Each state sets the rate of payment for services.
4. Each state administers its own program.

(Overview of the Medicaid Program, 2002)

Some of the healthcare benefits covered by Medicaid include the following:

•Inpatient and outpatient hospital care

•Physician services

•Laboratory and x-ray services

•Surgical dental services

•Nursing facility services

•Home healthcare (for persons eligible for a nursing facility)

Eligibility requirements generally vary from state to state, but are always determined by an evaluation of assets and income. In California, for example, a person can have a monthly income of 100 percent of the poverty level and be eligible for Medicaid benefits. California also mandates that total liquid assets not exceed $2000 ($3,000 for a couple). A person's residence and car are not included when being considered for eligibility. If you are interested in determining eligibility for your parent, contact the Health and Human Services department in your state for its guidelines.

The asset and income levels for qualifying for Medicaid are low. Because Medicaid offers such comprehensive coverage, the issue of giving away assets in order to qualify for coverage is frequently raised by my clients who are confronted with serious medical expenses but do not have significant financial resources. Understandably, they are fearful of having virtually everything they own eaten up by healthcare costs before they qualify for Medicaid coverage, thereby leaving them impoverished.

Unfortunately, this is an area of the law that is full of land mines. Generally, it is a criminal offense to attempt to meet eligibility levels by giving away assets. When a person applies for Medicaid, the government will "look back" at all gifts made by that person during the three years prior to the application. The amount of any gifts made during the look-back period will be recalculated into the person's estate to determine eligibility for Medicaid. For example, if your father gifted $10,000 to you twice during the three-year period prior to his application, the government would credit $20,000 to your father's estate for the purposes of determining his eligibility for Medicaid.

Advance planning for Medicaid benefits is not out of the question; however, when your parent is sick and in need of immediate care, it is too late to do significant planning. The time for planning is well in advance of the need. If you are concerned about your parent's possible qualification for Medicaid payments in the future, I strongly suggest that you consult your parent's attorney early in the planning process.

LONG-TERM CARE INSURANCE

No one is ever fully prepared for either the emotional or financial toll of placing an aging parent in a skilled nursing facility for an extended length of time. Unfortunately, as our population ages, the odds have greatly increased that an elderly person will indeed spend time in such a facility. Did you know that of adults age sixty-five and older, 40 percent will spend time in a nursing home? Or that the average stay in a nursing facility is 2.5 years? (Snyder, 2002). Or that the average cost of a nursing facility stay is $60,000 annually? (Oluwasanmi, 2002). Medicare covers only the first twenty days of a nursing facility stay in full. The next eighty days require a co-payment, and after one hundred days, coverage ends.

Medicaid provides full coverage for nursing facility care, but the means test for eligibility eliminates many people who have even modest assets. Furthermore, Medicaid-approved facilities are often the least desirable in terms of location and amenities. Patients and their families seldom have a choice of facilities; patients are often assigned to the nearest available bed.

What you should conclude from this is that a discussion of long-term care insurance should be part of the planning process for your parent's healthcare needs. Long-term care insurance is rapidly increasing in popularity, mainly because of the greater need for it now that people are living longer. It is the fastest-growing type of health insurance sold today. Although long-term care insurance usually refers to nursing-facility care, it actually covers a wide variety of circumstances associated with long, chronic illness. Coverage can include time spent in an assisted-living facility, an adult daycare facility or even home health-care services. Any conversation you have with your parent about long-term care should stress its inevitability. This might be difficult for some parents (or even you) to accept, but the statistics make a strong case for planning for this eventuality.

Predictably, premiums for long-term care insurance are higher the older your parent is. Once your parent passes age sixty, you can expect annual premiums to be around $2,000. After the age of seventy, premiums rise to around $4,000. Policies provide a daily benefit for nursing-facility care, but your parent must be careful to ensure that the policy includes a compounded inflation rider so that the daily benefit is adjusted upward with the rising costs of healthcare.

The most important help you can provide for your parent is to make sure you thoroughly dissect any policy your parent might be thinking about buying. Remember, insurance is a business, and the goal of any company selling long-term care policies is to make money. I've heard stories of folks who have been hit with huge premium increases when they were under the impression their premiums couldn't be raised. Many policies have exclusions, too, such as mental illness (aside from Alzheimer's disease) and suicide attempts. Still others don't compensate for inflationary increases in nursing-facility costs; thus, the benefits paid might hardly put a dent in the actual costs.

You would be well advised to have an attorney examine any policy your parent is thinking of purchasing. This may sound overly cautious, but if your parent is going to spend precious resources on an expensive item such as long-term care insurance, you'll want to be certain it's a fair and sound policy that will truly protect your parent. The goal is to provide a financial safeguard against the very real possibility of a future nursing-facility stay. You would be doing your parent a great service by making sure this is the goal being accomplished.

The federal government, realizing the importance of long-term insurance, has instituted a long-term care insurance program for federal employees, postal employees, active and retired military, and their relatives. If you think your parent might be eligible for long-term care coverage under this program, and you would like to verify eligibility, contact the U.S. Office of Personnel Management at (800) 582-3337 or www.opm.gov/insure/ltc/.

The U.S. Office of Personnel Management offers the following tips for anyone considering the purchase of a long-term care policy:

Top Considerations When Purchasing Long-term Care Insurance

1. **Don't assume your parent has this coverage.** Long-term care is not covered by most health insurance policies or disability insurance. Medicare generally pays limited amounts for skilled care (not custodial care) only following a hospital stay.
2. **Educate yourself.** Visit the web sites of reputable organizations related to aging or long-term care, or read articles in consumer or personal finance magazines related to this topic.
3. **Discuss long-term care plans with your family.** Consider whether or not you or other family members could provide care if your parent needs it and the extent to which you want to depend on family members.
4. **Consider a range of care options.** Decide if your parent needs a policy that includes coverage for a range of care options including home care, community-based services (like adult daycare), assisted-living facility and nursing home care, or care in limited settings such as facilities only.
5. **Don't be penny-wise and pound-foolish.** Sometimes the least expensive plan is not the wisest choice, because coverage may be limited and/or provide few options. Your parent may be better off spending more on a plan that ensures more choices about the level and type of care that might be needed.
6. **Buy only the coverage your parent needs.** For example, most people don't need a policy that covers nursing home care for many years. The average stay in a nursing home is two and one-half years. Consumers should also check local nursing home rates to determine the cost of care in their area, and decide how much of that cost they can pay for out-of-pocket. You don't need

to purchase insurance to cover all anticipated costs if you can pay part of them from your income or assets.

7. **Buy at a young age.** Long-term care insurance rates are based on your age when you first buy the coverage. Buy in your forties and fifties when you have rich plan designs to choose from for a fraction of the price you will pay later.

8. **Ensure that the coverage keeps pace with inflation.** Your parent may not need to use the benefits for many years, and the costs for long-term care will increase. Be sure plan benefits are protected against inflation and are adequate to meet future needs.

9. **Determine where the nursing home coverage is provided.** Some long-term care policies reserve the right to designate the nursing home where coverage is provided. This could mean that your parent is placed in a facility which may not be convenient for you or your family to visit easily.

10. **Establish who gets paid for home health services.** Some long-term care policies pay only licensed professionals and non family members for home health services; however, many policies will pay a family member for taking care of another family member. This can be especially important for a child who is contemplating leaving a job to take care of his or her parent.

11. **Don't overlook an employer or an affinity organization.** More are offering long-term care insurance that is usually carefully researched and may offer cost savings.

12. **Purchase from a financially stable company.** Compare company ratings and history of premium increases to ensure the company will be around when your parent needs benefits.

Navigating the complex maze of insurance possibilities can seem overwhelming. However, I cannot stress enough the importance of a thorough evaluation of your parent's healthcare needs and current insurance policies. Once you have established what your parent already has, you can reasonably judge what additional coverage might be beneficial or even essential. When your parent's needs have been assessed and insurance coverage issues have been settled, 90 percent of the work is out of the way. From that point forward, all you need to do is keep abreast of any changes in Medicare and/or whatever additional policies your parent has. You might need to make slight adjustments as time goes by but, for the most part, you can rest easy that your parent's needs will be met.

If undertaking an evaluation of your parent's insurance coverage seems too daunting or complex, consider consulting with an insurance counselor. Most states have established formal health insurance counseling programs in which volunteer counselors work with seniors to help them understand health insurance options. The counselors are trained to assist with Medicare, HMOs, long-term-care insurance and other related health insurance issues. Counselors also act as advocates for seniors in health insurance disputes. If you or your parent wishes to consult with a health insurance counselor, contact your local Aging and Independence Agency or a senior center in your neighborhood for a referral.

FINANCES

If, after completing your parent's insurance evaluation, you find that there simply aren't enough funds to provide the necessary care, there is a solution. Finances frequently seem to be an issue as people age. Especially when their health begins to decline, elderly people find that they are spending more and more of their limited income on doctors and prescriptions, and it becomes harder to make the money stretch. Unless your parent is financially well off, you might need to do some scrambling to help make ends meet.

Heavy losses in the stock market in recent years have severely reduced many older people's income stream. Portfolios have dwindled, certificates of deposit offer ridiculously low rates, and money-market accounts yield hardly anything at all. A significant downturn in income, coupled with reductions in Medicare benefits, increases in health insurance premiums, and astronomic increases in prescription drugs, and a finite source of funds can be seriously squeezed.

You may need to have a frank, heart-to-heart discussion with your parent if you suspect a financial bind. This could be difficult; parents can easily feel embarrassed or offended when questioned about their financial stability. But it may be necessary to air the issue so that you can then suggest some techniques for getting more money into your parent's hands without affecting quality of life. One such technique is the reverse mortgage.

Reverse Mortgages

Many seniors wondering where to turn in a difficult economic time are looking at reverse mortgages, especially those who are property rich but cash poor. A reverse mortgage is a loan available to homeowners age sixty-two and older. It is a loan against a home that converts part of the equity into tax-free income, and the loan does not have to be repaid until the home is sold, the borrower permanently moves out, or until the borrower's death. The primary benefit of a reverse mortgage is that the homeowner does not have to sell the home, relinquish title, or make a new monthly mortgage payment. Depending on the type of loan selected, it can provide a lump sum amount, a credit line that can be drawn upon as needed, or regular, predetermined payments to the homeowner.

Eligibility requirements for a reverse mortgage include the following:

•Everyone listed on the title of the home must apply for the reverse mortgage and must sign the loan papers.

•All borrowers must be at least sixty-two years old.

•Borrowers must occupy the home as their principal residence.

•Single-family residences are eligible, as are some condominiums and manufactured homes. Mobile homes and cooperatives usually are not eligible.

No restrictions exist on what the funds from a private-sector reverse mortgage can be used for. They can be used for home improvements, medical expenses, supplemental income, even vacations. Some reverse mortgages offered by state and local governments, however, do restrict use of the proceeds to specific purposes such as home repairs or property taxes.

Another benefit is that the amount owed can never exceed the value of the home. In other words, if your parent were to get a reverse mortgage that paid monthly sums, the amount owed would continue to grow as long as your parent was living and continued to receive payments. But if your parent lived for many years, the amount paid out could technically be larger than the value of the home. The loan cannot be called if this happens; the loan amount simply stops when it reaches the point of equaling the value of the house, but the payments do not stop. So your parent can never be forced to sell the home or to move simply because the loan value has exceeded the property value.

Typically this happens only rarely. The average term for a reverse mortgage is 11.2 years (Kelly, 2002). Also, during the term of the loan houses will usually appreciate in value, thus protecting the lender and giving the homeowner the advantage of even more borrowing power if it is needed.

The amount of cash available from a reverse mortgage depends on several factors:

•Your parent's age

•The value of the home

•The geographic location of the home

•The cost of the loan

Usually, the highest cash amounts available are for the oldest borrowers living in the most expensive homes. But even a modest home has the potential to provide your parent with an income boost that can reduce or eliminate financial pressure.

Now for the caveats. As with any financial program, there are unscrupulous lenders who charge enormous up-front fees, unconscionable interest rates, and shared-appreciation terms. One extreme example resulted in a recent class-action suit against a reverse-mortgage company called Financial Freedom. In this case, a woman received a total of $58,000 in reverse mortgage payments over a period of thirty-two months. When she died, her heirs were stunned to discover that the terms of the reverse mortgage required a repayment of $765,000! The lender had built in an egregious shared-appreciation clause that by far outdistanced the value of the loan amount.

As a result of abuses like this one, the government has stepped in. Most reverse mortgages are now insured by the Federal Housing Administration. However, there are still some private companies in the reverse-mortgage business who are creative about their lending terms, most often to their own benefit. Currently, the most popular (and least expensive) reverse-mortgage program insured by the FHA is called the Home Equity Conversion Mortgage.

If you and your parent think a reverse mortgage would be a good option to pursue, check with the National Reverse Mortgage Lenders Association (NRMLA), a trade organization for companies that provide reverse mortgages.

National Reverse Mortgage Lenders Association
www.reversemortgage.org
Telephone: (202) 939-1760

On NRMLA's web site you can find listings for companies that provide reverse mortgages in your area, along with a wealth of information about current news and legislation affecting reverse mortgages. Make sure your first question to any prospective lender is whether the loan will be insured by FHA. Most financial advisors point out that because the costs involved in securing a reverse mortgage are high (example: a $200,000 home could incur $9,600 or more in fees), these loans are not recommended as a short-term solution to income problems. But if your parent is planning to stay in the home for at least five years, a reverse mortgage might be the perfect solution.

One final word of warning about reverse mortgages: If your parent receives Medicaid assistance, be very careful about how funds from a reverse mortgage are dispersed. If, for example, your parent were to take a lump sum amount, that figure would be included as part of total liquid assets, which could adversely affect Medicaid eligibility. If, however, loan payments are issued monthly, and the funds are used up each month, there would be no addition to total liquid assets. As with anything you and your parent do that results in a significant change, be certain you understand as many of the possible ramifications as you can before you sign on the dotted line.

Most important of all, keep reminding yourself that there are remedies to help with nearly every situation, even if your parent's is desperate. The law itself may fall short of offering the necessary protection against elder abuse, but society is continually addressing the needs of our elder population. Creative solutions do exist.

CHAPTER 7

Weighing the Options

*E*scaping the confines of the lockdown unit and the hospital itself was a relief. It was a good feeling, being in the car with all the windows down, wind blowing in my face. It was no secret that I missed California. I had left San Diego in 1973, after graduating from law school and passing the California bar. My law practice took Pamela and me first to Atlanta, Georgia, and then to Washington, D.C. Once we had children, we traveled back to San Diego at least once a year so Dad, Mom, and the other family members could get to know Brett and Kimberly. Even though I had been gone for more than twenty-three years, I still had a special feeling of home whenever I was in San Diego.

Following K.C.'s directions, I headed toward Mountain View, the assisted-living facility we wanted to inspect. We had a lot to talk about as we headed north on the freeway. K.C. especially wanted to discuss Dr. Weaver. She believed he was competent despite his flagrant mistake during in-take. She also pointed out that Dr. Weaver seemed honestly concerned about Dad's condition. I couldn't argue these points. Plus, I knew my anger with Dr. Weaver was mostly caused by my unwillingness to accept the possibility that my dad did care for Grace more than his children. Other than this, I had no real beef with Dr. Weaver. It was the system, not the doctor, that was causing me grief. I shuddered at the thought that if Dad had not signed the involuntary commitment form, we would be taking him home today, ill-prepared for his care.

Even though we hoped that Dad would agree to stay in an assisted-living facility, we both knew this possibility wavered between remote and nonexistent. Therefore, we also had to make plans for the more likely probability of Dad's insistence on staying at home, which meant new caregivers needed to be hired. K.C. offered to telephone the agency that had recommended Jane Buchanan, the caregiver she had brought to the house the day before, to say we would hire her. Even though Dad had reacted badly to her, we agreed that his outburst was a result of the circumstances, not the person. K.C. also offered to speak with the agency about interviewing other caregivers in order to provide Dad with the around-the-clock care he needed.

We knew that twenty-four-hour care provided by professional caregivers was going to be considerably more expensive than the housekeepers Dad had promoted to caregivers over the years to take care of Mom, Sue, and himself. "You get what you pay for," I said.

"With Grace, this was certainly true," K.C. replied. "The cost of Grace during the past year alone could have supported Dad with a squad of caregivers for quite a while."

Cost was not the most important consideration when it came to Dad's care. While we were sensitive to the fact that we were making decisions on how Dad would be spending his money, we agreed that if he wanted to stay at home with twenty-four-hour care instead of the less-costly alternative of an assisted-living facility, then his money should be spent the way he wanted—as long as it was not spent on Grace.

Our conversation drifted into a philosophical reflection on the dramatic reversal of roles taking place. We had been the children, cared for by loving parents for many years until we could spread our wings and leave the nest. Now we were assuming the role of parents taking care of a child. We didn't mind the responsibility, because our father had always been there for us, but it still felt odd.

The simmering fury over the perverse influence of Grace on our father bubbled to the surface several times as we drove. We vented our hatred for the way she had abused Dad. "I hope she's sweating bullets, wondering about her fate," I said. "She has to know that she has committed several crimes that could expose her to jail time." My knowledge of criminal law was limited. But vague recollections of my criminal law class, some twenty-six years earlier, led me to believe that the embezzlement of Dad's money alone could send her up the river for many years. I assured K.C. that there were undoubtedly other charges that could be leveled against Grace, if Dad was inclined to press charges.

"Once Dad recovers, I hope he does," K.C. said.

I strongly believed that for criminal charges against Grace to stick, Dad would have to explain to a jury the evolution of their close relationship and how he ultimately had trusted her to be his loyal companion. K.C. and I both realized this was going to be a problem under the present circumstances, where he would say anything to keep Grace with him. We agreed Grace had committed the perfect crime. She had embezzled a boatload of Dad's money, even had her sights on the big payoff, but without Dad's testimony she would never spend a day in jail or be required to pay restitution. Even though we knew we were skating on thin ice legally, we didn't dismiss the possibility of threatening Grace with criminal charges if she tried to contact Dad.

The other incomprehensible issue that we kept returning to was Dad's deep feeling for Grace. We discussed it over and over again. What had we done wrong? What cues had there been that we had overlooked? It wasn't as though Dad was isolated from his children. I spoke to him often. More important, K.C. lived close by and visited frequently. Yet, she was as surprised by his commitment to Grace as I was. The promise Dad had extracted from me before he left the conference room spoke volumes on this point. Grace, not his children who loved him, was uppermost in Dad's mind. He had not let the opportunity pass to tell us his primary concern: Grace's staying with him.

I hoped and prayed that Dad would come around because he was in a good medical environment and seemed to be thinking more clearly. After all, during our conversation, Dad had given a plausible explanation for his call to his stockbroker. Also, he had commented on the high level of security in the unit. These were good signs that his memory was basically intact, providing some hope that, with stable meds and good food, my father would return to his old self.

One thing continued to trouble me. Why did the return of Dad's stable memory also have to involve Grace? I had hoped that once Dad was on the road to recovery, Grace would be history. But Dad was obviously dependent on Grace, like an addict who needs his regular fix even if it kills him. Dad was not going to forget about Grace, at least in the short term. This was now clear. Irrefutable evidence that she was an opportunistic criminal did not matter to Dad. Obviously, we were not going to be able to do anything about Grace until he was healthier. For now, the top priority was securing the best care for our father when he got out of the hospital, which is what we wanted most of all.

As we neared Mountain View, K.C. told me it was on the high end of elder-care facilities. It had come highly recommended by a friend whose mother was a resident. I pulled into the drive, parked the car in a visitors' space and looked around, noticing that the grounds appeared relatively new and well kept. The grass was green and nicely manicured, flowers were growing in beds of rich soil, and the parking lot was free of trash. To my critical eye, it was a good first impression.

A sign directed us to Admissions. We walked down a cement path, and through a set of automatic double doors to a reception desk in the middle of the room, where a woman directed us to the Admissions Office. Once inside the Admissions Office, K.C. asked for Connie Adams, who was expecting us. We took a seat in the waiting room, which had mauve-colored walls, complementary carpet, and tasteful office furniture.

I didn't have time to observe more of the waiting room before we were greeted by Ms. Adams. She was in her mid-forties, thin, well-dressed and coiffed, with a million-dollar smile. She escorted us to her office where she presented us with information about Mountain View.

"The facility is about seven years old," Ms. Adams said, "and has three different levels of care, each with increasing levels of supervision. Independent Living is like living in your own home, but you have cleaning and laundry service and dinner in the facility's dining room. Most of the independent-care residents have their own cars. The next level, Assisted Living, is also like living in your own apartment, but the residents take all three meals together." Ms. Adams continued. "Even though these residents do not have cars, they are free to take the Mountain View van to go shopping, out to eat, or on any of the many field trips that we offer each day. The third level is Full Custodial Care and is more like a hospital environment." I noted she did not use the words "nursing home" to describe the highest level of care.

On the basis of her discussion with K.C., Ms. Adams felt that the assisted-living housing was best for Dad. He would live in his own apartment, and a nurse would ensure that he took his meds. Further, he would eat with the rest of the assisted-living residents in a dining hall, where a nutritionist would be responsible for his eating a balanced diet every day.

It sounded like an ideal environment for my dad, but I was anxious to see the facility firsthand. I would reserve judgment until K.C. and I had had a chance to investigate for ourselves.

Ms. Adams offered to show us a typical assisted-living apartment. We followed her down a hallway, which looked like the hallway of a hotel, until she stopped at one door and knocked several times with the door knocker that was mounted at eye level. A printed name was affixed to the door, presumably the name of the occupant. After a few moments without an answer, Ms. Adams took out her passkey and unlocked the door. As she pushed the door opened, she called the name of the occupant, "Ms. Jaminson, are you home? It's Ms. Adams from admissions. Is anybody home?" Hearing no response, she explained that all of the assisted-living apartments were currently occupied, so she was showing us an apartment of one of their residents.

I thought it odd that Ms. Adams would let us into someone's apartment without the permission of the resident. I realized that she was trying to help us with our decision about the appropriate place for our father to stay, so I didn't question her about what seemed to be a blatant breach of privacy, but I filed it in my mind for later. I knew my dad would be incensed if someone came sashaying into his home without permission.

The layout of the rooms was typical of what one would expect of a one-bedroom apartment, except that it lacked a kitchen and it was small, very small. There were three rooms—a living room, bedroom and bathroom. I couldn't guess at the size of the rooms, but they seemed pretty confining to me. The claustrophobic feeling in the apartment was so pronounced that I asked if there were any bigger units. Ms. Adams said that this was the size of all the assisted-living apartments. She opened the drapes, suggesting that the room would look larger with natural light shining through the windows, which ran the full length of the living room. The light was nice, but it really did not help my feeling of the walls closing in on me when I imagined myself living in this apartment. I thought my father would probably feel the same way.

I explained to Ms. Adams that Dad spent a lot of time in his home, where he liked to roam from room to room. "Although his home is not particularly large by contemporary standards, it's considerably bigger then this apartment. I'm concerned that Dad might not be happy in such close surroundings. Also, there is an issue about Dad's furniture. If he were to make this move, it would be better for him to take as much as possible from his home so that he would feel less strange in this new place. I don't believe much of his furniture would fit here comfortably."

Ms. Adams seemed to understand my concern. She pointed out that this was a different environment from Dad's home. "Here, the residents should not be in the apartments during the day, except for maybe a few minutes to change for dinner. The apartments are used to sleep and rejuvenate from the busy Mountain View days. This is the 'Mountain View Vision.' So the apartment is not a place of refuge for the residents during the day. Every day Mountain View offers an extremely large menu of activities, which keeps the residents on the run and out of their apartments from morning until bedtime. Our goal is to help the residents overcome their initial fear of living in a new place and get them involved quickly in the many activities of the community. If a resident is holed up in the apartment, then we aren't doing our job."

She promised to give me a copy of the day's activities list when we returned to the Admissions Office. On the furniture issue she was honest. It was her opinion that the room looked smaller because it already contained someone else's furniture. It was possible that more of Dad's furniture would fit in the apartment than I imagined. If not, she felt that once Dad became immersed in the Mountain View routine, furniture would be less important than being with friends his own age who shared his interests. She said to bring lots of pictures to make it feel like home. Ms. Adams's explanation made sense to me, and I thanked her for the insight. She had given me a lot to think about, and her professionalism enhanced my confidence in her and the facility she represented.

Next Ms. Adams showed us a large dayroom with a big-screen TV, where some people were watching a soap opera. Others in the room were involved in playing cards or board games. All the residents had their hair neatly combed and were wearing clean, casual clothes. Many of them were smiling, which I thought was also a good sign. Ms. Adams explained that these residents were taking a partial day off from off-campus activities.

"The Mountain View social director is responsible for ensuring that residents don't spend too much time in front of the TV or playing board games. His goal is to strike a balance with each resident, so that he or she has a good mix of outside, off-campus activities combined with some local activities." She was right. Everyone needs a break from running, and these people were catching up. I was impressed by what I had seen so far.

The next stop was the dining room. Although our visit was not during a regularly scheduled meal, the room was not empty. On the perimeter of the room, near the windows, several groups of two or three people were engaged in conversation, some quite animated. They were seated around small coffee tables, and had access to soda and juice from a nearby refrigerator. On each table was a plate of what looked like freshly baked chocolate chip cookies. I asked Ms. Adams who took their meals in this large room. She said that the meals were taken "by both the assisted-living residents and the full-custodial-care residents who were capable of eating a meal at a table." A warning alarm resonated in my head. I pictured my father at a table for four shared by three custodial-care residents. I knew that residents requiring that level of care would not be good dining companions for my dad, and this prospect disturbed me.

Obviously I had inherited some of my father's skepticism about nursing-home care. I tried to raise my concern in a delicate manner to Ms. Adams, and she was ready with a reply that made perfect sense to me. Economics did not permit having separate kitchens and dining rooms for the assisted-living and full-custodial-care residents. Therefore, a decision had been made when the facility was built that both groups of residents would dine in the same room; however, the different groups took their meals in separate parts of the room, which was one reason the room was so large. The assisted-living residents ate with each other on one side of the room, and the custodial-care residents ate on the other side.

The tour ended in Ms. Adams's office. Overall, K.C. and I were pleased with what we had seen, especially the staff. I was still bothered by the size of the living accommodations but on balance Mountain View was a viable option. We told Ms. Adams we were interested in having Dad stay in an assisted-living apartment at Mountain View, but he would need to take a tour and make the decision for himself. As soon as he was able to make the trip, we would bring him to the facility.

While obviously pleased to hear we were interested, Ms. Adams explained that there was a short waiting list for an assisted-living apartment. She would be happy to put Dad's name on a waiting list if we would provide a refundable deposit. She believed that with his position assured at number two on the list, he would have an apartment in not more then a few months. She explained the pricing structure for the apartment and the other fees, which seemed reasonable.

Obviously this was not the environment our father had described to us when he was selling nursing homes on the virtues of linen supply. This place was free of any odor, especially the antiseptic odors I normally associated with the sick. In fact, the place had the feeling of a nice, modestly priced hotel.

I gave my credit card to Ms. Adams, who also recorded some preliminary information about Dad: his age, religious affiliation, medications (as best we could remember), allergies, food preferences, and treating doctors. Fortunately K.C. knew most of the medical information, and she promised to call Ms. Adams as soon as possible to fill in the gaps. Ms Adams then disappeared with my credit card, and after I signed the slip, Dad was officially on the waiting list.

Ms Adams asked when Dad would be able to tour Mountain View. K.C. explained that he was still in the hospital but was expected to be discharged in a few days. She reiterated that it was Dad's decision about whether he was willing to move, but we hoped to have him out visiting Mountain View soon. K.C. said she would call Ms. Adams as soon as she had a better idea of when he would be able to visit. Ms. Adams said she understood and that she was looking forward to meeting our father.

Our business concluded, we got up, said thank you, and were escorted by Ms. Adams to the entrance doors by the reception desk, where we had come in a little more then an hour before. She gave each of us one of her business cards and asked us to call her if we had any questions. We thanked her again, shook hands, and were out the door and halfway down the path to the parking lot when I heard Ms. Adams call my name.

We turned to see her not quite running but trying to move fast in her high-heeled shoes to catch us. Slightly winded, she extended a piece of paper to me and said, "I promised you a copy of the schedule of today's activities." I appreciated the fact that she had not only remembered her promise but had also made the extra effort to get this information to us.

As K.C. and I walked to the car, we agreed that we both felt good about Mountain View. Dad would be with people his age, he would be able to make friends who were not looking to put their hands in his pocket, he would get the medical and nutritional supervision he needed, there was a great variety of activities for him, he would be away from Grace, and it was only a forty-minute drive from K.C.'s home to Mountain View. We were both relieved to have found a facility run by professionals who cared about elder people.

While I drove, K.C. read from the list of the day's activities Ms. Adams had given me. We noted several that could be of interest to Dad: card playing at all levels of expertise—Dad always liked a friendly poker game; aerobic exercises—it would be good for him to exercise a little; and a field trip to La Jolla to go shopping—he could tell all of the other residents how he had built a business in La Jolla. Other field trips looked like they might interest him, too: a visit to the zoo, a concert in the park, watching the hang gliders in La Jolla, a trip to see an antique car collection, and a visit to Sea World. The list was long and impressive. We were convinced Dad could really enjoy this place, if he would give it a chance.

Despite the emotional high we had from visiting the Four Seasons of adult-care facilities, we couldn't stop reality from seeping in. We knew it was going to be a hard sell to get Dad to agree to stay at Mountain View or any assisted-care facility. In fact, hard sell might be an understatement. It would probably be easier to push a pebble up Mount Everest with the back of a spoon. But we could hope.

Even though it was only early afternoon, K.C. and I decided to skip a late lunch and go home instead. The events of the previous few days had exhausted both of us. I was thinking about a nap and an early evening, and I could tell that K.C. could use a break from the drama herself. I dropped her off at her house and promised to call before I picked her up the next day. K.C. said she would call Dad to see how he was doing, and she promised to call me at the house if there were any problems. I headed for home, looking forward to a peaceful evening.

Choosing a care facility: What you can do

Rarely does anyone choose to go into a nursing home. Nursing homes, or skilled-nursing facilities, as they are more commonly called today, are usually the option of last resort for someone who has a sudden illness or an illness that has become unmanageable at home. Many of today's elderly population still believe, as my father did, that nursing homes are places where patients are neglected, abused, and left to die. These beliefs have fostered a great fear of being abandoned in a horrible place, a fear that is unreasonable by today's standards but still pervasive among the elderly. Even though you will occasionally hear of nursing-home abuses, today such abuses are far more commonly the exception rather than the rule. As the number of senior citizens is rapidly increasing, government agencies and private watchdog groups such as AARP are paying closer attention to skilled-nursing facilities, scrutinizing them to make sure they provide their services in a sanitary environment with respectful and attentive care. And these groups are reporting their findings to the public.

When you are faced with the prospect of moving your parent to a care facility, the first thing you should know is that skilled-nursing care is the highest level of care offered. You will find facilities that are devoted exclusively to a single level of care, such as skilled nursing, but many are multi-level campuses, providing three levels of residential supervision:

1. Retirement or independent living
2. Assisted-care living
3. Skilled-nursing care

Whenever a move to any type of care facility is under consideration, the first thought that usually pops into everyone's mind is "nursing home." But you might find that a lower level of care would be more appropriate for your parent. This is the time to seek the input of trained professionals. Talk with your parent's doctors to find out exactly what kind of care your parent requires. Then, you can weigh your parent's needs against the services provided by each level of care and be able to make the best decision.

RETIREMENT OR INDEPENDENT LIVING

Retirement living is an option that many elderly people seek voluntarily. There are two different kinds of retirement living choices. You might be familiar with some of the highly publicized retirement communities, such as the Sun City retirement communities located throughout the United States. These communities offer homes and condominiums for residents to purchase outright, or apartments that can be rented. They are dedicated to an active senior lifestyle and offer an array of activities and clubs for residents who are independent and able to take care of their own needs. From the outside these facilities are no different from planned communities that we see for residents of all ages. The difference is that most of these communities require that their residents be at least fifty years old.

The second type of retirement community offers a full continuum of supervised living and care, ranging from independent living to skilled nursing. What distinguishes these communities from retirement communities such as Sun City is that all three levels of care are located on the same grounds, or campus. For our purposes here, we will focus on these types of retirement facilities.

As people age, they often look to a retirement community for several reasons.

1. They are in good general health but no longer want the burden of maintaining a house.
2. They have no family in their area who would be able to assist with future healthcare needs.
3. They crave the social interaction that a retirement community provides.

Retirement residents frequently find a new freedom in independent living. They no longer have to worry about things like mowing the lawn, shoveling snow, or home repairs. These facilities also provide the necessities-housekeeping, activities, transportation, and sometimes even meals, to name a few—which allows residents more time to pursue their interests, make new friends, and enjoy their retirement years. Residents at this level are usually allowed to have their own cars, and some facilities even allow pets.

Living units can range from small studio apartments to full-size apartments or cottages. Most retirement facilities have a health clinic that offers basic first aid, transportation to medical and dental appointments, and, most important, they maintain medical records and monitor the residents' general health. Fees for retirement living vary widely.

Some facilities require a large, lump-sum "investment" or "entrance" fee in addition to a monthly fee for rent and services. Others charge only a monthly fee. Still others allow residents to purchase living units outright, thus preserving their estate to pass along to heirs. If you are helping your parent select a retirement home, your first step is to determine what your parent can afford. Since this is a permanent move, your parent will probably want to sell his or her house to help finance the move.

A recent change in IRS regulations has made it easier to sell a home without the burden of paying capital gains taxes. As long as the house has been occupied by the owner for two of the five years prior to the sale, $250,000 of the profits ($500,000 for couples) is exempt from capital gains taxes, even if the gain is not reinvested in a new home. Thus, in most cases, the entire profit from the sale of a house can be preserved for future needs.

Most important is to select carefully. The following is a list of tips to guide you in choosing a facility that best meets your parent's needs.

•Make an appointment to visit the facility. If you and your parent have a favorable impression, drop by unannounced once or twice after your first visit.

•Find out what services are offered and included in the monthly fee.

•Ask for a list of the services not included in the monthly fee and the cost of those services.

•If the facility has a skilled-nursing unit, ask if the care is covered by Medicare, Medicaid, Medigap or Medicare HMOs. Retirement living is not covered by insurance, but most insurance plans do cover skilled-nursing care if the facility participates in Medicare, Medicaid, or other insurance programs. Not all do. (See chapter 6 for more information on insurance coverage.) If your parent should require skilled nursing at some point, it's easier and less unsettling to move to a different level in the same facility than to move to an entirely different facility.

•Check the facility and the living unit for safety features, including well-lit stairs and halls, handrails in the bathrooms, well-marked exits, and a way to call for help if needed.

•If communal dining is offered, join the residents for a meal. The quality of food is very important. Eating is one of the few pleasures elderly people can enjoy every day. If the food is not tasty or is lacking in variety, your parent's quality of life will be seriously diminished. Also, mealtime is a perfect opportunity to watch the residents and gauge their level of satisfaction.

•Try to speak with the residents without staff present. Ask if they like being there, and how plentiful and varied the activities are. Remember that the elderly may be somewhat more likely to complain. Don't discount all you hear, but consider their comments as part of your investigative effort.

•Try to get a sense of whether your parent would fit well with the type of residents in the facility.

•Observe how the staff interacts with the residents. Do they treat them like adults, with respect and dignity? Look for smiles on the faces of both staff and residents.

•Ask about the ratio of staff to residents. You can tell a facility is understaffed if the residents seem depressed or in a world of their own, or if staff is hurried and short-tempered with residents.

•Don't think that beautiful décor ensures perfect living conditions. It's easy to be impressed by what pleases the eye, but level of care and concern for the residents is more important than fancy wallpaper.

•Ask if your parent's furniture and personal belongings can be moved to the facility. The transition to a retirement facility will be easier if familiar objects can be taken along.

•Consider where the facility is, and if the location will allow for frequent visits from family and friends.

•Ask to see the most recent licensing inspection report. If it is relatively short and free of violations, the facility is likely to be a good one. Page after page of violations is a sure sign of trouble.

•Ask for a list of the last few months' activities. Make sure there are many that would interest your parent.

•Take the residential contract home with you and read it carefully. Make sure you understand what items are not covered in the care contract, the charges for those items and how often the charges are increased. This is critical because so-called ancillary charges can eat up money like a piranha if not anticipated. I strongly suggest that you ask an attorney experienced in reviewing such contracts to read it as well. This is too important a decision to have regrets over after your parent has moved to the facility.

Choosing to move to a retirement facility, of course, is an option usually decided early in your parent's senior years. Retirement living represents a stellar example of advance planning because your parent is probably concerned about the day when more assistance might be needed. My experience has been that once your parent is settled into a retirement facility it's much easier to make the transition upward to the assisted-living level of care, when such a move is warranted.

ASSISTED-LIVING CARE

The next level of care, assisted-living care, offers residents help with their daily activities, such as bathing, dressing, using the bathroom, and supervision of medications. As you have probably guessed, residents of assisted-living facilities are somewhere between being completely independent and requiring full-custodial care. They usually have medical conditions that require help on a daily basis, and many residents walk with canes or walkers, or even use wheelchairs. However, their overall health is not so bad that they require skilled-nursing care, and their quality of life can still be excellent with just a little bit of help.

Residents of assisted-living facilities usually live in rooms or small apartments within a building or group of buildings, and they typically take their meals together. Assisted-living care provides an array of services and activities similar to those offered by retirement living. Residents can choose from a full schedule of social and recreational activities with transportation provided. Assisted-living facilities should have health services on-site to provide first aid, supervise medications, and monitor the residents' general health. Some do not, however, so if this is important to you and your parent, be sure to make this your first question when seeking an assisted-living facility.

Overall, assisted living is much the same as retirement living but with a stepped-up level of supervision and assistance. And, like retirement living, the fee structure varies widely. Most common is a monthly fee for accommodations and services, with most personal services costing extra, such as laundry and dry cleaning, toiletries, and transportation to medical appointments. The search techniques for an assisted-living facility are similar to finding a retirement facility. But since the level of care needed is greater than in a retirement community, it's important for you and your parent to be even more scrupulous in evaluating possible facilities.

The following is a comprehensive checklist to help you in selecting an assisted-living care facility, which should be used in conjunction with the independent living checklist discussed in the previous section.

Daily Life

•Do the residents look content, well cared for, peaceful, and happy?

•Do the residents seem to enjoy being with staff?

•Are the residents clean and well groomed?

•Are the residents dressed appropriately for the season and time of day?

•Do staff members address residents by name?

•Do staff members respond quickly to residents' calls for assistance?

•Is there a written and posted schedule of activities?

•Are there nighttime and weekend activities?

•Does the facility provide a variety of activities, including music, art, and pet therapy, for example?

•Are religious services offered?

•Does staff make a concerted effort to interact socially with residents?

•Are meals tasty and served attractively?

•Are personal food likes and dislikes (or special diets) taken into consideration?

•Are snacks available?

•Can family members join residents for meals?

•How are "difficult" behaviors handled? Is the family always consulted?

•Does the facility have a family council? If it does, how does the council influence decisions about resident life?

•How are birthdays celebrated?

Residents' Care

•Do various staff and professional experts participate in evaluating each resident's needs and interests?

•Is a registered nurse available around the clock?

•How are medications administered and safeguarded?

•Does the facility have an arrangement with a nearby hospital?

•What is the availability of medical staff in the event of a problem or illness?

•How are medical emergencies handled?

Staff

•What is the staff to patient ratio? Does it differ on the various shifts?

•Is the staff licensed? (CNA, LVN, RN)

•Who is the staff accountable to?

•How is information about the residents shared among staff?

•How often are regular staff meetings held?

•What is the staff turnover rate?

•How long has the supervisory staff been at the facility?

•Is there a consistency of staff caring for the same residents?

•How does staff interact with the family?

•If there is a problem with a resident, how is this communicated?

•Is the family encouraged to visit at any time?

Facility

•What is the facility's philosophy or Mission Statement?

•Do the Administrator and other key staff members reflect the Mission Statement?

•What are the transfer/discharge policies?

•Does the facility look and smell clean?

•How often are the residents' rooms cleaned?

•What are the arrangements for laundry?

•Can the residents freely access the outdoors? Is there a requirement that the resident inform the staff before leaving the building?

•Are there places outside to sit comfortably in the shade? Is the outside area safe from traffic?

•Is the facility aesthetically pleasing inside and outside?

(Adapted, with permission, from *Questions to Ask When Looking for Assisted Living for Someone You Love* by Carol Mills, RN, MA)

Once you have visited a number of facilities and find one or more that you like, it's important to check with your state licensing agency or with the facility itself to find out about complaints and violations. Furthermore, every facility undergoes an annual survey, and the results of the survey are public. If you find a facility you like, but are concerned about certain items on the annual survey, a discussion with the facility's administrator will give you the opportunity to ask specific questions about violations. Ask the administrator what steps have been taken to correct any violations and what plans have been implemented to prevent future violations. Usually, a plan of corrective action must be submitted to the state licensing agency when a violation has been noted. Ask for a copy of the plan, which can be a useful tool to help you reach your decision.

SKILLED-NURSING FACILITIES

Skilled-nursing facilities, or nursing homes, provide care for both long-term and short-term patients. The level of care is much higher than that of an assisted-living facility and can include tube feeding, administration of intravenous fluids or medications, monitoring of vital signs or the effects of new medications, and wound care and dressing changes (Self, 2002).

As the number of Alzheimer's disease patients continues to increase, many nursing facilities have created separate Alzheimer's units or are devoted exclusively to such patients. If your parent has Alzheimer's disease, I highly recommend that you select a nursing home that has specific facilities for these patients. They are staffed and programmed to provide a secure, flexible, and activity-focused living environment that enhances the lives of those with Alzheimer's disease or related dementia.

If it is determined that your parent is best suited for full-nursing care, your search becomes even more critical. When you and your parent's doctors agree that a nursing facility is the best option, your parent obviously has health conditions severe enough to warrant constant medical supervision. Although your parent's doctors can undoubtedly refer you to any number of nursing homes, you will probably be on your own in a search for a facility because your parent is unlikely to be in a condition to help you. You might even be working against your parent's wishes, which places greater burden on you to find a facility your parent will like.

The task of finding a suitable facility can seem formidable, probably because of your lingering fears of nursing-home abuses. As I've said, such abuses have thankfully become much rarer, but they do still occur. So how can you be assured that the facility you choose for your parent will provide attentive and loving care? The following is a list of tips to help you begin your search. Once you have selected some possibilities, I'll show you how to find out if your selections have a good track record.

Skilled-nursing Facility Checklist

- •If your parent uses Medicare or Medicaid coverage, is the facility certified for either or both?

- •Does the facility provide the kind of custodial care your parent needs?

- •What services are provided by the facility, and what is the cost?

- •How long has the facility been in operation?

- •Is a bed available?

- •Is the facility located close enough for family and friends to visit?

•Do the residents appear clean, well-groomed, and appropriately dressed for the time of day and for the season?

•Is the facility free from unpleasant odors?

•Is the facility well-lit and is the temperature at a comfortable level?

•Is the relationship between staff and residents warm, polite, and respectful?

•Do the residents seem cheerful?

•Does the facility perform background checks on all staff members?

•Is there a registered nurse on the premises at all times?

•Do the same team of nurses and nursing assistants work with the same residents on a day-to-day basis?

•Is there an physician on staff?

•What is the staff turnover rate?

•May residents have personal belongings, including furniture, in their rooms?

•Do residents have their own telephones and televisions?

•Are the residents' religious and cultural needs given consideration?

•Are exits clearly marked?

•Do the bathrooms and hallways have handrails?

•Do residents have a choice of meal items?

•Are there planned activities for the residents?

•Can residents see their own personal physicians?

•Does the facility have an arrangement with a nearby hospital in case of emergencies?

•Are regular care-plan meetings held with staff, residents and family members?

Once you have narrowed your search to a few facilities that seem suitable, you'll probably start wondering if their operation is as good as it appears on the surface. Fortunately, the federal government has stepped in to help you secure the information you need to be certain. In a two-part program, the U.S. Department of Health and Human Services (HHS) has created a web site that allows you to compare the performances of skilled-nursing facilities in your community. By making this information public, HHS hopes that the second part of the program-increased quality of care-will come automatically. Officials expect that when nursing-home data is publicly listed, owners and operators will be motivated to increase the quality of services they provide.

This expectation is not unreasonable, as HHS has discovered. Health and Human Services began a pilot program in 2001 in six states—Colorado, Florida, Maryland, Ohio, Rhode Island, and Washington—to make skilled-nursing facility information available on the Internet. The results of the pilot program showed that facilities in those states responded to the standards of quality they had to report to HHS by improving patient services. (McDonald, 2002)

The drawback to the HHS program is that only facilities that are Medicare and Medicaid certified are included in the Internet comparison. Although such facilities comprise the majority of nursing homes, many fine facilities choose not to participate in Medicare or Medicaid programs. If you are considering a facility that does not participate in these programs, you will have to do your own data research. The task is made easier for you, though, because you can simply ask the facility to produce the same information the government requires of Medicare and Medicaid certified facilities. You can then make your own comparison.

What You Will Find on the Nursing-home Web Site

The web site address is www.medicare.gov/nhcompare/home.asp. The information contained on this web site can be invaluable in guiding you to the right skilled-nursing facility for your parent. It provides detailed information about the past performance of every Medicare- and Medicaid-certified skilled-nursing facility in the country. When you begin your online search, you will find the following sections:

About the Nursing Home. This information answers your basic questions about the facility itself, including the following.

1. **Total number of Medicare- and Medicaid-certified beds.** Some facilities have a combination of Medicare, Medicaid, and private-pay beds.
2. **Total number of residents in certified beds.** This number reflects the occupancy at the time of the inspection.
3. **Medicare/Medicaid participation.** This is important, because if your parent relies on Medicare coverage, it will run out after 100 days of skilled-nursing care. If your parent should then qualify for Medicaid coverage, but if the facility is not Medicaid certified, a move would be required.
4. **Type of ownership.** Nursing facilities can be owned by private, for-profit corporations; non-profit corporations; religious organizations, or government entities.

5. **Located within a hospital.** If a facility is located within a hospital or is affiliated with a hospital, the information will be found in this section.
6. **Resident and family councils.** The law requires that skilled-nursing facilities facilitate the organization of councils of residents and their families for the purpose of communicating with staff.

Quality Measures. Some of the quality measures for which data is listed include the following:

1. Percentage of residents with loss of ability in basic daily tasks
2. Percentage of residents with pressure sores
3. Percentage of residents with pain
4. Percentage of residents in physical restraints
5. Percentage of residents with infections
6. Percentage of residents with delirium

The percentages for each quality measure are listed in a column next to columns containing state and national average percentages, so that you can compare your facility's status.

Inspection Result Information. This information includes the health deficiencies found during the most recent inspection, as well as the results of complaint investigations. Each deficiency found is ranked on a scale of 1 to 4, in order of potential for harm to residents. If a deficiency has been corrected, the date of correction is noted. The areas scrutinized include the following:

1. Residents' rights
2. Nutrition and dietary
3. Environmental
4. Resident mistreatment

5. Quality care
6. Resident assessment
7. Pharmacy service
8. Administration

Staff Information. Data includes the average number of hours worked by registered nurses, licensed practical and vocational nurses, and certified nursing assistants per resident, per day. These figures are compared to state and national averages.

This is important data. Numerous studies have suggested that higher levels of staffing improve care. A recent study conducted by the University of California, San Francisco, reported that nursing homes that provide fewer then 4.1 hours of direct nursing care per resident per day are placing patients at risk (Wheeler, 2002).

I encourage you to visit the web site to see for yourself just how comprehensive the available information is. Even though it is limited to statistical data, you can still get an excellent overview of how a facility you might be considering compares with others. Once you have examined the data and visited possible facilities, you will have done nearly everything possible to be sure your parent will be safe and secure.

LONG-TERM CARE OMBUDSMAN PROGRAM

If you still have unanswered questions, there is one more step you can take. By federal law, every state is required to have a long-term care ombudsman program. Long-term care ombudsmen serve as advocates for assisted-living and skilled-nursing facility residents. They will give you personal guidance in finding a facility and ensuring your parent receives quality care. Further, ombudsmen are trained to resolve problems and assist with complaints.

The long-term care ombudsman program is administered by the federal Administration on Aging. The program has more than 1,000 paid staff members and 8,000 volunteers nationwide. These are the services ombudsmen provide:

- •They resolve complaints made by or for residents of long-term care facilities.

- •They educate consumers and long-term care providers about residents' rights and good care practices.

- •They promote community involvement through volunteer opportunities.

- •They provide information to the public on nursing homes and other long-term care facilities and services, residents' rights, and legislative and policy issues.

- •They advocate for residents' rights and quality care in nursing homes, personal care, residential care and other long-term care facilities.

- •They promote the development of citizen organizations, family councils, and resident councils.

For more information on the long-term care ombudsman program and how these trained professionals can help you, can contact the National Long-Term Care Ombudsman Resource Center (www.ltcombudsman .org (202) 332-2275).

As you are probably starting to realize, you are not alone in your quest to find quality care for your parent. The amount of information available to you has increased dramatically in recent years, and the avenues for guidance and assistance have greatly widened.

Your final hurdle is to help ease the transition to a facility for your parent. You might find it difficult to convince your parent that abuses are a thing of the past, so you probably will have to spend some time reassuring your parent that standards have greatly improved. To the extent your parent is able, a joint evaluation and decision about a facility is obviously preferable. But even if the task falls to you alone, with the guidelines provided in this chapter, you can rest assured that you will be able to find a facility that will provide your parent with high-quality care.

CHAPTER 8

Grace Resurfaces

*A*fter dropping K.C. at her house, I headed to a drive-through restaurant I had frequented as a kid, and ordered two large burgers with extra pickles and onions, fries, and a Coke. Not the most nutritious meal, I acknowledged, but I felt like indulging myself with a massive infusion of fat grams. Sitting in my car in the parking lot, I wolfed down my dinner, and then realized that I hadn't really tasted what I had eaten. At least I was no longer hungry, so I drove back to the house.

Inside, I checked the answering machine on the desk in the family room and found no messages, just the red digital 0. I remembered that I should collect the mail from outside, and, after doing so, I stacked it neatly next to the answering machine. I sat down in Dad's chair and called my wife to give her an update of the day's events and to tell her how much I missed her and the kids. Pamela caught me up on the family's events on the east coast. The conversation was shorter than it should have been, because I was exhausted. Exhaustion seemed to be my permanent state lately. I interrupted Pamela in mid-sentence so I could go to bed and get some much-needed sleep.

I probably should have followed my instincts and gone straight to bed. Instead, I looked through the stack of mail I had placed on the desk, which seemed like the usual letters one would expect. There was an envelope announcing that Dad had been approved for a credit card with a $5,000 credit limit and an advertisement for a not-to-be-missed sale on new cars.

Still sorting through the mail, I came upon an envelope that stopped me cold. It was addressed to "Ben Carnot, Guarantor." Across the front of the envelope in half-inch bold, red letters were the words OPEN IMMEDIATELY, LITIGATION PENDING. My heart started racing; I felt the vein in my forehead pulsing to presage a whopper of a headache. I knew from my legal training that a guarantor is someone who guarantees another person's debt if the borrower does not pay off the obligation.

This couldn't be right. Dad would never agree to guarantee someone else's debt. There had to be some mistake. I had heard about scams in which elderly people paid money for a debt they didn't owe simply because they had been threatened with litigation. Fearful that they had somehow made a mistake or forgotten the phantom debt, they would agree to pay. I wondered if the letter I was holding in my hand might be one of those scams.

I was in a bind. Should I leave the letter on the desk with Dad's other mail, or should I invade his privacy and open it? For several minutes I wrestled with the implications of opening my dad's mail versus leaving him vulnerable to a possible scam. Finally I decided to open the envelope. I was turning into a bit of a snoop, which made me decidedly uncomfortable. First I had eavesdropped on my father's telephone conversation, now I was opening his mail. Where had my ethics gone? Did my father's current situation warrant my invading his privacy like this? I didn't have the energy to dwell on the answers to these questions; instead, I followed my instincts. I felt in my heart that what I was doing was defensible because of Dad's circumstances. If this was indeed a scam or even a legitimate potential legal problem, I was in the best position to help Dad. Still, if put to the test, I would have to admit I was sticking my nose into my father's business affairs, something I had no right to do.

In the envelope was an official-looking letter from an entity called Federal Collections. I did not have to be a lawyer to understand this missive. It seemed that Dad had guaranteed a car loan for Grace, the borrower, who was now in serious default, despite repeated notices to her. Under the terms of the loan agreement, the lender had the option to accelerate the note and demand full payment from Dad, who had guaranteed the loan.

The letter was demanding the entire principal balance, late fees, accrued interest, and attorney's fees to date, totaling $14,235, to be paid within five days of the date of the letter—which I noticed was dated three days earlier. If the amount was not paid immediately, the letter threatened, the matter would be turned over to litigation attorneys for collection, which would no doubt increase the amount owed and seriously affect Dad's credit rating.

Even though I was alone in the house, I spoke out loud. "What is going on? Dad, what are you doing?" I tried to keep my anger from boiling over, but I was getting so worked up that I wanted to hit something. I was feeling a completely unfamiliar level of anger. The cumulative effect of everything that had happened with my dad was pushing me over the edge into rage. Obviously, Dad had guaranteed a car loan for Grace. Why? Why? Why? What was he thinking? I couldn't have been more shocked.

Dad had always been the person responsible for paying the bills at home when K.C. and I were growing up. We had seen him countless times sitting at the desk in the family room, writing checks, paying the bills the day they arrived. He did not believe in waiting to pay a bill until a few days before its due date; instead, he took great pride in paying all his bills immediately. He had taught his children to do the same. The reason he was so careful about paying bills was that he did not want to do anything to adversely affect his credit rating, which, Dad had taught us, would follow us around our entire life. "A bad credit rating is like a scar; it never goes away," was one of Dad's homilies.

Furthermore, Dad did not believe in borrowing money for a car. His rule when it came to borrowing was simple: If you can't afford the purchase, don't make it. A credit card purchase was fine as long as the total amount due was paid when the bill was received. Dad did not believe in supporting the credit card companies by paying finance charges, and he passed this belief on to his children. The only exceptions to Dad's no-debt rule were a mortgage on the house and loans for the business.

So why would Dad guarantee a car loan in violation of everything he had taught his children and the way he had been living until now? Even more incredible, Grace, who had no living expenses and was pulling down far more than her salary, had missed so many car payments that the loan was being called, and Dad was the deep pocket they were asking to pay off her debt. So now my big-hearted father was being screwed again, this time to the tune of $14,235.

Upset as I was, I knew that I wouldn't be able to sleep. I thought about calling K.C., but I didn't want to ruin her evening. I had no choice but to suck it up and come up with a plan for dealing with Grace's latest abuse, which I would discuss with K.C. in the morning.

I tossed and turned throughout the night. I knew that I couldn't do anything about the letter until morning, yet I couldn't sleep because of my anger with Dad for guaranteeing Grace's car loan. Compounding my restlessness was my anger with Grace for taking advantage of Dad yet again. No sleep for me, just an unending routine of looking at the clock, turning on the TV, hoping it would lull me to sleep, turning off the TV, looking at the clock. The night would not end.

I finally fell asleep after exhaustion won the battle with anger. I opened my eyes, stretched and looked at the clock, which read 7:00. I last remembered it being 5:30, so I had managed to sneak in at least a little sleep. Pushing back the covers to sit up, I realized I was nowhere near refreshed, but it was morning and time to get on with the day.

I got out of bed and headed for the shower, adjusting the temperature of the water to as cold as I could stand it, hoping to wake myself up. This was the same shower where I had learned the "lying lesson" years earlier. The shower stall was no different from how I remembered it, except that the lower showerhead had been removed entirely, and a cap of some sort was on the wall covering the spot where it used to be. I emerged from the shower feeling recharged and ready to go, got dressed, and repacked my suitcase and briefcase. I checked to make sure my airline ticket was in my jacket pocket, and then I moved my luggage to the family room next to the desk. If things went well with Dad today, I hoped to get out of Dodge and back to the east coast.

I made a cup of coffee, strong and black, and toasted a bagel. After my meager breakfast, I called my sister, and we agreed that I would pick her up. I grabbed my suitcase and briefcase, walked out the door, locking it behind me, and got into the rental car. As I pulled away, I realized that I had not left a light on in case I did need to stay another night, so

I drove back to the house to flip on the switch that illuminated the out-side stairway lights, and then left again to pick up my sister.

K.C. was standing in the front yard as I pulled up to her house. She had already spoken with Dr. Weaver, who said that Dad would be discharged tomorrow. His blood chemistry was closing in on the normal range, and he was eating his scheduled meals. We agreed that if all went well with our visit today, there was no reason for me to stay in San Diego any longer, and I should take the evening flight home. I told K.C. about the threatening letter from the collection agency. The idea that Dad had been sucked into guaranteeing a new car loan for Grace sickened K.C. as much as it had me. I offered to call the collection agency to get some information about the letter, even though it was already clear to me what had transpired. I considered arguing that Dad was not mentally compe-tent to sign as a guarantor. But that argument didn't seem too attractive in view of our recent education in the laws governing competence.

"Maybe I could use the incompetence argument as a red herring with the collection agency," I told K.C. "Ultimately, though, I need to con-vince the lien holder to take one of two options: Either seize the car, sell it at auction and use the proceeds to offset the amount Dad has to pay, or settle with Dad for a small lump sum." K.C. and I agreed that I should try to get the matter resolved at the lowest cost to Dad, which I was confident I could do because I had Dad's power of attorney. With this, I could make commitments for my father that were legally binding.

Our primary purpose in seeing Dad this morning, other than to see how he was doing, was to float a test balloon about Mountain View. We did-n't expect him to immediately sign on to the program, but we hoped he would not dismiss the suggestion out of hand. We discussed some strategies for raising this issue without alarming and angering Dad and agreed on an approach as we pulled into the hospital parking lot.

Our idea was to present the concept in as low key a manner as possible. Either of us could bring up Mountain View whenever we saw an opening. Once the topic was mentioned by one of us, the other would encourage Dad to take a pleasant drive out to the facility to see it. We wanted to push the pleasant drive to a destination, rather than the destination.

Being old pros in locating the lockdown unit, we went directly to the nurses' station outside the hall to the unit's door, where we identified ourselves as Ben Carnot's son and daughter. A different nurse was at the desk. After entering the appropriate data into the computer, she asked, "Do you need an escort to the unit door?" K.C. replied that we knew the way, so an escort wasn't necessary. She said that she would call the nursing station in the unit and ask the duty nurse to let us in. We waited at the unit's door for the nurse to let us in. While we were waiting, I looked through the small glass window and saw that the lockdown shuffle was in full swing, with maybe ten residents walking the elongated oval.

After a few minutes, I saw a nurse approaching the door with Dad shuffling behind her. She unlocked the door and pulled it open to let us in. While the nurse relocked the door, we hugged and kissed our dad, and, after an appropriate pause, she introduced herself as Teresa Jones. Nurse Jones indicated that she needed to escort the three of us to the conference room. Hospital policy was that visitors should not loiter in the hallway of the unit.

We followed her to the same conference room where we had met with Dr. Weaver the day before. She unlocked and opened the door for us to enter. Before leaving, she asked if we were familiar with the procedure for getting out of the conference room when we were ready to leave. Seeing our hesitation, she told us that we should pick up the telephone and dial 333 when we were ready to leave, which would ring the telephone at the nurse's station in the middle of the unit. A nurse would come to let us out of the conference room and escort us off the unit. We thanked Nurse Jones for her help and sat down at the conference table. After she left the room, I heard her lock the door from the other side.

With barely any preliminaries, Dad said he felt fine and was looking forward to getting home. I thought Dad looked markedly improved since the day before. He was cleanly-shaven and smelled of talcum powder. We both told him how great he looked. I asked him, "How were you able to shave?"

"I used an electric razor while one of the orderlies watched me." Dad added that he didn't like the idea of someone watching him prepare for the day, but it wasn't a big problem.

He wanted to know when he could go home, and we told him probably tomorrow. He was not happy with this news, but even though he desperately wanted to go home today, he reluctantly agreed to wait because that was what Dr. Weaver recommended. Despite Dad's disappointment he seemed relieved to know that he would be going home shortly. His ordeal in the hospital was finally coming to an end, and he breathed an audible sigh of relief. He told us again how much he wanted to get back to his home. We understood. It was hard for us to tell our dad that he couldn't go home today; it broke our hearts to deny him anything, especially something as seemingly innocuous as going home to the comforts he enjoyed and deserved.

I looked at Dad in his hospital gown and still could not get used to his skeletal-looking features. Malnutrition had caused his cheeks to cave in, the flesh on his arms was sagging, and his grey hair just added to the picture of an old man. This sad picture only reinforced my belief that Dad needed someone watching over him full time—someone who could be trusted. I bit the bullet, took a deep breath and told my father that K.C. and I had visited a wonderful "retirement community" that had an opening coming up, and we thought the place would be terrific for him. "Loads of people your age, all kinds of activities. The food looked good. Nice new apartment. Some nice-looking women." I explained that K.C. and I were so impressed with what we had seen that after he was settled in at home we wanted him to take a nice drive with K.C. to see the place.

Dad obviously understood what I was saying, but instead of responding, he asked something I was unprepared to hear. "Have you heard from Grace?"

In retrospect, I'm sure that my dad never anticipated that his question would cause a confrontation. But for me, it triggered the rage I had been carrying with me for days. I became visibly angry, unable to control myself. The frustration created by my father's obsession with Grace was causing a pressure in my chest that I had to relieve with a strong response. "Dad," I hissed in a low but assertive voice, "Grace is not coming back. Never. Ever. She is gone. Get on with your life, will you?" I was immediately sorry I had used this tone of voice with my sick father, but I just couldn't control myself.

K.C. interjected with the voice of reason: "Dad, Grace took advantage of your trust. We are never going to let her hurt you again." K.C. sounded so sweet and sincere, everyone stopped talking for a moment while her words hung in the air.

Dad seemed to be handling the stress of the exchange well. Clearly he did not want to get into a confrontation with me, especially if he was risking a longer stay in the unit. He obviously was exercising great restraint, certainly more then I had in the past few minutes. Still, his face was turning red and the pupils in his eyes were narrowing to pinpoints, but he didn't raise his voice. Dad lifted up his head and stuck out his chin, his eyes glaring at me, and said, "We will see about Grace." His tone of voice left no doubt what he meant: You will keep her away from me over my dead body. I knew then and there, with absolute certainty, that many more problems were in store for us with Grace.

When Dad made up his mind, he was a force that would not be stopped. I had drawn a deep line in the sand instructing my father to stay on the side of no contact with Grace. It was now clearer then ever before that when it came to Grace, Dad would cross the line at will. Furthermore, he was putting his kids on notice that he was in control of his destiny. In that instant I knew that our prayers for an easy move to Mountain View would go unanswered.

"Whatever you say, Dad," I sighed.

It was time to fall back to plan two and line up long-term caregivers for Dad's round-the-clock care when he came home. The conference room walls were closing in on me. The conversation with my dad was over, but I didn't know how to bring it to an end gracefully. Dad helped me out of my dilemma. He said he was tired and wanted to rest in his room. He didn't look tired; he looked fresh and perky. Obviously, Dad wanted to be far away from his kids, who were trampling on his independence and putting his life in turmoil. Dad also wanted out of the conference room, probably knowing his temper would soon take over.

"Ed, I'm tired. How do I get out of here?" It was the tone of the message, not the words, that cut deep into me. My father was burning with anger about his upstart kids trying to control his life. He wanted some space, quickly. Even though I too desperately wanted to get home, I needed to reach some closure before I left. I felt doubly bad because this was the last time I was going to see my dad for a while. I stood up and kissed my dad. I told him I was sorry for getting mad at him, but the past few days had been hell on me, especially since I had not slept well. "Will you forgive me, Dad?"

He said that he would, but I wasn't sure of his sincerity. I walked over to the telephone and dialed 333 and told the nurse who answered that we wanted to be let out of the conference room. We waited for the nurse in painful silence. I knew I had tried my best, but my father still didn't understand what had happened to him, how he had fallen victim to Grace. How could my father be so blind? I had saved my father's savings, I had ensured that he could continue to enjoy his money, and yet I was going home the bad guy. I honestly didn't understand what I had done that was so wrong.

After what seemed like an eternity, I heard the door lock retract and the same nurse who had let us in earlier held the door open for us to leave. Dad stiffly kissed us both, gave us each a small hug, and said goodbye. He shuffled into the hallway, head down as he turned to the right and we lost sight of him.

It was all I could do to fight back the tears that were threatening to spill over. Here was a person I loved dearly, and I had been cruel to him. Yelling at my dad, even about Grace, was unforgivable. Dad was sick, and I was having a very difficult time accepting this fact. I desperately wished I could turn back the clock to the beginning of today's visit.

With no more business at the hospital, we were escorted to the door of the lockdown unit. I was weeping softly. K.C. took my arm and told me, "Don't worry. It's not your fault. Dad will get better." Comforting words, but were they true or just a kind effort by my sister to make me feel better?

While she was unlocking the unit door for us, Nurse Jones commented on how nice it was that Dad had so many visitors. "What visitors?" we asked together. To the best of our knowledge, no one except Dad's doctors and we even knew he was in the hospital.

"I don't know their names, but it was a nice, middle-aged woman accompanied by several young men, who seemed to be her children, who visited him about an hour ago."

I asked, "Are you sure it was our father they visited?"

"Oh, yes, I am sure. They asked for him at the nursing station in front of the entrance to the unit, and I was asked to locate your father for a visit. I found him in the day room and I escorted him to the front door of the unit, just like I did when you came to visit. Then I escorted him and his visitors to the conference room."

Grace! It had to be! My legs were suddenly wobbling. Was there no way to protect Dad from exposure to this virus? I had thought that he was isolated from Grace, and I was feeling good about the past three days of separation, only to find that Grace and her children had simply sashayed into the unit to visit her prey.

"Has my father had any phone calls?" Nurse Jones did not know. "Well, is there a log of phone calls to the patients?"

No, no log is made of phone calls to the patients," she said.

"Is there a log of visitors?" I asked, even though I already knew who Dad's visitors had been.

"No, no log is made of visitors," the nurse replied.

"Is there some way that a patient can be insulated from certain visitors?'

"Of course," she said. "All that is needed is an order from his doctor. No one on the unit is allowed a visitor until the duty nurse checks the patient's file on the computer to see if there is an order from the doctor prohibiting specific visitors or even all visitors.

Now they tell us, I thought. It was frightening that anyone off the street—especially Grace—could have unlimited access to our dad unless someone had thought to tell us that we could protect him with a doctor's order. The nurse was obviously curious about my questions, but I didn't have the strength to give her the full story. Besides, it was too late. The damage was done.

My first instinct was to confront Dad again and find out why he'd had an audience with Grace and her sons. What had they talked about? Why was he talking to Grace at all, given what she had done to him? Did he *want* her to suck him dry of all of his money? My mood shifted in an instant from acute depression to loathing for Grace and, once again, anger at my dad. I knew, however, that another session with Dad in the conference room would be useless.

Also troubling was that not more then just a few minutes earlier, Dad had asked me whether I had heard from Grace. Why would he ask this question when he had just seen her and her crew? Had he been set up by Grace? Had Grace planted this question to get a rise out of me in front of my dad so that I would come off as the bad son while she was cast as the only one who really cared about Dad? I knew my dad had not forgotten about seeing her minutes before. Yes, a bear trap had been set, and I had walked right in and sprung the jaws. I had been trapped into getting into an argument with Dad that I could not win because of his strong feelings for Grace. Through guile, Grace had made me out to be the villain and herself the princess. Score one for Grace. I hated her more than ever.

Finding a Caregiver:
What You Can Do

When realization sets in that your parent needs supervision, you have many options to consider. As the child, you want your parent to receive the best care in the safest possible environment, which is why children tend to prefer community living options for their parents. As discussed in chapter 7, such facilities must be licensed by the state and undergo regular inspections and surveys, thereby providing the safe, regulated environment that children envision. Parents, on the other hand, almost always prefer to remain in the home. Unfortunately, a parent alone in the home with a paid caregiver creates the set of circumstances most likely to result in abuse. However, since this is the choice most parents prefer (and often insist on), and because most children truly want their parents to continue to have at least a modicum of independence and decision-making ability, home care is an option that is selected more and more frequently.

The key to establishing a successful caregiver-parent relationship lies in careful planning. How does one go about finding a caregiver? Who should it be? Should you hire the housekeeper? Should an adult child move in with the parent? Or is it best to work with an agency? As you can see, many options are available, and we'll look at each in turn, weighing the pros and cons.

HOUSEKEEPER BECOMES CAREGIVER

Grace became my father's caregiver simply by virtue of her longtime status as the family's housekeeper. Because she had helped care for my mother and also for Sue when they were ill, it seemed only natural for

Grace to move into the position of caregiver when my father began to need some supervision. Neither K.C. nor I ever considered that Grace might not be the appropriate person to care for our father. After all, she had a long and trusted association with our family, our father liked and respected her, and we believed he didn't have any medical conditions serious enough to warrant nursing care rather than just supervisory care. Never in a million years would it have occurred to us that Grace might evolve into a predatory opportunist. What K.C. and I learned from our experience, and what I wish to pass along to you, is that you should always expect the worst, especially in a housekeeper-turned-caregiver situation. If you take steps ahead of time to circumvent the worst-case scenario, you will rest easy knowing you have done your best to ward off the potential for abuse.

A housekeeper can evolve into a caregiver almost by default, without anyone in the family noticing. If this situation reminds you of your parent's circumstances, the time to formalize the transition is now. Even if a housekeeper has already assumed the role of caregiver, it is never too late to have a formal discussion about the role change. You have two major considerations when thinking of legitimizing a transition from housekeeper to caregiver:

1. To what extent does your parent need trained, professional caregiving? Caregiving can range from tasks as simple as monitoring medications for a fairly healthy person to full nursing care for a bedridden person.
2. Do the abilities and training of the housekeeper match the needs of your parent? Often, caregivers will quickly exceed the scope of their abilities, and they might try to accommodate your parent's needs in ways that are inappropriate.

Keep in mind that a housekeeper-turned-caregiver is prone to exaggerate abilities and cover up a lack of expertise in order to keep from losing the job. Also, neither your parent nor the housekeeper is likely to be objective about whether the housekeeper's ability matches your parent's needs, because both are probably intent on maintaining the current relationship, for better or worse. Consult with your parent's doctors. They are in the best position to give you an objective evaluation of your parent's needs. Only then can you assess whether a housekeeper is capable of providing the kind of care your parent requires.

FORMALIZING THE TRANSITION

If you decide that promoting a housekeeper to caregiver is the best solution for your parent, two important protective measures should be taken immediately:

1. Formalize the arrangement with a contract.
2. Set up a system of accountability.

Contract

When you hire a contractor to perform repairs on your house, you sign a contract detailing the scope of the work and how much it will cost. In fact, anytime you enter into an agreement for services, you undoubtedly sign a contract of some sort, even if you just scribble your name at the bottom of an estimate. When you sign a contract, both parties are expected to perform as agreed. If a subsequent dispute arises, a written contract eliminates any doubt about what each person was obligated to do.

I can't think of another set of circumstances that cry out for a legal agreement more than that of a housekeeper-turned-caregiver. You wouldn't trust a carpenter to come in and start tearing out walls without a contract, so why would you trust the care of your parent to someone with whom you do not have a document spelling out precisely what is expected? Some of my clients have felt uncomfortable broaching this subject with their parents' housekeepers, thinking that requesting a contract would be insulting. My suggested approach is to point out that a contract protects not just your parent but also the caregiver, and that a verbal agreement is just not enough. The idea that both parties are being protected is always an appealing way to broach this subject.

You can obtain a simple employment agreement from an office supply store that you can then adapt for your use. There is one clause that your contract should contain that I want to talk about here. Be sure to include a clause that addresses gifts and gratuities. It should state that the caregiver agrees not to accept any gifts, gratuities, additional compensation, or bonuses from the employer (parent). It should further state that in the event the caregiver accepts any such gifts, gratuities, compensation, or bonuses, the caregiver agrees to relinquish any claim to them and return them to the parent. If we had had a contract with Grace containing this clause, we would have had legal recourse against her for accepting so many "gifts" from my father.

Unfortunately, this paragraph is not a perfect solution to the problem of the caregiver accepting gifts from your parent. If, for example, the caregiver spends additional money received from your parent and has no other assets (house, car, bank account, etc.), you are without a remedy. You can sue and get a judgment against the caregiver, but you will collect nothing under these circumstances. Nevertheless, my feeling is that it is infinitely better to have a written agreement prohibiting the caregiver from accepting gifts from your parent than to have no agreement at all. Maintaining the right to sue can serve as an effective deterrent. Also, if your parent is aware of this paragraph, he or she will be less likely to attempt to give a gift to the caregiver knowing that the caregiver could be fired for accepting a gift.

You're probably wondering what you would do to reward a conscientious caregiver should you want to give a bonus or a gift for outstanding service. You can give gifts on behalf of your parent, which allows you the flexibility of recognizing exceptional service without exposing your parent to possible extortion by the caregiver.

Accountability

The next protective measure you need to establish is a system of accountability. The family should assign someone to be the "point person," the one who is responsible for communicating with and giving directions to the caregiver. As a family you need to decide how much information you want to know about your parent's care, and develop a tracking sheet for the caregiver to complete and submit to the point person on an agreed-upon schedule.

The following is a list of some of the behaviors and activities you might include on a daily tracking sheet:

1. Sleeping
   Bedtime
   Number of times awakened during the night
   Reasons for waking
   Measures taken to get back to sleep
   Time awakened in the morning
   Naps taken (times and duration)

2. Hygiene
   Bath or shower
   Grooming of hair, nails
   Oral care
   Shaving
   Condition of skin
3. Medications
   Schedule of necessary meds
   Times meds were administered
   Unusual reactions to meds
4. Meals
   When eaten
   Foods consumed
   Snacks eaten during the day/evening
   Alcoholic beverages consumed
5. General mood and well-being
   Mood
   Confusion
   Restlessness, agitation, paranoia
   Alertness
   Pain
   Health complaints
6. Activities
   Indoor activities (television, reading, phone calls, etc.)
   Trips outside the house
   Ambulatory ability
   Balance
   Enjoyment level
   Guests/visitors

7. Doctor/Dentist visits
    Reason for visit
    Doctor's comments
    Parent's concerns/complaints
8. General housekeeping
    Sheets changed
    Laundry
    House cleaning
    Grocery shopping
9. Comments or complaints from parent
10. Comments and observations from caregiver

If your parent has a specific medical condition, obviously you should include tracking information to keep the point person abreast of its progress and any changes. Your tracking sheet can be as simple or as complex as you feel is appropriate. The key to making this a successful endeavor is to maintain a regular reporting schedule and for the caregiver to know that the information is taken seriously. For these reasons, it is essential that you question the caregiver periodically about the report so that the caregiver will know the report is important to you and that the caregiver is being evaluated in part on submitting a complete report.

One final word about housekeepers-turned-caregivers: Having a full-time, live-in caregiver can present a unique problem. These folks often don't have much of a life of their own. Once they settle into your parent's home, what little life they may have had is likely to disappear almost completely. As a result, the caregiver can easily become overly involved with your parent's life, particularly since the caregiver is the one who is now physically closest to your parent and most responsible for fulfilling your parent's needs. The caregiver can begin subtly to manipulate your parent's life, just as Grace did with my father. Moreover, attempts by family members to be involved in the parent's care can be viewed as interference, and, as was the case with my father and Grace, they can team up to form an "us against them" alliance.

The best way to prevent this from happening is vigilance on the part of the point person and other family members. Continuous contact, both in person and by telephone, is essential. K.C. and I were not sensitive to the signs of abuse, and even though we were in constant contact with Dad, we missed many red flags. If you educate yourself and become aware of possible trouble signs, you will recognize them should they occur. Scrupulous adherence to your personalized tracking routine is equally important. As long as the caregiver knows that the parent's family is intimately involved and the caregiver's activities are being closely monitored, the opportunity for the caregiver to "take over" is greatly diminished.

CHILD BECOMES CAREGIVER

In many cases, children of aging parents believe it is their responsibility to assume the caregiving role. For some, this can be a richly rewarding experience, a beautiful gift to the parent and a testament to a close and loving relationship that no professional caregiver could ever provide. For others, having one family member take on caregiver duties can become the entire family's worst nightmare. Only you can decide whether you or another family member has the kind of relationship with your parent that would allow for the successful reversal of roles that caregiving entails.

Children who become the primary caregiver for a parent usually do so because of a desire to provide loving, quality care in a familiar setting. However, anyone who is thinking of assuming the role of caregiver should take an honest look at the situation, ideally in conjunction with other family members. As a family (or even on your own, if there is no one else to help you with the decision), ask these questions:

1. How much help does your parent need, and how much time is required to provide the necessary care? Is the amount of time likely to increase or decrease as time goes by?
2. Do you have the necessary skill level to provide adequate care for your parent?
3. Are there other family members or friends who might be able to relieve you from time to time?
4. How does your parent feel about having a child as caregiver? Is it possible your parent might resent your presence and see it as interference in his or her life?

If you decide that the best solution to providing for your parent's needs is for you to assume the role of caregiver, please know that there is no greater gift you can give. However, you must understand that you will not do either your parent or yourself any good by allowing yourself to become overburdened, overwhelmed, and burned out. Primary caregiving is most successful when it is limited in scope and for a short period of time. If your parent has a long-term, chronic (but not life-threatening) condition that requires substantial care, you would be well advised to seek an alternative care plan. You must consider your own needs as well.

You might be surprised to learn that, according to statistics provided by the National Center on Elder Abuse, more than two-thirds of elder-abuse perpetrators are family members of the victim (2003). Many of these abusers find themselves to be caregivers almost by accident, first by lending a hand for a couple of hours a day, and then realizing that the needs of the parent have increased so greatly, they are suddenly in a primary caregiver role. They feel trapped and resentful and see no way out of their situation. Abuse is most likely to occur under circumstances such as these.

As long as we're discussing the pitfalls of the child as caregiver, let's look at one more. Even if other family members are involved in your decision to be caregiver and occasionally help you with your parent's care, the burden of caregiving will still be almost entirely on your shoulders. Since you are the one closest to your parent, you will obviously feel that you know what's best, and input from other family members might tend to create resentment. Furthermore, it would be natural for you to believe that other family members aren't doing as much as they could-another breeding ground for resentment. From the perspective of the rest of the family, they could easily begin to feel left out of the decision-making process, feel as though you are taking over, and then start to resent you.

I have seen situations in which one child moved into the house to assume the role of primary caregiver and shortly became resentful of the other siblings for not helping with their parent's care. Under these circumstances, it's not uncommon for the parent to give large sums of money to the caregiving child, not unlike what happened with my dad and Grace. This can lead ultimately to the caregiving child being favored in the will. Mediating such disputes has consumed many hours of my time. From my experience, I am convinced that it takes a special child to assume the role of live-in or principal caregiver who does not begin to feel animosity toward other siblings. I strongly suggest that you consider whether your circumstances could lead to a family fracture because of the personalities involved. If you conclude that it could, or even might, then hire a professional to take care of your parent.

As you can see, the child-as-caregiver scenario is fraught with potential land mines. It is doable, though, as statistics show. More than one in four American households includes someone who provides care for an aging loved one (Seff, 2002). The most important thing for you to remember is that it is equally important for you to take care of yourself as it is to take care of your parent. The following is an Action Plan for Caregivers, developed by Carol Mills, R.N., M.A. I recommend that you post a copy of this somewhere where it will constantly remind you of the importance of addressing your own needs as well as those of your parent.

ACTION PLAN FOR CAREGIVERS

- •Involve your family from the beginning by sharing your concerns with them.

- •Access all the information you can about your parent's condition, and educate yourself as much as possible about what to expect.

- •Have an awareness of the losses to come, both concrete and symbolic, so they are not totally unexpected.

- •Recognize the hidden grief component of your anger, anxiety, guilt and depression. Expect adaptation, but not resolution, of your grief.

- •Appreciate your grief and seek out someone who understands it.

- •Recognize the signs of denial; for example, "I don't need any help," "Nothing's wrong-everything's okay." "The doctors made a mistake—he doesn't have _____." "I'm keeping him home, no matter what."

- •Acknowledge your right to feel emotionally off balance sometimes.

- •Learn to "let go" from the start and share your caregiving burden with others.

- •Forgive yourself for not being perfect.

•Stop trying to be perfect. Caring for someone with a chronic illness means your world has been turned upside down, and you will probably have to compromise some of your personal standards of housekeeping, cooking, and other activities.

•Join a support group early.

•Take care of yourself physically and emotionally. Have regular check-ups. Get as much rest and respite as possible. Eat well-balanced meals. Give yourself time to cry. Don't feel guilty for having a good time.

•Hang onto your sense of self. Keep up your regular activities as much as possible to help preserve your identity.

•Take one day at a time, but don't neglect the need to plan for the future, including consulting with an attorney, making funeral arrangements, etc.

•Learn how to communicate differently with your parent if cognitive and language abilities decline. Good communication strategies help to avoid frustration.

•Accept yourself for being human. Even if you "lose it" sometimes, give yourself a pat on the back for doing the best you can under very difficult circumstances.

FINDING A PROFESSIONAL CAREGIVER

If you do not already have a housekeeper who can be promoted, and you don't have a family member able to assume the responsibilities of caregiver for your parent, you must begin to search for a professional. You can conduct this search in one of two ways: on your own or through an agency.

Each approach has its pros and cons. If you hire on your own, the cost is likely to be less, which could be a major consideration. In some cases, Medicare will partially cover home healthcare, as will long-term care insurance policies, but only in rare cases will 100 percent of the cost be covered by either. The cons of a private hire are that you are responsible for payroll, payroll taxes, workers' compensation insurance, and all reporting requirements. Also, if the caregiver becomes ill or fails to show up, you don't have an automatic backup.

Using an agency has several pros:

1. The agency is responsible for payroll and reporting requirements.
2. Agencies will perform their own background checks on caregivers.
3. Agencies will provide a backup if the primary caregiver is ill.

The drawback to using an agency is that it is almost always more expensive than a private hire.

Hiring on Your Own

The first step in finding a private hire is to establish a schedule. How many hours per day and days per week does your parent need assistance? If you determine that full-time care is necessary, you should look for someone who is willing to live in, or you could hire several caregivers to maintain regular shifts around the clock. Get an application form (or design your own) that will supply you with the information you need to conduct a background check, a crucial step in making sure the potential caregiver does not have a criminal history. At a minimum, you'll need the applicant's name, address, telephone number and social security number. Many companies provide background checks for a nominal fee—search on the Internet or look in your Yellow Pages under "Investigators."

The next step is to find applicants. You can place an ad in your local newspaper, or you can contact retirement communities and senior centers in your area for referrals. Another good way to find caregivers is through word of mouth. Ask your friends and neighbors if they know of anyone who works as a caregiver and might be seeking a position. This can be a surprisingly effective method. Once you have a group of good applicants, schedule a day for interviewing. The ideal profile of a caregiver is someone with a solid employment history, relevant training and experience, flexibility, an aptitude for working with the elderly and strong references. The following is a list of questions to ask a potential hire:

1. What is your training? (A Certified Nursing Assistant would be ideal.)
2. What licenses and/or certificates do you hold?
3. Are you bonded and insured? If not, are you bondable and can you secure insurance?
4. How long have you been a professional caregiver?
5. How long did your previous job last? Why did you leave each job?
6. What range of medical conditions have your previous clients had?
7. Have you worked with clients who have dementia?
8. Do you have a driver's license for transportation to doctor's appointments and social activities?
9. Are you willing to cook and perform housekeeping chores?
10. What do you like most about being a caregiver?
11. What is your strongest skill?
12. Where are you weakest when it comes to the care of the elderly? (This question is essential; don't be afraid to ask it. You are asking a person who may ultimately have primary responsibility for the care of your parent to put his or her cards on the table about any possible shortcomings.)

Ask for a list of references for each job and follow up on them. If possible, have your parent participate in the interview process. It's vital that the caregiver you hire build a good relationship with your parent, but the chemistry you feel for a particular applicant might not be shared by your parent. Be clear about your expectations, and keep your eyes open for negative body language in reaction to the chores or duties you describe. Don't eliminate a likely candidate simply because he or she hates to do laundry. This is where you and other family members can fill in, with the added benefit of bringing you to the premises regularly to observe how things are going. Finally, ask the applicant if there are any questions you haven't answered.

Once you have decided on your caregiver(s), remember to take the same proactive steps suggested earlier, in the section on housekeeper-turned-caregiver. Draw up a contract that details the scope of the work (don't forget the no-gift clause!), and make sure you both have a signed copy. Create your tracking sheets, select a point person and establish a reporting schedule. Finally, maintain a scrupulous routine of communication, both by telephone and in person. Drop by unannounced and frequently in the early days of the caregiver's employment. Establish a firm employer-employee relationship, and let the caregiver know that you are supervising at all times.

Hiring Through an Agency

The primary advantage of using an agency to provide a caregiver is that the agency will do much of the work for you, including background checks, licensing, bonding, payroll, insurance, and reporting. The biggest disadvantage is the cost. Fees vary widely depending on your geographic location. Most agencies charge between $10 and $18 per hour for caregivers, with either a three-hour or a four-hour minimum shift. A twelve-hour nighttime shift ranges from $50 to $150 (again, depending on location). Round-the-clock, live-in care can fall anywhere between $100 and $200 per day. So the obvious first step is to determine the extent of care needed by your parent and whether or not the budget will allow for it.

To find an agency you can look in the Yellow Pages under "Home Health Services." Or you might contact your local commission or agency on Aging and Independence Services for a referral. If your parent is being discharged from the hospital, ask the hospital's discharge planner for a recommendation to an agency. Once you have decided on an agency, ask the following questions before you sign the agency's contract:

1. How long has your agency been in business?
2. Is your agency licensed, insured, and bonded?
3. Are all of your caregivers licensed, insured, and bonded?
4. Do you require special training or certificates for your caregivers? (Certified Nursing Assistant is highly desirable.)
5. Do you perform background checks on your caregivers?
6. Do you have caregivers who drive? Do you verify their driver's licenses?
7. Do you provide backup support in case a caregiver becomes ill?
8. Do you have a minimum shift requirement?
9. Do you provide live-in caregivers?
10. Do you monitor care documentation?
11. What are the fees?
12. Are there additional charges for services other than the basic caregiving? (For example, light housekeeping, transportation, laundry, etc.)
13. Are the fees the same for weekends and holidays?

14. Is there a sign-up fee or a deposit required?
15. Do you accept Medicare or payment from long-term care insurance?

If the agency answers all your questions satisfactorily, and you decide to use its services, don't automatically accept whomever they send to you. Insist on meeting your assigned caregiver before agreeing to hire that person. Your parent will want to meet the caregiver, too, to make sure they can work together. Also, even though the agency should have screened their caregivers for the appropriate qualifications, you still should ask some interview questions yourself. Don't simply take for granted that the agency will recommend only qualified candidates with no blemishes in their background. Agencies can get sloppy in their hiring practices. So you should do some leg work as if you were hiring the caregiver directly. Review the list of questions under "Hiring on your own," and select those that you would like a personal answer to.

Even if you hire from an agency, you will still want to be reassured that your parent's condition and progress is continuously monitored, so be sure to ask about care documentation. Ask if the agency is willing to work with you to develop a personalized tracking sheet that the caregiver will submit to both you and the agency. As with a private caregiver, you must be scrupulous in overseeing the relationship that develops between your parent and the caregiver. Accountability will always be an issue, regardless of who becomes your parent's caregiver.

LIVE-IN COMPANIONS

Another alternative merits a brief mention. In many cities throughout the United States, senior service agencies are setting up programs designed to match seniors with rent-paying roommates, other adults who need a place to stay. If your parent doesn't need hands-on care, but could use companionship or maybe just another person to keep an eye on things, this might be a solution worth investigating. The agencies that sponsor such programs carefully screen potential roommates. Each arrangement is tailored to fit the needs of both the homeowner and the roommate, with roommates often providing services such as shopping and light housekeeping in exchange for a break in rent. The average stay is two years. If you wish to investigate this program further, contact your local Aging and Independence Services to find out if it is available in your area.

A final word: Don't feel overwhelmed by the task of finding a caregiver for your parent. I've given you a lot of information here, and you might be thinking that it's a task too daunting for you. The reason I've given you so much advice is that it's important for you to dot all your i's and cross all your t's. The task is really not that much different from finding a nanny or a baby-sitter for a child. Once the initial work of hiring is out of the way, your success will depend only on your being ever watchful and vigilant, a task that should be relatively easy if you follow the accountability steps I've given you.

CHAPTER 9

Worst Fears Realized

I thought we had been making some progress in distancing Dad from Grace, only to find that, under our very noses, she and her brood, undoubtedly including the good minister, had waltzed into the hospital and had a little tête-à-tête with their favorite mark.

I had visions of Dad, Grace, and her children in the hospital conference room joining hands in prayer, led by the minister, who would thank God for the safe return of Grace from China and ask Him to help Dad return to good health. After everyone was prayed out, I imagined hugs and handshakes, and maybe some tears for good measure. Then the trap would be sprung. Looking into Dad's eyes, Grace would say something about how nice it would be if Dad showed his appreciation for the church, or maybe she would just cut to the chase and tell Dad she was tapped out because of unexpected travel expenses and ask for an "advance" on her salary. Of course, Dad would be jubilant, surrounded by his new family and rejuvenated by the prayers of the minister. I could picture Dad saying, "Certainly, I would love to help out, but my checkbook is at home." As luck would have it, Grace thinks she just might have one or two of Dad's blank checks, which she carries around for him for "emergencies." My imagination was getting the better of me as I pondered the endless possibilities for Grace to take advantage of Dad.

"Can you believe this?" I asked my sister after the door to the unit closed behind us. She was as shocked as I. Once into the hallway we started analyzing what had just happened. We began to understand a little better why Dad had reacted so heatedly to my declaration that Grace was gone forever. When we learned that she had paid Dad a visit, it became clear that she obviously was not going to simply fade away. Grace had now drawn her own line in the sand, staking out her ground, and, sadly, Dad was on her side. "You have to give her credit; she is a force to be dealt with," I said to K.C. But what could we do?

We now understood the restraint Dad had exhibited. Grace was visiting him. In the past, if Dad got mad, you got out of his way. He was a person who vented his anger, and then the anger was forgotten. Today we had seen him internalize his anger for the first time in our memory. He obviously knew the score: An outburst in the conference room might mean a longer stay in the hospital. Amazingly, Dad had enough presence of mind not to do anything that might jeopardize his departure date. He understood that after getting out, he had options, whereas in the lockdown unit he had none. I wouldn't have been surprised if his remarkable restraint was the result of a conspiracy between him and Grace, which was hatched during their visit.

Perhaps the only positive outcome of our visit with Dad was the proof that, with stable meds and good meals, our father's cognitive abilities had returned, with one notable exception: He was still hung up on

Grace. Whether Dad was thinking on an even keel or even listing a little, Grace was still paramount in his thought process. Of course, since
she had reappeared to reinfect the healing wound, this was somewhat
understandable but still depressing. The old adage "out of sight is out of
mind" was not working with Dad. Grace may have been out of our
sight, but not Dad's. Unfortunately, Dad's frame of mind did not include
anger for being bilked out of thousands and thousands of dollars.

K.C. and I concluded that even if we successfully kept Grace out of
Dad's sight, she would never be out of his mind, at least not for a long
time. There were too many ways for her to get in touch with him. She
could call. We were well aware that Dad insisted on answering the telephone when it rang. She could write. Dad was adamant about going to
the mailbox to get the mail; it was sort of a treat for him. She could send
a gift by messenger, knowing that Dad always answered the door. And,
of course, she could visit. Who was going to stop Grace if she paid Dad
a visit? Her options were limited only by her creativity. We were at the
distinct disadvantage of having to come up with a plan that would effectively insulate our father from Grace.

We were frustrated beyond belief. How were we going to get this par-
asite out of our dad's system? Where was the "magic bullet" we so desperately needed? We sat in the car and talked through our possible legal
options: A criminal complaint was out of the question because Dad
would not testify against Grace. Neither a civil complaint nor an injunc-
tion forbidding Grace from having contact with Dad would work
because Dad would not testify in support of such a measure. We could
not get control of Dad or his estate through a guardianship procedure,
because legally he was not a harm to himself or others. We were stuck,
left to our own resources. In the absence of Dad's support, the law was
absolutely no help.

Then I had a flash of inspiration. "Why don't I take Dad to Maryland to live with me? Maybe putting some serious distance between the principals would help."

"That won't work, Ed," K.C. said softly. "If Dad won't consider living in Mountain View, he most assuredly will not go to Maryland to live. Also, it would be impossible to get Dad to Maryland even on the pretext of a short visit with your family."

She was right. Dad did not fly anymore because airplane trips caused his feet to swell and hurt him for several days. So an airplane trip was out of the question.

It was painfully clear that the burden of keeping things running smoothly at Dad's house was going to fall on K.C. She would be responsible for doing everything humanly possible to keep Grace away from him. All I could do was reassure her that I would be available by telephone for anything I could do from a distance.

K.C. reminded me of one thing she could do immediately: call Dr. Weaver. Using her cell phone, she left a detailed message about Grace visiting Dad in the hospital, and she asked that Dr. Weaver issue two orders: one prohibiting Dad from having phone contact with anyone except his children, and the second order prohibiting Dad from having any visitors at the hospital except his children. She closed by saying she hoped Doctor Weaver could issue the orders immediately.

I then called my lawyer friend in San Diego and left a message requesting his suggestions about what could be done to insulate Dad from Grace, considering Dad's probable refusal to testify against her. I wasn't optimistic he would come up with anything, but I felt better asking an expert's opinion on the subject.

K.C. then called the agency that had recommended Jane Buchanan. She told the agency representative that, commencing tomorrow morning, our father would need twenty-four-hour care at the house and requested that Jane be assigned to care for Dad if she was still available. She also asked that each caregiver be given written instructions that Grace and all members of her family were not to have contact with Dad—no phone contact, no personal contact, absolutely no contact at all. After hanging up, K.C. said, "Well, the agency didn't blanch at the request, so maybe we can get around the law for a while, and keep Grace away from Dad." We knew her request to the agency was probably futile if push came to shove with Dad, but at least they were willing to make some effort to help us.

Dr. Weaver could issue orders prohibiting contact with Grace, which could be justified as necessary for Dad's medical care. However, once Dad was discharged, we were once again up against the "harm to self or harm to others" standard, which meant that Dad was in sole control if he chose to flex his muscles. I doubted that anyone could legally restrict Dad's visitors once he got home.

Finally, K.C. called the bank. Her favorite branch manager was in, so she asked her to put a hold on any of Dad's checks that were presented to the bank made out to Grace or cash. The banker seemed amenable to cooperating after K.C. filled her in on some of the events with Grace since her "return from China." After K.C. hung up, she said the banker was very willing to help out because she thought the world of Dad.

I realized that my work in San Diego had come to an end. I had done all I could. It was time for me to go home. K.C. agreed. I had checked with the airline earlier, and learned that a flight to Dulles Airport was leaving in about two hours. I called from the car and was able to reserve a seat. So K.C. and I headed straight to the airport after she graciously offered to drop me off, return my rental car, and take a taxi home.

As we were driving to the airport, my heart felt heavy. I kept thinking about my final words with my father, which brought fresh tears to my eyes. Also, I was leaving my sister with an awesome responsibility. Single-handedly, she had to take on the parenting responsibility for our father. Of course, I would always be available to help her, but I would be 3,000 miles away. She was the front line in ensuring that Dad got good care and was isolated from Grace. Since the law was no help to us, K.C. was the only defense we had. I felt sad about not being able to help her more.

Both K.C. and I got out of the car at the airport so that she could switch to the driver's seat. I wrapped her in a bear hug, and we simultaneously said how much we loved each other. As I walked away toward the ticket counter, I realized that the situation with our father had forged an incredibly strong bond between us—one that would never be broken.

It seemed like an eternity since I had been strapped into an airplane seat, even though I had arrived in San Diego only a few days earlier. As the plane gained altitude, I thought of an expression my father had used often: "The sun will always rise in the east and set in the west, no matter the problem." Dad was right. Life would go on, but I wondered, when the next day dawned, what would life hold for my father and his children?

K.C. and I had accomplished a lot during my time in San Diego, although not as much as I had hoped when I had boarded the airplane at Dulles. We had stopped Grace from getting all of Dad's assets, we had fired Grace, we had hired new caregivers, we had gotten Dad's meds stabilized and gotten him back on a healthy diet. We had even found a lovely place for Dad to stay at Mountain View, should Dad ever decide he could accept such a move. We had accomplished a lot, but I knew an awful lot of work was left undone.

Our obvious failure was that Grace was still lurking around essentially unrestrained and able to strike at a time and place of her choosing. I couldn't get over her brazenness in visiting Dad in the hospital.

What was her agenda now? What did she hope to accomplish by these contacts? Was she still targeting the big payoff, hoping Dad would turn over all of his assets to her? These were troubling questions, and the answers eluded me.

Most troubling of all was the inability of the law to help. The "harm to self or harm to others" standard was simply out of touch with the realities of modern-day life. I had never before realized how vulnerable a single, aged parent is to influence by a caregiver. I had heard stories from clients about caregivers taking pocketbooks, jewelry, and loose cash from the aged. But I had always believed that the law was the ultimate deterrent to this petty theft. I was wrong, decidedly wrong. The law was of no help, whether the theft was small or large, unless the victim was willing to stand up and testify.

The second shortcoming of the law is its failure to recognize that, over time, the parent actually can fall in love with the caregiver, as seemed to be the case with my father. When such a bond is forged between the parent and the caregiver, it is not broken easily. Certainly, the parent is unwilling to do anything to break up the relationship. It makes sense that the parent would do nothing to upset the friendship the caregiver has deliberately nurtured. When a caregiver is with the parent day in and day out, it is unrealistic to think that they would not become extremely close. I now realized, all too clearly, that K.C. and I were really powerless to stop our father if he chose to live his life with Grace, so as long as he was marginally competent. This was a frightening prospect.

The next few weeks brought a series of intense mood swings. I was happy to be back at work because work was a distraction, albeit temporary, from thoughts about my father. In California, things started off well. K.C. reported that Dad seemed to be getting along with his new caregivers. They were attending to his needs, making sure that he was taking his meds and serving him good, wholesome food; however, he was eating only liquid food because of the problem with his esophagus, which made it difficult for him to swallow. Apparently, when Dad swallowed his food, it had a tendency to go to his lungs rather than his stomach. This was one of the reasons he had a weak appetite. Dad's doctors suggested surgery to correct the problem which was scheduled for the following week.

The swallowing problem notwithstanding, Dad seemed to be doing fine. K.C. was "on watch" at the house at least twice a day and called often to speak with Dad and the caregivers. Dad seemed happy and all was well. His doctors were satisfied with his improving health.

Then, things started unraveling. One of the caregivers caught Dad speaking on the phone with Grace late one night. When he tried to intercede to stop the conversation, a shouting match ensued, and the caregiver threatened to leave. The caregiver called K.C. in the middle of the night, and K.C. went to the house to make peace. K.C. said she felt like a diplomat, shuttling between the caregiver holed up in the kitchen and Dad in the family room, trying to get everything back on an even keel. Dad insisted that he could speak to whomever he wanted, whenever he wanted. K.C. glossed over the conflict, suggesting that they discuss it the next day, when everyone would be in a better mood. The caregiver was still on the job when K.C. left, but she knew the fragile peace she had negotiated was not going to last long.

K.C. telephoned me and asked, "What should I do?"

I didn't have any answers, other than, "Just tell the caregiver to follow your instructions to keep Dad from having contact with Grace, and hope for the best." It was a weak offering, but it was all I had.

The end of our drama began a few days later when the caregiver caught Dad packing his suitcase. He wouldn't say where he was going, just that someone was coming by to pick him up for a short drive. The two got into a shoving match when the caregiver tried to take the suitcase from Dad. In anger, Dad slapped the caregiver, who was not injured but was very upset. The caregiver called the police and ultimately walked off the job as soon as K.C. arrived. K.C. stayed with Dad. She assumed that he was planning his escape with Grace, although Dad refused to say where he was going or with whom. Whoever was going to pick him up was probably scared off by the police car parked in the driveway. Turn View Drive was becoming a high-crime area on the police blotter.

Given my Dad's combative behavior during this incident, which was well documented by the police report, Dr. Weaver once again admitted him to the hospital for observation. At that point, Dad dug in his heels. He refused to take his meds and resisted all forms of nourishment. Also, because his swallowing problem had gotten worse, Dr. French recommended that a stomach tube be inserted to feed Dad until he got stronger. Dad was angry and rebellious, stating adamantly that he didn't want a tube. He simply wanted to go home to the place he loved and be left alone, without anyone looking over his shoulder telling him what to do. He wanted peace and quiet and an end to this horrible nightmare.

After the tube was inserted into his stomach, a procedure that required minor surgery, Dad became even more hostile and immediately pulled the tube out. The tube was reinserted and Dad pulled it out again. Finally, the tube went back in and Dad was restrained so it would stay in place. K.C. and I were horrified by the use of restraints, but there seemed no other way to get nourishment into Dad.

After a few days of feeding Dad via tube, while he was tied to a hospital bed, Dr. Weaver informed K.C. that Dad could not stay at the hospital much longer, because his medical condition didn't require a hospital's level of care. Essentially, he wanted her to know that Dad had to leave, and soon. Now we were really in a bind. It was obvious that Dad could not go home, because he would pull out the feeding tube or become combative with the caregivers, who were not trained to care for someone who was willing to throw his fists around.

When sedated, Dad was out of it, talking in incomprehensible blabber. Continued sedation wasn't good for him, physically or mentally, according to his doctors. But when the sedatives were reduced, the combative man emerged. During the times Dad was coherent, he begged K.C. to let him go home and live his own life. So simple a wish from a man who deserved to live the rest of his life in peace—however, going home was simply not possible for someone in his condition.

K.C. told me how painful it was to see our father, literally tied down to his bed, fighting his restraints or floating in the ozone layer from strong drugs. I could not imagine the guilt K.C. must have felt telling Dad that going home wasn't possible until he got better. Dad needed to go where he could get a higher level of care then she or home caregivers were able to provide. K.C. had to deliver this message, without my help, to a person who had always been there for her, regardless of the circumstances. My heart ached for her. I knew this ordeal was taking a severe toll on K.C.

I was upset about our father's rapid deterioration, as well. He was sick, and all I wanted was for him to get well. This was my goal, but each day it seemed to get further and further away. K.C.'s twice-daily reports confirmed that Dad's condition was becoming progressively worse.

Since Dad was being discharged from the hospital with a tube sewed into his stomach, our only choice was to put him in a nursing home. We could no longer consider a residential, hotel-type environment like the one we had seen at Mountain View. After talking with several nursing homes, K.C. discovered only a limited number of homes willing to take a combative person with a feeding tube. Fortunately, K.C. found one that met Dad's needs and had an available bed.

We knew we had no choice, but still we agonized over this decision because of Dad's strong opposition to nursing homes. But what else could we do? We simply could not arrange for him to receive the care he needed at home.

It was with a heavy heart that K.C. made arrangements to have Dad admitted to a nursing home. He was transported by ambulance. From the start, it was a terrible experience for everyone. As he was wheeled into the nursing home on a gurney, it was as if a big red button had been pushed inside Dad's head. This was the place Dad feared most, the place he dreaded both in his dreams and during his every waking moment as the worst kind of torture imaginable. Over the years, he had repeatedly made K.C. and me promise never to put him into a nursing home. Now he was being wheeled, flat on his back and held down by restraints, into the worst place he could imagine, the hell of hells. Dad was unwilling to accept that this nursing home was radically different from those he had regularly visited in the 1950s and 1960s. K.C. spent a lot of time talking to him about the differences, but it didn't matter. This was a nursing home. This was the place he feared most.

K.C. and Jane Buchanan were with Dad when he was admitted. Jane had been one of his caregivers during the short time at home between his stay in the lockdown unit and his return to the hospital. We reasoned that Jane should continue staying with Dad, even though the nursing home had ample nurses and aides. We wanted Dad always to have a familiar person nearby when K.C. could not be with him. When Jane was not at Dad's side, K.C. had arranged for one of the other caregivers who had attended to Dad at the house to be with him.

Despite our best intentions for his welfare, it was obvious that Dad was not going to stay in the nursing home for long. K.C. described how he was deteriorating virtually in front of her eyes. Paradoxically, he was obviously getting weaker, but at the same time his resolve to fight was getting stronger. All he wanted was to go home and see Grace. Time after time, even in a stupor, he asked for Grace. "Where is Grace? Have you heard from Grace? When is Grace coming?" He was either begging K.C. to let him go home or wanting to know when Grace was coming to see him. Painfully, K.C. had to tell him that Grace was not coming to see him ever again.

Dad was doing everything possible to make things difficult for himself at the nursing home. His anger with K.C. and me was unabated. His beloved children had broken their blood oath to him, and he was tormented by his surroundings. Despite the best care that money could buy, he wanted out, even if the only way out was to end his life.

Two days after Dad was admitted to the nursing home, I was in the conference room, talking to a client, when there was a knock on the door. My legal assistant had come to tell me that my wife was on the telephone. Pamela said it was urgent and asked that I be interrupted. I excused myself from the meeting and walked to my office with my legs trembling. I knew that my wife would not have good news.

"Hi, dear," I said into the telephone.

"Hi," she responded, and then after a long pause, "It's over."

"Oh, God, are you sure?"

"Yes, your sister just called."

I couldn't speak further. I had to get home to confront this terrible news. My heart was broken; I started to weep. Dad had lived in the nursing home, the place he feared most, for less than forty-eight hours.

Depression and Loneliness in Your Parent: What You Can Do

As I reflected on the final weeks of my father's life, I realized that he undoubtedly had been suffering from depression, probably for quite some time. Depression can occur at any age, but it is becoming increasingly common among our older population. According to the National Institute of Mental Health, approximately 2 million adults over the age of 65 have diagnosable depression (Narrow, 1998). The reasons for these large numbers should not be surprising. Elderly people, especially those who live into their eighties and nineties, frequently experience great losses during their lives. My father was no exception. As my father did, elderly people lose their spouses and friends; oftentimes their children live far away. Frequently they suffer physical changes that limit their mobility and reduce the activities they once enjoyed. Older people often feel socially isolated and have difficulty adapting to the changes in their lives, changes that can easily trigger the onset of depression. Often, too, a biochemical change in the brain causes depression.

Another loss often experienced by older people—less tangible but just as real—is the sense that they have lost their place in society. Throughout their lives your parents were focused on being productive. They worked hard, they enjoyed their families and friends, and they looked forward to the day they could retire. However, unless they made a conscious effort to extend their productivity or level of activity into retirement years, it shouldn't be surprising that they might begin to feel irrelevant. Many older people feel as though society does not value them and that younger people view them with disdain. Although this perception is changing—believe me, we baby boomers demand attention—the feelings of being discarded have some merit.

Couple this sense of devalued self-worth with the losses of loved ones and health problems, and you've painted a picture of a person who has a greatly increased propensity to be depressed. Further complicating the problem is that depression sometimes can be misinterpreted as dementia because some of the behaviors are similar. Diagnosis of depression can be even more difficult because many of the symptoms—such as loss of appetite and trouble sleeping—are considered part of the normal aging process. As a result, depression in the aged is often not diagnosed, and therefore it is frequently undertreated.

HOW TO SPOT DEPRESSION

If your parent is exhibiting behavioral changes that don't seem to be related to a medical condition, consider that depression might be the culprit. If you think your parent may be experiencing the onset of dementia, it's particularly important to rule out depression. Depression is absolutely treatable, whereas treatment for dementia is far less successful (see chapter 3). If three or more of the following signs persist for longer than two weeks, it is a clear sign that your parent may be depressed.

•Feelings of sadness or worthlessness

•Loss of enthusiasm for daily activities that were once pleasurable

•Excessive concern about body aches and pains

•Difficulty sleeping

•Weight loss or decreased appetite

•Feeling fatigued even though rest is adequate

•Memory loss

•Feelings of agitation or restlessness

•Diminished ability to think or concentrate

•Expressing thoughts about death or suicide

The difficulty of detecting depression is compounded by the fact that older people are often reluctant to admit to feeling depressed because of pride. Furthermore, physicians sometimes don't think to ask their older patients if they are depressed. If you suspect your parent might be suffering from depression, a conversation with the doctor might spur him or her to discuss the symptoms you observed with your parent. It's often easier for parents to speak frankly with their doctors than with family members about such delicate, personal issues.

You should also consider that your parent could have an undiagnosed medical condition that is causing depression. If your parent is showing signs of depression, the first course of action should be a thorough check-up. A blood test can pinpoint any problems your parent might be having with thyroid, liver, or kidney function. Oftentimes the treatment or alleviation of a medical problem can go a long way in helping to reduce depression.

Once depression is diagnosed, it can be alleviated in a number of ways. Many mental health professionals, including psychiatrists, psychologists, and clinical social workers, are now specializing in geriatric mental health. They have a unique understanding of the challenges facing the elderly and can prescribe therapeutic treatment that can be remarkably successful.

COUNSELING AND MEDICATION

If your parent is suffering from depression, enlist the aid of a mental health professional. This may be a difficult task because your parent may be of a generation that attached great stigma to mental health problems. Even though that stigma has been greatly diminished in modern society, it might be a tough sell to convince your parent that a visit to a "shrink" might be in order. A recommendation by your parent's doctor would probably be better received than one coming from you.

Aging parents tend to have a healthy respect for their physicians. If a doctor tells your parent to see another doctor (in this case, a mental health professional), you might not see the same level of protest that you would if the suggestion was yours. Of course, you'll have to recruit your parent's doctor as an accomplice, but that shouldn't be difficult if the doctor agrees that treatment for depression is necessary.

Just as my father had a morbid fear of nursing homes, many older people harbor a misperception of the work done by mental health professionals. They still cling to the notion that treatment routinely consists of powerful, mind-altering drugs, or extreme procedures like lobotomies and electroshock therapy. Research has produced quantum changes in mental health treatments, and the drugs used today add to quality of life rather than take away from it. The treatment prescribed for your parent will, of course, depend on the cause and severity of the depression and how much it is adversely affecting your parent's life.

A mental health professional will perform a thorough evaluation of your parent's condition before deciding on a course of treatment. Sometimes a short-term program of talk therapy will be sufficient to guide your parent back to a happy and fulfilling life. Occasionally medication will be prescribed to work as a mood elevator or an antidepressant. Often, mental health professionals will advise a combination of therapy and medication.

Even if your parent is amenable to seeing a mental health professional, the prospect of taking medication for depression can be frightening, given the powerful drugs that used to be commonly prescribed. It's helpful for older people to learn that the new generation of medications is entirely different. Understanding some rudimentary biology of the brain might help your parent be more receptive to the prospect of taking medication.

Researchers have discovered that the brain contains chemicals called neurotransmitters, and if the level of these neurotransmitters gets too low, people can feel depressed. Today's medications simply elevate the neurotransmitter levels back to normal, thus eliminating the depression. You've probably heard of some of the more common medications, drugs such as Paxil, Prozac, and Zoloft. There are many others, and if it is determined that medication might be helpful to your parent, the doctor will prescribe the one that seems best suited to your parent's needs. Initial dosages for the elderly are usually lower than those prescribed for other adults, and modifications in dosage are made at a slower rate. Sometimes it takes a while to get the dosage right, and often one medication will be abandoned in favor of another. Even if it takes some time to find the right medication and get the dosage right, the good news is that this new generation of drugs is remarkably effective and produces relatively few side effects. Persuading your parent to try medication, if that is what the doctor recommends, will be well worth the effort.

MENTAL HEALTH CARE PROFESSIONALS

People often express confusion about the differences between mental health professionals. What makes a psychiatrist different from a psychologist? And how can a clinical social worker be an appropriate person to treat mental health issues? Should your parent need the services of such a professional, how do you determine which professional is best for your parent's situation? The following is a brief description of the various mental health professionals you will most commonly encounter.

Psychiatrist

A psychiatrist is a fully licensed medical doctor who has completed four years of residency training in psychiatry in addition to graduating from medical school. Psychiatrists are the only mental health professionals who can prescribe medication and order medical tests, although there is an effort underway to give psychologists the ability to prescribe medication under certain circumstances. In recent years, psychiatrists have moved away from therapeutic counseling and have focused more on the biological and scientific aspects of mental illness. Although many psychiatrists still engage their patients in talk therapy, most one-on-one counseling has been shifted to psychologists and licensed clinical social workers.

Psychologist

A psychologist has undertaken an intensive educational program in the behavioral sciences. Some states require clinical psychologists to have a Ph.D. or a Psy.D. (doctor of psychology) in order to practice as psychologists; others require only a master's degree. All states, however, require testing and licensing of psychologists, and they must follow a strict code of ethics. Psychologists treat mental, behavioral, and emotional disorders using psychological principles. They also conduct psychological testing, using a wide array of tests that have been refined through the years to spot problem areas that people sometimes have trouble articulating. Although psychologists cannot currently prescribe medications, most work in conjunction with psychiatrists or other medical doctors to provide a combined treatment program for patients (or "clients" as they are more commonly called today).

Licensed Clinical Social Worker (LCSW)

An LCSW is trained in psychotherapy and usually has a master's degree. These professionals help individuals learn to manage a variety of mental health problems with the goal of improving overall daily life. Although it may sound odd to consider a clinical social worker as someone to turn to for mental health care, LCSWs are well trained in cognitive and behavioral therapies. Like psychologists, they often work with psychiatrists or other medical doctors if medication is deemed part of an appropriate treatment plan.

Finding a Mental Health Professional

Selecting a mental health professional for your parent should be done with care. Your search should follow the same methodology you would use to find a physician specialist. In other words, if your parent is diagnosed with cancer, you would look for an oncologist, not a general practitioner. So if your parent is depressed, you should find a mental health professional who specializes in depression. Even better, the ideal candidate would specialize in geriatric mental health as well as depression.

The trickier issue is deciding between a psychiatrist, psychologist, or LCSW. Psychiatrists can prescribe medication, but they often don't engage in cognitive or behavioral therapy. Psychologists and LCSWs have a broad spectrum of cognitive and behavioral tools to help guide your parent back to a happy and satisfying life. If medication is recommended, a psychiatrist or another doctor would have to be brought into the treatment plan, which requires additional doctors' visits. Fortunately, in some instances, a psychologist will consult with your parent's primary physician, who will prescribe the recommended medication, and then both will monitor your parent's progress, watching for any side effects and adaptation to the medication.

Recommendations and referrals can come from a number of different sources. Psychiatrists, psychologists, and LCSWs all have professional organizations with chapters in every state and most major cities. As a service to the public, these organizations will provide you with referrals to licensed professionals with a specialty in specific disorders. If you live in a town or city that does not have a local chapter of one of these organizations, you can contact one of the national groups listed below, which will help you find the appropriate state or regional chapter that can provide you with a referral.

American Association for Geriatric Psychiatry
www.aagponline.org
(301) 654-7850

American Psychiatric Association
www.psych.org
(703) 907-7300

American Psychological Association
www.apa.org
(800) 964-2000

National Association for Social Workers
www.naswdc.org
(202) 408-8600

WHAT YOU CAN DO TO HELP

There are many things you can do to help a depressed parent. Often depression can be mitigated by social intervention—involving your parent in group outings or volunteer work to lessen the feelings of isolation and loneliness and increase their feeling of self-worth. Here are some suggestions:

Community Connections. I have often suggested to my retired business clients that they go out into the community and offer their services to help people who are starting up companies. Giving helpful solutions to an entrepreneur is great for the ego, and everyone benefits from the experience. One nationwide group that specializes in matching retirees with new businesses is called SCORE, an organization that partners with the Small Business Administration to provide counsel and advice to people starting up businesses. The years of expertise and knowledge provided by senior citizens participating in the SCORE program are highly valued by these entrepreneurs.

This is just one example of a volunteer opportunity. There are countless others. The change in a retiree's outlook on life when he or she has an opportunity to perform a community service is truly amazing. I'm certain that if I had been able to persuade Dad to get involved with an organization such as SCORE, his outlook on life would have been more positive. I suggested it from time to time, and he always said, "I'll think about it," which I knew meant the discussion was closed. Sometimes you have to be crafty to give parents the necessary push to get out and get involved. You might have to literally lead them by the hand to an opportunity you think they would enjoy, but it's worth it if they connect.

Most senior centers have loads of information about volunteer and social opportunities, and the range is almost endless. I know of a group of senior women who get together once a week to knit blankets for underprivileged babies. They not only provide a needed service, but they also enjoy the social interaction. Another group of seniors hosts a weekly "philosophy" discussion at a local coffee house that is open to all who are interested. I don't know how many weighty philosophical topics are actually discussed, but the attendees truly love the chance to get together with others of their age and experience.

Keep in mind that simply encouraging your parent to get involved may not be enough. If your parent is indeed even mildly depressed, don't expect the necessary enthusiasm to materialize simply because you've thought of something that might be appealing. Scout out several activities or volunteer opportunities you think your parent might enjoy. Plan to accompany your parent, or enlist the aid of another active senior who would be willing to act as a "buddy" until your parent reaches a comfort level with a new group. Be persistent. The end result will be worth it.

Religious Connections. Encourage your loved ones to maintain contact with their religion or religious institution. I strongly believe that older adults with a lifelong tradition of involvement with a church, temple, or synagogue need that spiritual nourishment, even when frailty prevents them from attending services. For many years congregations around the country have been developing programs to reach out to homebound elders and their caregivers (Powers, 1996). One church I know of has organized a regular visitation program. Once a week, after services, they visit the homebound. These volunteers share thoughts and inspirations from the weekly sermon and spend time socializing, as well. This opportunity for renewed connection with God and others in their religious community can provide much help in alleviating depression.

Outreach Programs. Most religious organizations, senior centers, and eldercare agencies have outreach programs for the elderly, which include socials, field trips, and regularly scheduled telephone calls. The goal is contact and social interaction. Even if your parent is housebound, outreach programs exist that can connect your parent with others. Regular visits, even by someone who is not a family member or a caregiver, can open the door once more to the outside world.

Pet Therapy. Pet therapy has proven to be amazingly successful with the elderly. Volunteers bring specially trained pets to nursing homes and sometimes for home visits, too, and the animals lavish love and affection on the objects of their attention. Check with your local humane society or animal shelter to see if such a program is available in your area. Remember, if your parent lives alone, he or she probably does not get to enjoy the sensation of touching very often. The hugs, kisses, and affectionate touching that once may have been a big part of your parent's daily life may now be woefully insufficient. No matter how old they are, most people crave the sensation of physical contact. Animals are a wonderful outlet to help satisfy this need. Who can resist a soft, fuzzy cat purring away in your lap? Or a dog licking a hand in gratitude for an affectionate head scratch?

PRACTICAL ADVICE FOR THE CAREGIVER

It isn't easy being around a depressed person. However, there are some steps you can take to help a depressed parent, and you can become a valuable ally in the journey back to mental health. First and foremost, it's important to remember that depression is an illness, not a voluntary state. Your parent doesn't want to be depressed and may well have no control over the illness, especially if the depression is a result of a biochemical imbalance in the brain. It's equally important for you to understand that chronic or long-term depression rarely goes away without treatment. Don't think that you alone can rescue your parent from the blues without professional help. However, you can certainly be a strong advocate for your parent. The following suggestions might be helpful to you if you're dealing with a depressed parent. Remember, though, that these suggestions are not a substitute for professional help; rather, they are tools for you to employ to help your parent throughout the recovery process.

1. **Recognize and acknowledge the symptoms of depression.** Your parent's behavior may be extremely frustrating for you. You might think that if only your parent would make an effort to do something positive, or make an attitude change, then depression wouldn't be an issue. Acknowledge that inertia is a symptom of depression. Your parent doesn't want to be depressed, but you must accept that he or she probably doesn't have the power to rise above it alone, no matter how much encouragement you provide. Don't nag your parent to get out of the house, or just do something, or snap out of it. Depression is a disabling disorder that can sap both energy and will. No amount of cajoling on your part is going to change that. Your empathy and understanding are critical.

2. **Allow your parent to talk or cry.** To you, it might sound as if your parent is engaging in a bad case of "Woe is me." For your parent, having someone to simply lend a sympathetic ear, without judgment or criticism, can be a loving reminder that you truly care and want your parent to feel better. Ideally, exposing such emotion is most productive when done with a therapist because professionals know how to direct such thinking into positive outcomes. Still, your parent wants to be reassured that you care enough to listen, even if you don't have any answers.

3. **To the extent you can, help your parent to be active.** Plan a movie date. Arrange a lunch or dinner with a friend or two. Go for a drive. It is unlikely your parent will plan activities and outings while feeling depressed, so do it yourself. Make short-term plans that are doable for your parent. A daylong shopping trip might be too much, but a short drive to the beach to watch the seagulls for half an hour might be perfect. An hour or two away from the house won't cure depression, but sometimes a change of scenery can provide a welcome respite. In the long run, activity is essential to conquering depression, so it's helpful for you to set the pattern and, with luck, increase the level of activity as your parent progresses.

4. **Make humor a daily part of your parent's life.** It's hard to be sad or depressed when you're laughing. Collect funny jokes or cartoons that you know your parent will enjoy. Relive humorous moments from when you were growing up. Watch old comedies on television with your parent, or rent a funny movie. Again, although laughter is wonderfully therapeutic, don't think of it as a cure-all.

5. **Try to counter black-and-white thinking.** Does your parent say things like "I'll never be happy again?" Or, "Bad things always happen to me?" It's very difficult to effectively use logic and reason with a person who is depressed, but if you counter with a combination of acknowledgment and hope, you might help stem the tide of negative thinking. For example, you could say, "Yes, I understand you're very unhappy right now, but I believe you will be happy again one day soon." Or, "Yes, you're experiencing a very bad time right now, but I have hope that good things will soon come your way."

SENIOR CENTERS

As I said earlier, activity is a key factor in mitigating loneliness and depression. One of the best places to find continual activity geared toward seniors is at your local senior center. Most neighborhoods have active senior centers, but many elderly people do not take advantage of them, probably because they aren't aware of how much these centers have to offer. Your parent's neighborhood senior center can provide a critical lifeline to the rest of the world, providing services and social opportunities for virtually every need and interest.

Senior centers are usually funded by local Aging and Independence Service agencies, and the staff members are specially trained in issues affecting the elderly. Following a national trend, most senior center organizations are beginning to use the name Multipurpose Senior Centers (MSCs) to describe the all-inclusiveness of the services provided.

The challenge, of course, is convincing your parent that a senior center is more than just a place to play bingo and get a free lunch. Centers typically offer nutritious meals, social activities, and a range of programs such as health screenings, creative arts, exercise, and special events unique to individual centers. Even beyond meals and social activities, MSC staffers can be powerful advocates in addressing the specific needs of your parent. The following is a list of senior issues for which centers can offer guidance, advice and referrals:

•**Health and mental health,** including assessments and health screening, medical services, depression screening, Social Security and Medicare information, Alzheimer's Association, suicide intervention, support groups, low-vision clinics, deaf and disabled services

- **Assistance to remain independent,** including in-home care services, housekeeping, companionship, day care, and telephone calls

- **Food,** including nutrition centers, food stamps, and Meals-on-Wheels

- **Transportation,** including medical appointments, activities, escort programs, lift-van programs, public transportation passes, and taxi coupons

- **Personal security,** including home security checks, lock repair, installation of grab bars and handrails

- **Legal services and public advocacy,** including legal assistance, tenants' rights advocacy, health insurance counseling, and dispute resolution

- **Housing,** including alternative living arrangements, low-income and subsidized housing, retirement homes, assisted-living facilities, and nursing homes.

As you can see, an MSC can be a starting point for nearly every issue I have addressed in these pages. But even if your parent has no special needs other than social interaction, the local senior center can provide the spark of interest that returns your parent to an active, involved life.

There certainly is a problem of perception, though. Many elderly people are reluctant to go to senior centers because of a mistaken belief that they are for "poor" people who can't afford to buy their own food. Take a look inside any senior center, however, and you'll probably find a vibrant, noisy place, filled with people laughing, sharing meals, exercising, working on computers, taking classes, dancing, listening to lectures, and countless other activities. Organized groups take full advantage of senior centers, and you'll find everything from the local Kiwanis to arts and crafts associations, and from Alcoholics Anonymous to book discussion groups.

Visit the senior center in your parent's neighborhood to find out what it has to offer that would be of interest to your parent. Gather as much information as you can to help tempt your parent to participate. If you find a few activities or services your parent would be interested in, accompany him or her the first few times. You'll probably find that your presence will quickly become unnecessary (and maybe even unwanted!). The benefit to you is the knowledge that your parent has a contact with the outside world, one that will provide pleasure as well as assistance.

Many centers, particularly those in large cities, are developing outreach programs for people who are housebound. The goal is to provide a sense of connectedness to the rest of the world that isolated seniors so often feel, as well as to make sure needs are being met. If you are a long-distance caregiver, the senior center in your parent's neighborhood could become your strongest ally in monitoring your parent.

DIAL 211: ACCESS TO HEALTH AND HUMAN SERVICES

In July 2000, the Federal Communications Commission reserved the telephone number 211 for a nationwide service to provide callers with health and human services information and referrals. Among the participating members of this service are the National Association of Area Agencies on Aging and the National Mental Health Association (NMHA). As of early 2003 the service was already operating in twenty states, serving more than 51 million people. The remaining thirty states are in either the planning or the implementation stage.

This valuable service offers referrals for all the eldercare services I have mentioned in every chapter of this book, including referrals for mental health care. As you have undoubtedly noticed, throughout these pages I have advised you to contact various agencies, associations, and volunteer organizations to find the information you need. When 211 is activated in all 50 states, it promises to provide a one-stop referral source to help you find services for your elderly parent. If, for example, you're seeking a mental health professional for your parent, calling 211 would be your natural starting point.

It's significant that the National Mental Health Association is one of the founding members of the coalition to implement 211. The NMHA's participation demonstrates the clear need for reliable information about mental health issues.

Dealing with a depressed person can seem like a thankless task. But if your parent is also getting help from a mental health professional, the extra steps you take to aid and encourage recovery will pay off enormously. Again, I must stress that you should not try to go it alone. Depression is a physical disorder, and if it is long term, your parent needs professional intervention.

Think of all the possible physical conditions that can disable an aging person. Then think about depression and understand that it alone has more power to disable than any other physical disorder. Showing compassion and helping your parent get the necessary treatment for depression can make all the difference in his or her quality of life.

Some Final Thoughts

*M*y father was laid to rest on June 12, 1996.

When I delivered his eulogy, the most important quality about my father that I wanted to convey was his capacity for love. I can't ever remember hanging up the telephone without us saying "I love you" to each other. And I know we both said it because we meant it. Dad taught me the importance of love. Whenever we were together we would greet each other with a hug and a kiss on the cheek. I loved him for the wonderful things he did to mold my personality. I loved him for the way he took care of and stayed strong for my mother who was ill for so many years.

Dad loved people and people loved him. He truly had the ability to walk with kings but keep the common touch. He taught me how important it is to learn about life from everyone I meet. His many lessons continue to guide me, and I have tried to teach them to my children.

The expression "Time heals all wounds" is actually an inappropriate description of what has happened since Dad's passing. Perhaps more appropriate is the idea that time teaches you to live with your wounds, even if they never completely heal.

Grace declared bankruptcy. In the bankruptcy petition she did not list any of the income she had received from Dad; however, she did agree to pay off the car loan, which I assume she did because I never again heard from the finance company. To this day I don't know where she is or if she has found someone else to manipulate and abuse.

When K.C., my wife, and I were cleaning out the house after Dad's death, Pamela found an unexecuted, undated, do-it-yourself will with a paper-clipped note attached from Grace stating that she would take care of Dad forever in exchange for being named his beneficiary. I do not know when the will had been presented to Dad for his consideration and signature, but it was obvious that Grace had visions of being the only heir upon Dad's demise. She came so very close to hitting it big, but she didn't quite grab the gold ring. I still believe she never got the punishment she deserved.

I never made an effort to locate the church or Grace's son, the minister, who also played a role in bilking my father. I knew I had no legal recourse against the church, so it seemed pointless to try to find it. I only hope that it has taken a new spiritual direction. I would be upset if Grace's son were still using his church ostensibly to deliver God's message while deceiving another victim with deep pockets.

I have had a difficult time since the passing of my father. Pamela and I have moved from Maryland to La Jolla, near where Dad used to have his laundry, and we are happy here. I "speak" to my father regularly from my heart. K.C. and I visit Dad and Mom at the mausoleum where they are interred. Perhaps I don't go as often as I should; however, even when not visiting I think of my family often.

The hardest part of coming to grips with Dad's death, other than the loss of someone I loved, has been dealing with several levels of guilt. The last time I saw my father was in the lockdown unit, just before I left San Diego. In addition to the distress I was feeling at that time, I also experienced a strange sensation, a feeling of power. In some perverse way, I almost enjoyed seeing my father no longer in control. The power had shifted to me, and the decisions were mine, not his. It was a strange feeling.

My father was an extremely strong-willed person. He often imposed his will on me even when I was a young married adult. The lockdown unit was the proving ground for my one and only opportunity to assume all the reins of control, and for that brief moment or two, I actually relished having power over my dad. I am sure the mental health professionals could explain the power trip I experienced. For some reason I am not yet ready for the explanation.

My biggest source of guilt, however, is not knowing whether my actions hastened Dad's death. This turmoil remains with me today. As events were unfolding during my stay in San Diego, I believed I was acting only in Dad's best interest to protect his assets and remove him from Grace's malevolent influence. In retrospect, I am not so sure if my actions truly were in his best interest. If I had let Dad give everything to Grace, perhaps she would have stayed around to take care of him. It's possible he could have returned home and Grace would have continued to care for him there, which was clearly what he wanted. In my eyes, this was improbable. Grace had proven by her actions that she was more interested in securing Dad's assets than monitoring his health and well-being.

Even assuming Grace would have taken the money and headed for the hills, without my intervention Dad would not have endured the many shocks to his system that might have hastened his demise. I think about everything that happened to Dad during the short time I was in San Diego: my unceremonious termination of Grace, his stressful encounter with the police, being committed involuntarily to the psychiatric unit of the hospital, having new caregivers forced on him, and the loss of his comfortable lifestyle at home. And then, after I left, the ultimate insult, indignity, and shock of being forced into a nursing home, the place he feared most and the place his children had promised he would never go.

I have discussed with K.C. and Pamela my guilt about how I handled my father during his time of need. Even though they say all of the right things to reassure me that my actions were in Dad's best interest, I am not sure they are right. For me, time has not tempered the guilt associated with the possibility that my actions hastened his death.

How the Law Should Change

We have come a long way. By now you have learned the many warning signs of elder abuse. Let me take a moment to step on my soap box and talk a little about the dramatic change that is needed in order to bring the law up to speed with the reality that our parents are—thankfully—living much longer.

Change in the law is absolutely necessary so adult children can protect their parents from abuse and neglect. From my experience, I acknowledge that there is no perfect solution. Also, regardless of what the law is, you can never let your guard down when it comes to protecting your parent. After all, the law is no help until there is a problem, and there cannot be a problem until you discover that your parent is the victim of abuse. This being said, however, I believe that the law must relax the harm-to-self-or-harm-to-others standard so that a child can more easily assume at least minimal control of the parent's affairs. This standard poses such an impossible hurdle to jump that, as you have seen in this story, my father's abuser was able to continue her conduct unabated because Dad was unwilling to testify against Grace.

I believe a simple facts-and-circumstances test is the only appropriate standard for these cases. A facts-and-circumstances test means that the judge would decide the issue of whether abuse is occurring or might occur based on the facts and circumstances of the case. After hearing testimony from the child who wants to take control of the parent's estate and all of his or her witnesses, and the parent and all of his or her witnesses, the judge would make a determination based on the facts and circumstances as presented by the parties. The harm-to-self-or-others standard would not apply to these cases. It would be irrelevant. Using a facts-and-circumstances test is a much more logical and simple way to conduct the law's business, and this change in the law is overdue.

I admit this is not a perfect solution. The law rarely provides perfect solutions. Some would argue that giving the child control over the parent's assets, could allow the child to abuse this position by taking lavish payments from the parent's estate. Or, on the other side of the spectrum, some might argue that the child could be so stingy with payments for the benefit of the parent that the parent would suffer.

My response is twofold. I believe that most children are basically trustworthy because of the bond between them and their parents. However, to the extent that the court believes there is the potential for abuse, an independent guardian of the parent's property could be appointed instead of the child. Alternatively, an independent guardian could be appointed as cosigner of all checks. In the capacity of cosigner, the independent guardian would be a watchdog, only cosigning checks that he or she believed were in the best interest of the parent. Second, regardless of whether the child or a guardian is appointed, the court's order should require monthly reporting in sufficient detail that the court could easily detect abuse.

I believe any adult child would think twice about taking advantage of a parent when the child knew that his or her activities were being closely monitored by the court, and that there could be severe sanctions for abuse, including incarceration. Indeed, the type of monthly reporting to the court that I envision would not only address financial issues but also include a detailed report of the parent's quality of life. This latter report would provide much of the same tracking information I have suggested you require from a caregiver (see chapter 8). With the monthly submission of both a financial report and a quality-of-life report, the judge would get a complete picture of the care being provided to the parent. Once the legal standard for appointment of a guardian is changed, the court would have great latitude to issue orders that both ensure the parent's quality of life will stay the same, if not get better, and protect the parent's assets from abuse.

A facts-and-circumstances test is clearly better then the harm-to-self-or-others standard. This is an easy fix to a difficult problem. It is my belief that the long-term effect of a facts-and-circumstances test would be a dramatic plummeting of the instances of abuse.

I have tried to move the ball forward on the adoption of a facts-and-circumstances test by talking to people of influence. Alone, however, mine is a small voice in a large ocean of voices. You can help. E-mail or write your state legislators and your local judges. Ask them to challenge the law to change. Perhaps our collective voices will be heard, and we can help our parents now and ourselves as we get older.

Conclusion

From ancient times to the middle of the twentieth century, the elders of most cultures were treated with respect that bordered on adulation. Their experience and wisdom were treasured, and their every need was met with a sense of honor and devotion. The tradition of honoring the elderly members of a population disappeared in the mid-1900s, probably because of huge changes in the way we live. During the past several decades the needs of these people have been largely ignored. Thankfully, we have emerged from that trend, and our elderly loved ones are once again beginning to receive the attention they so richly deserve.

We have built-in obstacles to meeting our aged citizens' needs, however, simply because of societal changes. We no longer have several generations of families living under the same roof, which, in the past, provided a natural caregiving environment with several family members acting as caregivers. Most seniors now live on their own or in group communities. We rejoice in the fact that scientific advances have greatly extended the average life expectancy, but these advances have also created an aged population that requires a heightened level of supervision. Fortunately, society has recognized this need and is actively addressing this problem.

As you have learned from reading these pages, neither society nor the law can single-handedly protect your parent from the growing number of opportunists who are lying in wait to take advantage of someone who lacks the savvy to recognize the more subtle forms of abuse. Thus, the responsibility falls upon you, the child, to take the necessary steps to protect your parent. Take advantage of all the good programs that are available. Be creative in your measures. Have lots of patience. Plan well. Ultimately your goal is to provide the perfect balance of protection and quality of life that your parent deserves.

References

Alzheimer's Association, "About Alzheimer's," 1 Oct 2002, www.alz.org/aboutad/ statistics.htm (retrieved 24 Oct, 2002).

Bayer, Ada-Helen and Leon Harper. "Fixing to Stay: A National Survey on Housing and Home Modification Issues." Fielded by Mathew Greenwald & Assoc. Washington, DC: AARP Research Group & AARP Programs/Applied Gerontology Group. May 2000, pp. 24-25.

Bell, Russell T., Ed. "Dementia in the elderly: Is it Alzheimer's?" *Patient Care.* Nov 1996, vol. 30:18, pp. 18-38.

Driscoll, Eileen H. *Alzheimer's: A Handbook for the Caretaker.* Wellesley, MA: Branden Publishing, 1994.

Elder Abuse Prosecution Unit, San Diego District Attorney's Office. www.daoffice.signonsandiego.com/2.html (Retrieved 11 Nov 2002).

Harney, Kenneth. "Pending settlement reveals predators." *The San Diego Union-Tribune,* 9 Feb 2003, pp. 1-13.

Heath, Angela. *Long Distance Caregiving: A Survival Guide for Far Away Caregivers.* Atascadero, CA: Impact Publishers, 1993, p. 76.

Kelly, Tom. "Seniors look to reverse mortgages for monthly income." *The San Diego Union-Tribune,* 8 Dec 2002, p. 1-13.

Kornstein, Susan G. "Dementia." *The National Women's Health Information Center,* August 2002, www.4woman.gov/faq/dementia.htm (retrieved 24 Oct 2002).

McDonald, Jeff. "Nursing home report card released." *The San Diego Union-Tribune,* 13 Nov 2002, pp. A-1, A-17.

Narrow, W.E. "One-year prevalence of depressive disorders among adults 18 and over in the U.S." NIMH ECA prospective data, 1 Jul 1998, Unpublished.

"Nursing home compare." The Official U.S. Government Site for People with Medicare. www.medicare.gov/nhcompare/home.asp (Retrieved 28 Dec 2002).

Oluwasanmi, Nkiru A. "Aging Parents' Needs." *The San Diego Union-Tribune,* 1 Dec 2002, p. H-9.

"Overview of the Medicaid Program," Centers for Medicare & Medicaid Services, 6 September 2002, http://cms.hhs.gov/Medicaid/mover.asp (retrieved 11 Dec 2002).

Powers, Marie. "Homebound Elders Still Need Spiritual Connection." *Aging Today,* Sept/Oct 1996, vol. 17:5, p. 13.

Seff, Marsha K. "Long-distance caring takes some work." *The San Diego Union-Tribune,* 31 Aug 2002, p, E-5.

——, ed., *San Diego Eldercare Directory.* San Diego: Union Tribune Publishing, 2002, p. 52.

Snyder, Edgar & Assoc. "Nursing Home Facts," Nursing Home Residents Legal Center, www.nursinghomeabuseresourcecenter.com/facts/ 2002, (Retrieved 12 Dec 2002).

Stiegel, Lori. "Abuse and Neglect of Older People," *Generations: In-Depth Views of Issues in Aging.* Summer 2000, vol. XXIV:2 p. 62.

"Three Stages of AD." *ARICEPT(r) (donepezil HC1) (Eisi Co., Ltd.),* www.aricept.com/three_stages_of_ad.htm (Retrieved 13 Nov 2002).

"What are the major types of elder abuse?" National Center on Elder Abuse, Washington, D.C. http://www.elderabusecenter.or/basic/index.html (Retrieved 28 Jan 2003).

"What Is Medicare?" Department of Health and Human Services, Centers for Medicare & Medicaid Services. www.medicare.gov/Basics/WahtIs.asp (Retrieved 11 Dec 2002).

Wheeler, Larry. "U.S. nursing homes under order to post staffing levels, but..." *Arizona Republic,* 29 Dec 2002, p. A-14. 1 272 Parents - References

Index

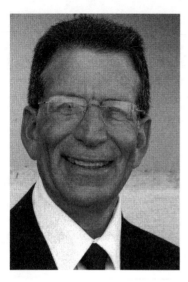

*E*dward J. Carnot has practiced law for almost thirty years. As the former managing partner of a Washington, D.C. area law firm, he has been co-lead counsel on class action lawsuits involving healthcare issues against insurance companies, some partly funded by the American Psychiatric Association and the American Medical Association. For many years he provided *pro bono* service as counselor and member of the Board of Governors of the Hebrew Home of Greater Washington, one of the largest such facilities in the country. He is a frequent speaker on techniques for protecting the elderly from abuse and asset protection strategies. Edward and his wife of 32 years, Pamela, moved to La Jolla, California in 2001, where he is a partner in the law firm of Karp Frosh Lapidus Wigodsky & Norwind, P.A. and continues to help protect the elderly from abuse.

If you have personal stories about abuse of the elderly you would like to share or want insight on problems you are having with an aging parent, Ed can be reached at *isyourparentingoodhands@juno.com.*

JENNIFER LEVINE

A NOVEL

SUMMER SECRETS

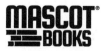

MASCOT® BOOKS

Countless people encouraged my writing over the years, all have my heartfelt love and appreciation.

Summer Secrets, my debut novel, is dedicated to Jill Carpenter. It's hard to put into words how instrumental her friendship and support have been to my development as an author. She encouraged me during my first NaNoWriMo marathon, which ultimately led to this book. Over the subsequent five years, she has always been up for conversation over coffee and "gently nudged" me to send this manuscript out. She even accompanied me on a 1200-mile road trip to find Writing Dog. Jill remains steadfast in her belief in this book which does amazing things for a writer's confidence.

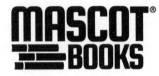

www.mascotbooks.com

Summer Secrets

For more information, please contact:
Mascot Books
560 Herndon Parkway #120
Herndon, VA 20170
info@mascotbooks.com

Library of Congress Control Number: 2016903408

CPSIA Code: PRBVG0416A
ISBN: 978-1-63177-694-6

Printed in the United States

JENNIFER LEVINE

A NOVEL

SUMMER SECRETS

CHAPTER 1

Lauren wiped away tears of rage with her sleeve. Her throat constricted as she fought the hurt, anger, and humiliation building up inside her chest. She slammed the phone down on the counter, barely registering the clatter of the battery as it fell to the floor.

As she turned off the stove-top heat and slammed various utensils into the sink, the rage settled down into her usual state of being: silent frustration. This was not the life she expected or would even tolerate. Her family was falling apart. Actually, it was being blown apart with a force greater than the Big Bang. Everyone going off in different directions with little more than a glance back at what was commonly referred to as home.

"Home," she muttered half out loud. "People spend more time in a drive-through line." Tears welled up in Lauren's eyes again as she put away the stew she'd so lovingly prepared in anticipation of a family dinner. She tossed the pot holders into the drawer and walked out of the kitchen. *Screw it,* she thought. Certainly her invisible husband wouldn't be home for hours.

Lauren fell in love with David Breckenridge the moment she laid eyes on him in college. She was in her second year, experimenting with a variety of majors but without any real direction. As clear as day, her first vision of David was there for instant recall. She hadn't expected lightning bolts as she walked back to her dorm with a few friends after astronomy class. It was mid-afternoon and freezing cold with a dusting of flurries in the air. There stood this beautiful, shirtless—albeit exceptionally stupid—boy playing football in the snow.

David was running straight for them, looking over his shoulder, stretching out his arms and leaping for the rock-hard football. It glanced off his fingertips and spiraled into a snow bank. David, now covered in snow, landed at Lauren's feet. Lauren's breath left her body as the gangly boy sat up, snowflakes clinging to his eyelashes as his intense brown eyes met hers.

"Overthrown." Such were the first words he ever said to Lauren.

"Idiot." Lauren laughed as she stepped over his legs and continued trudging through the fresh snow on her way to her dorm room. The girls laughed and ignored the taunts from the boys, but Lauren's heart was racing.

At a class reunion many years later, Lauren found out David had begged his frat brother to toss the ball in her direction. "Chams," aka Charles Allen Mooney III, was David's best friend, best man at their wedding, and godfather to the kids. She didn't believe he could have kept this secret for nearly a quarter of a century. In fact, it took many shots of tequila at the bar they used to frequent in college before the truth came spilling out as a series of challenges unfolded, and the inevitable debate continued as to whether or not the catch had been completed.

David, his memory ever so flawed, was convinced he had made a brilliant catch worthy of his beloved San Francisco 49ers—Montana to Rice. The debate continues to this day.

The memories made Lauren long for the passion which once existed in their relationship, instead by 10 p.m. that night, neither David nor the kids were home, so Lauren climbed into bed alone. Lonely and frustrated, she hugged her pillow for comfort, wondering if this was the way life was supposed to be or if there was something more out there for her somewhere. She was no longer needed by her family, banished to a life of irrelevance and invisibility.

Breakfast the next morning was the usual chaotic event: the kids running through the kitchen asking where one thing or another could be, reminding Lauren about an after-school activity or money needed for some event, when to be picked up or dropped off, grabbing a muffin or one of the ever-present sandwiches pre-made to order the night before and flying out the door in a flurry to the bus. All the while, David barking out his list of the to-dos he expects Lauren to accomplish while they're gone. She wonders if anyone actually listens to the rhythm of the morning, the song of demands and needs sung by the Breckenridge Family Choral Society.

A peaceful quiet fell over the house after everyone had gone. Lauren dutifully picked up the debris left in the path to the door. It was the only evidence that people actually lived in this house. She deposited the aforementioned items at the appropriate locations on her way to her sanctuary—her office and craft room.

An hour later, the front door opened with the usual clatter, and a voice called out, "Hey sweetie, what kind of muffin did you bake for your ravenous neighbor to swoop down and scarf?" No answer was required.

In typical Alice Lane fashion, Lauren's friend headed straight for the kitchen and poured a cup of coffee, helped herself to the remnants of breakfast, and sat down in the sunroom to wait for her compatriot to join her. Alice was flamboyant, exceedingly cheerful, but with a vein of sarcasm that ran deep. Despite her larger-than-life personality, she was beautiful in a natural sort of way. Her long, wavy, strawberry-blond hair and blue eyes captured the attention of all around. Elegant and graceful when needed, she preferred to live in jeans year-round.

"Ahhh, my other child has decided to join me for breakfast, I see," Lauren said with great sarcasm. "Did you finish your homework last night, and do you have any after-school activities I need to be aware of?"

"Oh dear, tough morning?" Alice looked up from her coffee cake.

"What could possibly be tough? I stand here, listen to the commands, and then do as ordered."

"Wake up on the wrong side of the bed this morning, sweet pea?"

"No, it's not that, and yes, I know it's always like this. And yes, I also know this is the life of a mother with a couple teenagers." Lauren sighed. "I just feel like a piece of furniture, or maybe a robot, like Rosie on *The Jetsons*, important to the family's well-being and happiness but God forbid I have a feeling or need of my own. I'm there for others, but certainly there can be no reciprocation."

Alice sat back and studied her friend. They'd both been near the end of their pregnancies when they first met, moving into the new neighborhood within a month of each other. Their firstborn children were eight days apart, and a deep friendship formed over breast-feeding, subsequent children, and the trials of being a suburban house mom. The women hated the term housewife, because neither had said, "I do" to a pile of bricks and wood.

Looking at her best friend, Alice saw deep pain oozing to the surface. Not something easily cured by a moms' night out, or MNO as they preferred to call it. She took a swig of coffee while considering her next sentence, wanting to get to the root of her friend's frustration without seeming superficial.

"How is David's work going?" Alice murmured, her words guided with laser-like precision.

The question penetrated all of Lauren's walls and tears etched her cheeks as Alice handed her a paper napkin within reach.

David was a scientist at heart. A true geek, studying Physics and Chemistry in college. After the first baby came, he managed to complete his MBA at night and was working on his PhD when they had their second child. He had wanted to complete his doctoral work, but somehow life kept happening and he was never quite able to finish. Lauren knew this bothered him; however, he never complained about it. David was a man's man, proud of his family life and accomplishments. Taking care of his family and providing for their needs was his primary goal.

For the past seven years, David had been working at NanoTech, a research subsidiary to a medical conglomerate. His primary work had been managing a department of biotechnology engineers who used both chemistry and engineering to produce artificial appliances to assist people with severe disabilities. The group had been studying the chemical and electrical impulses of the brain in order to better control biomechanical appliances.

Lauren held the napkin to her eyes, absorbing the tears and pushing harder to absorb the frustration she felt. "The FDA is holding up some sort of approval which David's group needs in order to continue the project. It looks like the approval and the budget won't come through until the fall, and David is stressing badly. They can't continue until the funding goes forward. It looks like the whole group will be furloughed from mid-June through September." Lauren paused for a few seconds. Alice remained quiet. She knew her friend well enough to keep her mouth shut on occasion.

"David can't deal with the idea of being out of work for months, and the stress in this house is unbearable with nobody talking... Or maybe everyone is talking but nobody is listening. And the kids. Oh my God, the kids! It's out of control. I can't imagine how we'll survive as a family if this actually happens this summer."

The two women sat in silence, each contemplating life, their kids, husbands, and the general disposition of their worlds. Neither of them had the answers, and both had endless questions. Without further words, they finished their coffee and threw on sweatshirts, heading out the door for their morning run.

The air was brisk, and there had been a light dusting of snow the night before which crunched softly beneath their running shoes. In upstate New York, there was always one late snowfall before spring seemed to burst from the ground. It was as if the buds on the trees needed that extra bit of moisture before the first flowers poked through. Spring was in the air and just around the corner.

The women took it slow, jogging their usual mile-and-a-half route without saying a word. Sometimes on their run, when they were feeling playful, they would sprint past the old cemetery while holding their breath in a kid-like fashion, mimicking the game children play in the car. This morning was not one of those days.

As they returned home, pausing at the two driveways to catch their breath, Alice broke the silence.

"Lauren, this is an opportunity of a lifetime." Alice's breath came out in puffs like a steam train, slowing to normal as they stood at the mailboxes. "I think you should find a summer cabin and get away from it all. Take the entire family and go." She paused long enough for Lauren to start in with objections.

"Are you kidding me, what planet did you come from?" Lauren scoffed. "You think I could peel Jason away from lifeguarding at the pool? And Audrey barely registers my existence. How do I get them to agree to this? Not to mention the master himself, as if he would agree to something so frivolous."

"That's the point, Lauren, don't give them a choice." Alice continued her train of thought. "You are the keeper of the schedule. Do you ask anyone about when they would like to have dental appointments, or do you just make the appointments? All the PTA meetings, father/daughter dances, plumbers, car maintenance, teacher conferences... Don't you just schedule them and post it on the board?"

"Yeah, but—"

Alice continued as if she hadn't said a word. "You decide on when and where the vacations are, based on the kids' school schedules and seasons and interests. Sure, you suggest things and you all come to an agreement, but isn't it your general idea in the first place?" The question was more rhetorical than anything else. Both women knew the answer.

"I dare you, no, I even double-dog dare you. Just do it! Think Nike." Alice had a gleam in her eye while she elbowed her friend in the ribs.

Lauren reached up and brushed the snow off the mailbox into the hood and collar of Alice's sweatshirt. The two giggled madly as a snow fight erupted with the powder.

Alice waved as she turned up her drive and called out her last words of the morning. "Think about it, or better yet, just do it. If you're not on your computer in twenty minutes, I'll annoy you until you get it done."

Lauren had to laugh. She felt much better, so much so that last night and this morning seemed more like a hazy dream. She couldn't imagine not having Alice in her life. Lauren jogged up her drive and into the house. After a quick shower, she sat down at the computer to check her e-mail.

The first message was from Alice. "YOU BETTER START LOOKING FOR A SUMMER PLACE NOW OR I WILL DO IT FOR YOU! LOL." All caps. Truly ominous.

CHAPTER 2

The Lexington Club was founded by a group of wealthy businessmen in the late 1800s when Northern Michigan was a popular resort destination. Located on Lake Charlevoix near what later became known as Hemingway Point, the club housed forty or so summer cottages which were larger than most houses. The elite would escape the heat of the south for the more temperate summer climate near the Upper Peninsula in Michigan.

With The Grand Hotel on Mackinac Island and the nearby resort communities of Harbor Springs and Petoskey, The Lexington Club stood apart from the rest with its family-driven exclusive membership. One couldn't just buy or sell a house within the grounds; a new membership was only awarded after years of visits and rentals, along with the requisite vote by the stockholder members. Of the original forty member-families, eight current members could trace their memberships back six generations. Twenty-five families' lineages fell in the three or four generation range. Only seven members were considered new to the club, having purchased a home within the past decade or so.

There have been many marriages between the families, so much so it seemed everyone was related somehow. New blood was not always welcomed with open arms.

Lake Charlevoix connected to Lake Michigan via Round Lake, an intimate harbor, home to the town of Charlevoix as well as a Coast Guard station. Summer tourist activities included excursions to Beaver Island, abundant golf courses, world-class tennis facilities—including the opportunity to play on clay courts—as well as fishing and sailing. The town had all sorts of shops tourists loved, selling everything from T-shirts to truly unique items hand made by local craftsmen. And, of course, there was the ubiquitous Murdick's Fudge, which had operated a confectionery in various towns throughout Northern Michigan since 1877. Locals referred to tourists as "fudgies," taking into account an overwhelming love for the handmade, intensely creamy fudge.

For over one hundred years, the wealthy traveled north during the summer months to enjoy their prosperity and make business connections. By the 1970s, most of the men were no longer able to spend their entire summer up north but would commute via private jet, landing at a local airport on the outskirts of town. They would fly in on Thursday night and spend a long weekend relaxing with their families, returning to work early Monday morning. The wives and children would stay at the club for the entire summer. Nannies and counselors would take care of the kids while the mothers had their tennis lessons and cocktail parties.

The Danforth family of Lexington, Kentucky, could chart their membership to the club's beginnings. William Danforth was a distant relative of Mary Todd Lincoln, who was born and raised in Lexington, and for all practical purposes this made him nearly American royalty. And, as with most wealthy families, the origin of his considerable wealth was questionable by today's standards.

Liza Danforth was fifth generation Lexington Club and a legacy to the Chi Omega women's fraternity, one of the more prestigious college fraternal organizations. She was often heard explaining, in her strong southern drawl, that the "Chi O" national headquarters was located in Lexington from 1915 through 1926, in a building owned by her granddaddy. The veracity of the statement has never been questioned.

As is common with "old money" families, their resources have dwindled over the generations, and Liza found herself owning a 5000 square foot summer cottage for which the club dues now exceeded twenty thousand dollars per year. The dues did not include any of the social or dining activities that could add thousands of dollars to the tab.

Those who did not know Liza personally would have called her a snob or pretentious, but in reality she was career-minded and determined to rebuild her family wealth without sacrificing their good name. Practical by nature, she considered the family cottage to be a huge drain on her resources, but she was unable to bring herself to part with it. Plus, taking a summer off from her career was simply not an option at the time.

After careful scrutiny of The Lexington Club's bylaws, Liza found a way to rent the cottage for the summer without breaking the trust. And so, in early spring, she listed the property on the website vacationrentals.com.

CHAPTER 3

A few days later, during their morning jog, Alice asked if Lauren had started looking for a vacation home.

"Jesus, Alice, would you give it a rest? It's never going to happen. What part of my life don't you get?" Lauren snapped. The immediacy of her situation had not changed, nor had the week gotten any better. But even as the words were coming out of her mouth, her imagination was going into overdrive.

She pictured everything from a beach villa on a remote island to a weathered house nestled within the pine trees on the coast of Oregon. They would be one big happy family living in a house with minimal electronic connection to the rest of the world. A life without TV or Wii or YouTube. She even imagined the only newspaper being a weekly rag filled with local gossip about the monstrous trout caught the day before or the summer fruit canning festival. If only.

Lauren promptly put the idea out of her mind. She'd been volunteered to organize the PTA's booth at the New York State Maple Festival at the Dutchess County Fairgrounds. The event was two weeks away, and she had not heard from the chair of the decorating committee or from the women who were making the maple scented candles they sold every year. It was more than enough of a distraction for the next week or so.

Lauren sat down at her desk to check in on the morning e-mail. Chams had sent a joke. A few of the PTA volunteers had traded shifts. Susan Davis was suggesting the prices of the candles be raised. Of course there was the usual junk e-mail from various websites.

Alice's e-mail had four links to vacation properties for rent. There was one on Paradise Island near Nassau—a luxury home complete with servants. Not to overshadow the mega yacht available for cruising the Greek Isles during the month of August. Alice had a sense of humor.

Lauren responded to Chams' joke by updating him on David's work situation. A few minutes after sending the e-mail, an instant message popped up on her screen.

"You okay?" Charles asked.

"Sure, why do you ask?" was Lauren's reply.

"Tone in your e-mail... what's up with Dinky?"

"Dunno, he barely talks to me anymore."

"Not good, you guys around this weekend?"

"Yup. Jase has a water polo practice, and Audrey has the usual homework and a sleepover planned."

"How about I pop up on Saturday and take Dinky out to get him stinking drunk? That should cure him. Maybe he'll pull his head out of his ass and take a look at the hot babe he snagged."

"You're a shameless flirt."

"Yeah, and Dinks got lucky beyond measure."

"LOL... See you Saturday and plan to stay for dinner."

"Deal... Wait, who's cooking?"

"Go away, Chams! LOL"

"Later babe."

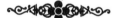

Uncle Chams showed up midday on Saturday as anticipated and not without the requisite gifts for each family member. He was a frequent visitor, never missing a performance or sporting event, and was forever lavishing the kids and Lauren with gifts.

"Hey Jase, my man," Charles called out as he walked into the kitchen.

Jason, the oldest son, was sixteen and was the jock of the family. Already five feet eleven with broad shoulders, he excelled in most sports but had a strong preference for swimming, water polo and sailing.

Pisces to the core, he preferred to keep his home life separate from his personal life. The only way to gauge what was going on with his friends was to study his general mood when he walked through the house. Lauren suspected he had recently met a girl, as his disposition had taken on a new exuberance hard to attribute to anything but infatuation. His hazel eyes danced with light, and for the past couple weeks, he'd taken to swinging his mama around the room for no apparent reason. Lauren was delighted by the energy but wished she knew the details.

Jason stood up, embracing his pseudo-uncle with one of those man-hug back thumps. "Yo, Chams. 'Sup?" This was their common, casual greeting, belying the deep bond the two have had since the beginning.

Charles put his backpack on the kitchen table and dug out a package of homemade turkey jerky. "Jase, go long!" Chams called out as he backed up into an imaginary pocket looking for receivers.

Jason bolted past the kitchen island and leaped to catch the bag, then hurdled the coffee table in the living room and fell backward onto the couch, hands in the air to signal a touchdown. "The crowd goes wild, and the chicky cheerleaders are doing their thing as I win the game in the final seconds," Jason yelled at the top of his lungs. "Thanks, Uncle Chams."

Jason ripped open the bag and tore into one of his favorite snacks. "Mama Mia, I'm heading out da door... to the pool and then to a friend's. Later!" And he was out the front door and gone before anyone could respond.

Charles walked up behind Lauren, playfully throwing his arms around her and smashing his face into her neck and hair. "Oh, if only I had been the one running for the pass, you would have been mine, all mine."

"And change the course of history? You still had dozens of hearts to break," Lauren responded with a sarcastic twinge.

"You are a wicked woman. I should take you over my knee and spank you right here and now, but you would enjoy that too much, so I'll keep my distance. By the way, Molly sends her best and told me to tell you she would like to meet you for lunch in Saugerties next week."

"Tell your lovely wife message received and lunch confirmed. Perhaps she and I will finally understand why we put up with the likes of you two for so long... or come up with the perfect murder plan. It's not as easy as it looks, you know."

The two laughed easily as David entered the kitchen. "Unhand my woman, you hound, or I will kick your ass all the way to Albany and back."

Lauren felt a deep sense of relief seeing the two college buddies act like little boys. The laughter and joking was music to her ears, and she could feel the tension melting away.

When the two got together, more often than not, they became twenty-two or twenty-three again. Within minutes, the guys were laughing and arguing about some football game. Lauren shooed them into the living room with a couple Heinekens, hoping that a day of play would remind David he was human and had a life.

Twenty minutes later, David announced they were heading out across the river to Saugerties. Lauren knew they would head to The Dutch Alehouse, a dive bar with great burgers where the locals hung out, played darts or pool, and listened to local musicians trying out new material before a recording session at Bearsville Sound in Woodstock.

Alone once again, Lauren decided to take a bubble bath and finish her novel in peace.

CHAPTER 4

A white GMC Yukon sat parked in a strip mall about a mile away from the Breckenridge home. Jason jogged to the car with ease; his heart rate did not increase any measureable amount. At least not from the run. He slid into the passenger side, tossing his gym bag into the back seat. The woman behind the wheel handed him a pipe loaded with pot and pulled out onto Clinton Corners Road.

Jason lit the pipe and took a couple hits before handing it back to her. They drove a few miles in complete silence before turning off onto a dirt road which headed back into the woods. Once off the main road, the woman reached over and put her hand on Jason's thigh. His heart raced with anticipation. After a few minutes, they reached a secluded cabin and headed inside.

Karen Alderson was twenty-five years old and a teaching assistant at nearby Marist College. She was almost five feet nine with curves that would make any man drive off the road. When she wore heels, she stood eye to eye with Jason. It was her bold assertiveness and playful nature that attracted his attention. She was not at all like the twittering high school girls his age.

Jason and his buddy Alec from the water polo team had gotten hooked up with fake IDs a couple months earlier and had started hitching rides or taking the bus to bars in Poughkeepsie. Late one night, the two of them were sitting in Gino's Pizza drinking beer and scarfing down a deluxe Sicilian-style pie when a group of girls came in and sat down at the table opposite them. Jason could not take his eyes off Karen, who was flattered by the attention. She could tell he was younger than she was, but since New York's drinking age was twenty-one, she figured what the hell. The physical chemistry was magnetic. She didn't ask to see his ID.

The group bantered for an hour or so, closing down the joint, and then walked to a bar down the street. The three women and two boys strolled passed the bouncer, and nobody questioned their ages.

Jason had arranged to spend the night at a friend's house, so he was good to go. From there, nature took its course.

After a night of drinking and flirting, Karen was astonished that Jason had been a complete gentleman. She expected to have to fend off the usual grabby hands, as she had on most of her recent dates. Instead, he was a little reserved, playing with her hair and telling her she was the most beautiful person he had ever seen. By the end of the evening, Karen wanted him badly; instead, Jason pulled back, asking if she wanted to hang out again the following Friday.

Karen did not recognize the signs of youth or inexperience. She was blinded by desire, attraction, and a deep yearning to be in a relationship. She had been lonely far too long, and her neediness outpaced her sensibilities.

After three weeks of making out in the back of a car or in a movie theater like teenagers, Karen was hooked. Their dates became more frequent, and it seemed like they were texting or talking on the phone continuously. Karen was intensely flattered at his interest in her. Most of the men she dated had been so self-centered; this was a refreshing change.

Jason could not believe his luck. Here was this hot chick who was smart and completely into him. Karen was funny and interesting. Compared to the high school girls who had few interests other than being seen with a jock, it was like he'd hit the jackpot. He was floating on air, happy beyond reason, and unable to concentrate on anything around him. At the same time, there was the fear of getting busted. The adrenaline rush was a kick.

He wanted to scream at the top of his lungs, telling everyone about his relationship. But deep down, he knew he had to keep this all a secret. Somehow it was wrong, and he knew if Karen found out his real age, his whole world would burst like a bubble. The element of danger added to the excitement.

The sexual chemistry was growing stronger. During one of their heated moments, Karen asked if there was someplace they could go. Jason was afraid he would blow it, he was still a virgin. Blowjobs from high school cheerleaders didn't count. Thinking fast, he said he could make arrangements for the weekend at a cabin in the woods where they could be alone together. The suggestion made Karen melt in his arms.

Over the next couple days, Jason scrambled to arrange the details without getting caught. Saturday morning came, and he explained to Karen that he had to take his car to the shop. He asked if she'd meet him at a strip mall. Would she be willing to drive?

Breathless with anticipation, Karen agreed without hesitation. Relieved, Jason was again able to duck his lack of a driver's license or car.

Once inside the cabin, Jason pulled Karen to him and kissed her deeply, grinding his hips into her. He could feel the pull of her heat through their clothes.

She was every bit as ready as he was.

For the past month he had blown off everything, including school and his team practices, as their sexual relationship progressed at a rapid pace. There were no other obstacles in the way, and he was about to lose his virginity to the sexiest woman he had ever known. Someone who knew what he liked, not unlike the little girls who gagged and pulled away when he came in their mouth.

Nope, he wanted to take his time and enjoy this moment, which was taking enormous restraint and self-control. "Slow down, babe, we have all night," Jason whispered in her ear. "I want this to be special."

Karen's knees buckled under her, but she wanted the same thing, though for completely different reasons.

"Go get us some beer. The fridge is stocked," he whispered into her neck, taking a nip at her collar bone. "I'll start the fire and warm it up in here."

"Jase," Karen moaned, "I believe that fire is already lit, and I am hot."

Jason laughed. "Yes, you are." He pulled back and slapped her on the ass to get her moving.

The one-room cabin was sparsely furnished. In the center of the room stood an iron potbellied stove. In front of the stove was an oversized daybed covered with pillows and a down comforter. The far wall had a linear kitchenette with a fridge. Jason had stocked it with beer and food— enough to last them until Monday morning. His parents didn't expect him home until Sunday. He hadn't quite figured out how to get away for a second night—a school night, no less.

As he stood up from the wood-burning stove which had started to crackle, all thoughts of his parents and responsibilities flew out the window. Karen had stripped down to a flimsy tank top held loosely in place by her rounded tits and nipples straining against the fabric. One of the spaghetti straps had fallen off her shoulder. She had unbuttoned her jeans, and Jason saw her panties matched the top. It took his breath away, and he stood there admiring the view.

"You like?" Karen asked playfully.

"Uh huh." Jason gulped, hoping he wouldn't cum in his pants before he even touched her. "Come here."

CHAPTER 5

Charles and David settled into a booth and ordered burgers and a pitcher of beer. Having caught up on the week's worth of events, Charles turned to his friend with a serious look on his face.

"Okay, bro, spill it," Charles prodded.

David looked at his friend and tried to duck the issue, pretending not to understand.

"Come on, don't make me work at this. You know, I know, you know…" Charles laughed.

David couldn't help but smirk. "You are an immature mofo," he said, teasing his friend. Of course, the prodding and joking did loosen him up, and David explained his situation at work. He shared his concerns about being out of work for a few months, and while it wasn't really a financial issue for him, due to his contract with the company, the people who worked for him were not as protected. He was afraid he would lose his best engineers due to the uncertainty of the whole situation.

"So, what are the odds the Feds won't approve your work or delay it further?" Charles asked.

"Actually, almost none. I spoke with our contact this week, and they've already given tentative approval. The formal documents take six to eight weeks to process. Once we have the docs, our investor will release the next chunk of money which will fund us for three to five years. I just don't like counting chickens, if you know what I mean."

Chams sat back and looked at his friend without saying anything. He reached out and refilled their glasses and signaled the waiter for a refill on the pitcher. Taking a deep slug of the amber liquid, Chams put down his glass and leaned forward, looking David in the eye.

"Dinky, you're my best friend," Charles began in an uncharacteristic show of emotion and seriousness, "but right now you're being a jackass, and you're going to screw up your entire life if you don't pull your head out of your ass and take a look around at what you're about to lose."

David sat there stunned, not knowing how to respond. "Fuck off, Chams" was all he could muster.

Charles slammed his hand down on the wooden table, startling David and attracting annoyed glances from a slew of patrons. "Dickhead, I'm only going to tell you this once. You have exceptional kids and a wife who loves you more than you deserve... and you know I'm speaking the truth about that one."

Charles nodded without saying a word, his eyes glued to the glass of beer as if he might miss a drop of condensation and screw up his count.

"You have the opportunity of a lifetime staring you in the face, and you're so damn stupid you don't even see it."

David shot a semi-quizzical look at his friend, clearly not seeing the truth of the situation.

Charles continued. "Don't you remember when we were kids in college and would rent a cottage on Martha's Vineyard for the summer? We swore that when we were adults we would get to a point where we could do that with our kids."

A hint of recognition flashed across David's face. He was transported back in time, back to their youth, to the carefree time when the biggest worry they had was how to avoid spending all the rent money on pizza, beer, and weed. They worked at various summer jobs around Oak Bluffs, spending the vast majority of their time cruising around the island on their bikes, meeting at sunset for clam bakes on beaches only known to locals. There they would build bonfires and hang out with the girls all summer long. It was the happiest time he could remember.

At the first signs of fall, the gang would have one last bash near Gay Head Point before they headed off to their various colleges. Dinky, Chams, Lauren, and Molly would head back to Boston University to settle down to their studies.

"Those were great times, Chams," David muttered wistfully, "but you can't go back."

"That's my point, Dinks," Charles whispered. "That opportunity is in the palm of your hands. You don't have to go backward, but you *can* go forward. Rent a house on the beach for the summer and relax with your kids before they grow up and leave the nest. Spend the summer admiring your beautiful wife in a bikini. Be a kid again..."

The two friends sat in wistful silence, remembering the past and pondering the possibilities that awaited them.

Chapter 6

Liza Danforth sat in her office staring at her monitor. Not a single hit on vacationrentals.com. "This is ridiculous," she said out loud to nobody in particular. Well past dark, she was contemplating her finances for the summer and how to budget for the club payment. As much as the members all called themselves family, the fact remained that as soon as someone fell behind on their dues, the wolves came out and tore into each other.

She was appalled when the family who owned the house up the hill from her summer home was denied access to their house until the dues were paid. She could see both sides of the equation. The club needed the money to keep up the property, but everyone had financial trouble from time to time, and this feeding frenzy did not seem particularly loving or understanding.

More proof that you can pick your friends but not your family. And to Liza, this was her extended family. It was easy to overlook character flaws when you spent idle summer days playing or doing whatever you pleased whenever the mood hit you.

Liza, no longer a kid and now fully responsible for her cottage, was unwilling to admit to the board that she didn't have the cash available to pay the dues. Her plan had been to tell the club she was renting her cottage, as work requirements would keep her in Manhattan over the summer. She planned to visit Charlevoix over Venetian Weekend and assumed she would be able to stay at any number of her friends' homes.

Charlevoix has held this festival on the third weekend of July since 1930. In theory, it was based on the pre-Lenten Carnavale held in Venice and cities around Europe since the 1700s. How it came to be a summer tradition in Northern Michigan was anybody's guess. Any reason for a party. The weekend festivities grew in popularity every year, and the event mushroomed into an eight-day extravaganza, including such things as a boat parade, multiple nights of fireworks and music in the park at night, and Battle of the Bands competitions. Although the town became overcrowded, it was not an event she wanted to skip. Everyone who was anyone would be there.

Liza Danforth learned an important lesson from her grandfather very early in life. "You need to take the bull by the horns, little miss, and don't you forget that," he often said. Liza adored William Danforth, the third generation of her family's involvement at The Lexington Club. He always had an obscure or old-fashioned saying to share. But what Liza loved most were his stories. In the evenings, she would crawl onto his lap, and he would tell her tales of self-made men or his own perspective on the news of the day. It was his stories and guidance that sowed the seeds of entrepreneurialism deep within her soul.

Her brothers—and many other family members—took the easy way out and lived off the trust funds. Liza was Grandpa Willy's spiritual clone and as she grew up she saw the hidden disdain he held for the rest of the family's laziness. Not that he would ever say anything negative, in fact, nobody would ever believe her if she said Grandpa Willy was anything but proud of his entire brood.

Liza relished the look in his eyes and the extra attention she got whenever she brought home a project from school. William Danforth would drop whatever he was doing to help her with a problem or answer a question. Anytime she came up with some harebrained scheme involving commerce, he was in.

When she was six, Liza had her Barbies set up a lemonade stand in the front entrance of his estate before one of the many elaborate banquets they held. Rather than being embarrassed or angry, Grandpa Willy, dressed in his tux, sat down on the slate with her and assisted with the sales and customer service as his guests arrived. Liza was, without a doubt, the only person who could have gotten away with this sort of behavior, as in those days, children were to be seen but not heard—and barely seen, at that. Wallis Danforth, her grandmother, was mortified, although the couples' guests were amused by the little girl who had charmed her powerful and enormously successful grandfather into playing with dolls.

Liza was raised to be an entrepreneur in the spirit of her family heritage. With this thought in mind, she focused her attention on how to get her cottage rented. Pulling her knowledge of marketing to the forefront of her brain, she concluded using the internet and social marketing tactics would be the most efficient way to complete her task.

Heading to the website and alumni boards of her college, Liza posted the listing, describing the summers of her youth, those lazy days of childhood when the hardest decision she ever had to make was whether to play tennis or go to the beach. She described the protective nature of the club and how the family members socialized together during beach picnics, formal Sunday night dinners, and friendly softball games with the other clubs around the lake.

She also posted the information on her sorority website. Finally, heading to Facebook, she posted the information to her wall, asking if friends of friends of friends would spread the word. Hopefully someone would become enticed and contact her quickly.

She wondered if Grandpa Willy would be proud of her efforts or appalled by the uncivilized use of technology which made her appear desperate.

"It's the modern world, Willy." Liza looked to the heavens and spoke out loud. "This is how it works now. Just like the flyers you helped me hang when I was fourteen and decided I was going to run a car wash over the summer."

It had been seven years since Willy died, but Liza still talked to him every day. He was her mentor and her rock. Without him she felt alone, adrift in the world with no beacon to guide her.

CHAPTER 7

Lauren woke to the sounds of Audrey in the kitchen. David was sound asleep in the bed next to her. She had no idea what time he got home last night, but from the pieces of clothing tossed in random places, she knew it had been pretty late. Years of experience had taught her that clothes droppings meant David would sleep until noon and be relatively cheerful for the rest of the day.

Throwing on some sweats, she went downstairs to greet the day and see if Audrey was in the mood to talk to her.

Audrey was a rebel. She fought against everything suggested to her and was now dabbling in a punky-goth sort of look. So far, Lauren had managed to prevent piercings and tats, convincing her daughter to make temporary changes rather than permanent ones in her effort to have fun and express her creativity. It was a last-ditch effort to prevent the permanent desecration of her body... and it worked—though now she had to bite her tongue and let her daughter express herself.

Long term, Lauren won the war; short term, she lost a few minor battles. She assumed Audrey would grow out of this phase eventually.

"Morning, sweetie." Lauren bent and kissed her daughter's head. "I see you found a new 'do' for your hair." Lauren knew better than to compliment a style. Audrey glanced warily at her mother and grunted, unsure of what was coming next. For the past year, a change in style had often turned into a screaming match. This acceptance thing her mother was doing seemed weird and fake. It almost made Audrey want to push it just to see what would happen.

Lauren sat down at the table, getting her first true look at her daughter's hair. Actually it wasn't that bad... or maybe she was just getting used to Audrey's hair being a form of conceptual art. The cut was completely asymmetrical, dyed jet black with one streak of a neon blue in the front. The blue chunk was the longest part of the cut.

"Where did you get your hair done?" Lauren asked calmly without making eye contact. She tried not to laugh as she heard the voice of Marlin Perkins in her head: *Approach the wild animal slowly and with caution. Sudden movement or noise will cause fear, and the beast will be sure to attack.*

"Ra and I went across the river yesterday," Audrey answered nonchalantly. "Her mom dropped us off in town while she went to some meeting at SUNY New Paltz. Then we hung out on campus for the rest of the day."

Oh great. "When did Ashley change her name to Ra?"

"We went to the library and looked up new names. Since Ra was born under a sun sign, we figured she should be the sun goddess. I'm Satis, an early war and hunting goddess responsible for flooding. I'm known as 'She Who Runs Like an Arrow.'"

"Sounds interesting. Did you get your homework done while you were in the library?" Lauren asked cautiously.

"Not really. I don't have much, so I'll get it done later. Ra and I are gonna walk up to Franklin and see if anyone is around."

"Sounds good. Can you be home by 4:30 today, please?" Lauren tried not to show too much emotion. "I'd like to have a family dinner tonight and a quiet evening."

"Sure, Mom," Audrey responded as she disappeared down the hallway.

An hour later, Lauren got a text from Jason. "In Philly... road trip 2 Temple 4 swim meet. Back Mon. Thx!" Her heart sank. So much for a family dinner.

CHAPTER 8

Jason slipped back into bed, trying not to wake Karen, at least not yet. He didn't want her to see him texting, fearing it would bring up questions he was not prepared to answer.

Wrapping his naked body around hers, he was rock hard, raring to go again. Karen stirred, feeling the heat of the man behind her, and smiled—half-asleep, half-awake. She was completely happy for the first time in a long time. She'd finally found someone who was considerate, kind, and compelling. In many ways, this man was mysterious and yet so open, allowing himself to be vulnerable and playful all at once. She felt none of the pretense of having to prove himself. Karen knew she was falling deeply in love with this person.

She took a deep breath and sighed with happiness. Making love for the first time last night was the most amazing experience. Up until now, her first time with a man came with nervous tension and a certain amount of performance anxiety. She always worried whether she was pretty enough, her body sexy enough, and whether her partner would enjoy her and the things they did together.

Last night was completely different. Jason undressed her in a deliberately unhurried fashion, lingering over her like a long-anticipated Christmas gift. It was as if he was touching a woman's body for the first time. And the kissing. Oh the endless kissing! He explored every inch of her body with his hands and mouth, leaving her breathless and begging for him to take her.

"Not yet," he whispered as he alternated between rubbing his fingers around her clit and thrusting them deep inside her, making her cum over and over again. After one particularly strong orgasm, he lay on top of her, grinding but not entering. "You squirt!" Jason said with delight and surprise.

Karen, at that point, was only able to nod her head in response.

He pulled up, straddling her face, and rocked his dick in her mouth. When he asked if he could cum in her face, she answered with a flick of her tongue against his bulging head. She held his hips as he stroked his dick with increasing speed, reaching up with her tongue for an occasional lick until his semen warmed her face and neck. He picked up a towel from the floor and wiped her clean with tender care, kissing and touching all the while.

To Karen's surprise, he was still hard and spread her legs with his knees. Looking down as he entered her for the first time, his entire body quivered in anticipation. He didn't move for a moment, staring into her eyes, surprised by the warmth surrounding his penis. The look of delight was as if he were a kid in a candy store. She rocked her hips, gently at first, and then the two moved in unison, gaining speed until he was grunting, his head swelling with each stroke. Karen came again, her muscles gripping and pulling him from deep within, his release into her came with an uncontrolled force he had never felt; he wanted more.

Night became early morning before either of them fell asleep. His ability to become hard mere moments after climax was something she had never experienced before. Karen felt totally consumed by her lover. Appreciated like never before, wanted like no man had ever wanted her.

And now, in the middle of a Sunday afternoon, this man was pushing up against her again, clearly wanting more. Karen was in love or in lust or possibly both.

"Babe," Karen whispered, half-asleep, "would you like some food or coffee or something?"

Jason's stomach rumbled in response. "See? You do need fuel for energy. Relax, I'll make us something and bring it to you in bed." Karen kissed him softly as she moved over his body, grabbing the shirt he'd tossed aside and slipping it over her head.

"Damn, you look hot in that tee, girl!" Jason took a last grab at Karen's tits and thrusted up at her as she straddled him.

"Easy, big fella. We have all day, right?" They hadn't talked about when they would return to the real world or if there were any place either of them had to go.

"You better believe it, babe! I'm yours until you drop me off Monday morning at the place where you picked me up." Jason hesitated a beat too long. "You know, the place where my car is being fixed," he added in a hurry.

His comment struck Karen as odd, but she decided to ignore it. There were many mysteries to this man. Perhaps she was destined to spend a lifetime figuring them out. "Stop it," she muttered to herself. *I hardly know this guy. I can't be in love. It's not possible!*

CHAPTER 9

Lauren looked around the kitchen in dismay. Her plans of a relaxing day spent with the family, topped by a pleasant Sunday dinner, came crashing down around her. How moronic of her to think her teenaged children would want to spend time with her. And David, of course, he didn't seem any more interested than the kids.

She looked out the window searching for the first signs of spring, but the backyard was grey and slushy. Her eyes focused on the play set, long since forgotten, a symbol of the more joyous days of youth.

They'd lived in Manhattan after getting married, in an inexpensive place on East 37th Street. Not a "cool" part of town but certainly accessible to everywhere via subways. When David got his first job at a pharmaceutical company in the suburbs, he actually did a reverse commute up to Westchester County. They didn't want to give up the active life of the city. Friday and Saturday nights consisted of late dinners before heading to the clubs downtown. They went dancing and to jazz bars. Took in plays or Knicks games at The Garden. Life was full and active.

Lauren graduated with a degree in history and English literature. Companies were not clamoring for her experience as they were with David. Nevertheless, she was able to find a job as a publications editor for a consulting firm. Her days were spent correcting the grammar on poorly written articles regarding some up-and-coming company whose IPO would redefine the world. Apparently, every new company recreated fire and applied it to sliced bread in a new and improved way.

It became clear that the company was ripping off its clients by stroking the egos of the owners. It seemed to Lauren that some of the product launches would have less than a zero percent chance of success, but here were these well-educated Harvard and Stanford MBAs telling the well-educated USC and Yale graduates their companies would be the next big thing. And, because of the impressive degrees being tossed around, innocent people listened and invested their hard-earned money on products that would never make it to market.

Lauren kept her mouth shut, made the edits to the white papers, collected her paycheck, and went on with her life. She never thought about it being a career, so much as making a decent living and saving as much money as possible while exploring the city.

By the time she got pregnant, she and David had saved enough for a house in the suburbs. They found a nice house, on a decent-sized piece of land in Millbrook— close enough for David to drive to work and for Lauren to start settling into the idea of being a mom and a wife. During the end of her pregnancy and when Jason was first born, Lauren did freelance writing and editing. She actually earned more doing the work from home, in fewer hours, than she had when she was working full time. With the arrival of Audrey four years later, she stopped working altogether.

The days were long but the years flew by, the kids were teenagers, and they were living the suburban lifestyle—complete with a picket fence. Lauren kept herself busy volunteering on various committees and charity boards while keeping track of the family movements.

Sometimes it seemed that people were no different from ants, scurrying here and there with no apparent purpose. In fact, it all seemed pointless. On any given day, half the county drove in one direction while the other half did the exact opposite, only to reverse directions eight or nine hours later.

Kitchen cleaned and the dishes put away, Lauren tried to clear her head and focus on the day ahead.

She was annoyed with Jason who had taken off without a word of notice, and she would discuss this with him on Monday when he returned. This was completely out of character for Jason; he was her good child, after all. Jason was the star athlete with excellent grades and a part-time job to save money for college. Her responsible one. So, if he and his buddies took a road trip to watch a college swim meet, what was the real harm in that? Jason had probably been thinking about which college team he wanted to swim for in a little over a year and forgot about asking for permission, which more than likely he would have gotten anyway. Lauren was quite good at rationalizing for her boy lately. Maybe it was a new girlfriend who was keeping his head in the clouds.

Lauren poured coffee for herself and David, toasted a bagel, and grabbed the *Sunday Times*. Maybe it would be like Sundays of old, when they spent half the day reading the paper in bed. Putting the tray on the nightstand, Lauren slipped out of her sweats and between the sheets.

Out of instinct and decades of being together, David rolled into her, cupping her breast. Only half-awake and without opening his eyes, he mumbled, "Morning. You feel nice." She smiled at the compliment. It had been awhile since they'd been together. "Where are the kids?" David asked, a little more awake now.

As Lauren gave the report, David reached between her legs. Feeling moisture, he became instantly aroused and began caressing her with purpose. With years of study and the precision of a scientist, he knew exactly how to get her going. Six minutes later, they sat in bed, coffee in hand. "That was nice," David said. "We need to do it more often."

"Mmmm," Lauren responded, not exactly dissatisfied sexually, but yearning for something more. Functional. That's the way she'd described their sex life to Alice, who responded by saying, "Well, at least you have sex!"

Is this really what marriage becomes? Lauren couldn't help but wonder.

The two of them sat in bed, flipping through separate sections of the paper, with a running dialogue about the information contained within. Something only accomplished after a lifetime together. Half listening to each other, yet comprehending all.

"David, can we talk about this summer?"

David looked up from the business section without speaking and waited for his wife to continue.

"I'm not sure how to bring this up. In fact, I don't even know if it's a good idea or not, but I was talking to Alice about your—I mean our—situation..."

"This is something new?" David teased.

"I'm serious!" She gave him a playful shove on his midsection.

"Then please, by all means, continue. I'm all ears." David laughed as he pushed the paper on the floor and nuzzled Lauren's breasts, his tongue teasing her nipple playfully.

"Would you please pay attention?" She giggled and pushed him away.

"Okay, okay, I'll listen. What did you and the Mad Hatter come up with?" It was David's pet name for his neighbor, a reference to the *Alice in Wonderland* character and her seemingly endless energy and stream of ideas.

Lauren rolled her eyes. "She thinks we should go away together as a family and spend a summer doing something fun. Different. Together. You know, just get away for a break."

David paused and looked at his wife for a minute in disbelief, thinking about the conversation he'd had with Chams last night. He wondered if the girls had listened in somehow. He studied his wife, her knees tucked up to her chest, her expression quite earnest.

"You want to do this?" he whispered.

Lauren nodded.

David paused for what felt like an eternity to Lauren. "Okay, babe, if you think it's a good idea, then let's do it," he said as he kissed her temple, climbed out of bed, and headed for the shower. "Have you considered where you'd like to spend the summer? Or do you want to see if we can rent that old broken-down house on the Vineyard?"

Stunned, Lauren realized David was serious. He had agreed without any hesitation. She sat there with a warmth in her heart she had not felt in years. He remembered their years at the Vineyard! As the reality sank in and her mind started to churn with the planning process, her mood lifted dramatically.

Redrum flashed through her head, and she laughed out loud at the silliness of the reference to the Stephen King novel about a family going insane through the winter at the Overlook Hotel. "Goofball," she muttered. "It'll be summer; you really need to find better material. Amityville, perhaps?"

CHAPTER 10

The rest of the weekend went as planned. On Monday morning, once Audrey was off to school, Lauren sat down at her computer to look for their summer home. She and Jason had spoken that morning when he flew in the house to take a quick shower and change clothes.

Jason was appropriately apologetic, telling her it wasn't his idea, just sort of a last minute thing with a bunch of guys, and he'd have felt "awkward calling his mommy." She sat back and listened to him explain the situation and came to the conclusion that he was maturing rapidly. He seemed more young man than boy, particularly when he took complete responsibility for his actions before she could even start in on him.

He promised it would never happen again and kissed her on the cheek as he dashed out the door to school. Lauren surmised kids grow up faster and at a younger age than she did and forgave him.

"No punishment, just don't do it again."

"I promise, Mama Mia, I won't let you down." The words hung in the air and in her heart all morning long.

She and Alice exchanged e-mail about the weekend events. Sure, they were right next door to each other, but texting and e-mail gave them instant and continuous communication with each other, highly efficient when you have a busy schedule. Alice was still pushing an exotic foreign destination, but it was mostly tongue in cheek. In fact, Alice was searching websites for her family as well, thinking in the back of her mind that they might join Lauren's for a week or two.

Several hours into the search, Lauren had sent out a dozen e-mails requesting further information. The possibilities were endless: everything from Southern California to a remote island off the coast of Maine. Her one absolute requirement was ocean. She wanted—no, needed—to be able to have beach barbeques and watch the sun set into the water.

She even decided to post her request on Craig's list. Perhaps there would be some takers there. If nothing came of these requests, she'd ask David how he felt about offering their house in trade, hoping to find an Italian family who would want to experience America and New York City in exchange for the use of their villa.

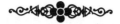

Liza kept checking her e-mail for responses to her various posts. She was so stressed about the cottage, it consumed her; therefore, she couldn't focus on work at all. *Not good,* she thought. *Think, think, think. What else can I do?* Lost in her dream world, she didn't notice her boss's boss, the president of her company, standing in her office.

"I assume you're deep in thought about your summer sales forecast, due last week?"

Liza jumped, obviously startled. "Holy shit, Ted, you scared the crap out of me!"

"Clearly." Ted Sagan sat down in one of the guest chairs. "George and I need your numbers, but I'm also wondering what's going on with you. Something must be up, because in eight years you have yet to miss a deadline. I almost expected to see a dead body slumped at your desk." They both laughed, the tension broken.

Liza worked in a man's world. She was the national sales manager for a building supply company. She handled national retail chains like Home Depot, as well as large construction companies with multi-state housing projects. Her company had a diverse product line, and she was responsible for fifteen salespeople and twice as many sales assistants located in field offices across the country. Her position got her a window on the eighteenth floor of the building on lower Park Avenue in Manhattan.

Ted Sagan was twenty years older than Liza and had worked for her grandfather for most of his career. He had the utmost respect for William Danforth, who had built his company from the ground up. In fact, when it became clear that Willy's life was ending, he called Ted to his home in Lexington and specifically requested he watch over Liza, mentor her until she was ready to take the reins of the company. Willy made sure Ted was taken care of financially for the rest of his life, so the idea of training his replacement did not seem threatening in any way.

"Spill your guts, Little Miss, or Willy is going to have something to say about it," Ted said with a smile. Liza ducked her head and looked skyward, as if expecting a lightning bolt out of nowhere. She gave him the situation in a nutshell.

"Craig's List?" He shook his head as he walked out of her office. "And get me the numbers by Tuesday morning."

Lauren looked up at the ceiling. "Duh. Are you laughing at me, Willy, 'cause I am!" How could she miss something so obvious?

CHAPTER 11

Craig's List: the great facilitator on the Internet. If it was possible to exchange an item for cash or prizes, this was the place to go. There, people listed wants, needs, or desires, and there was no shortage of people willing to fill the bill.

Lauren posted the need for a summer retreat, a place where a family could become close again, complete with plenty of activities to choose from. And water. It had to be near the water. She was asking for a slice of heaven and figured if she came close, then it would be perfect. She wanted to get away from it all, yet still be able to have a social life. The idea of a resort seemed too crowded and forced and the idea of an isolated house too remote or lonely. What she really wanted was the sense of a small community she'd had during summer break at college—but without the work of meeting people.

She stared at her computer screen in amazement. There were dozens of e-mails to go through.

The first twenty-five responses left her discouraged. Maybe this was a bad idea or perhaps just not meant to be. After all, fate does tend to play with your life every once in a while. She warmed up her coffee and decided to give it one more shot before calling a travel agent.

It was the forty-fifth response that caught her attention.

"Hi, I just read your post. My cottage is not exactly what you're looking for, but I thought perhaps you would consider it. There is a place called The Lexington Club in Northern Michigan. It is located on Lake Charlevoix which is pretty big and directly connected to Lake Michigan. Not quite an ocean, but I can tell you from personal experience that watching sunsets from a boat on the lake is divine. The only difference is the size of the waves and fresh water rather than salt.

"My family has owned the cottage for generations. For most of my life, I have headed north every summer to what I consider heaven on earth. Stress-free days where the hardest decision you have to make is whether to go waterskiing or play tennis and what to wear to dinner on Sunday night. The club has a beach, tennis courts, and a clubhouse with a dining hall and chef serving breakfast and dinner every day. On Sunday, there's a formal buffet dinner followed by a nondenominational "hymn sing," left over from the formality of society 100 years ago.

"The club hires an activities director and staff to supervise the beach and give sailing or tennis lessons. Every week there's a family beach picnic, along with themed parties, and friendly softball games played against some of the other clubs in the area.

"As I write this note to you, it all sounds unbelievable—even to me, and I've been there! I would love to spend yet another summer with the people I consider my extended family; however, my commitments at work will keep me away, and I would rather another family enjoy the summer than leave the cottage empty.

"The club dues are significant, and I have to pay them regardless, so if I can offset the cost via a rental it makes financial sense. But I must be honest with you. I cannot rent the house to just anybody. The board needs to approve the rental. There is something about your request that resonates with me, and my instinct says it's a match. If you're interested in continuing this discussion, please respond to my private e-mail."

Lauren read the response several times. It was unusually long and well written, considering the source. The line about dues being "significant" made her apprehensive. That could mean anything.

As usual, Lauren picked up the phone and pressed the number one. David said they should just tie two cans to a string.

"Yo," said the familiar voice, "not in the mood today. Wanna grab lunch in town later?" Alice began the conversation assuming Lauren was asking about their run.

"Nope. Let me read something to you," Lauren responded.

"Ready, go."

Lauren and Alice spoke in shorthand. Formalities like "how was your day" were a waste of time, as the communication was practically continual. Not only did they finish each other's thoughts, but frequently they started in the middle of a conversation. The husbands would tease that the relationship bordered on incestuous.

Lauren read the e-mail aloud, forwarding it at the same time, and the two dissected the document, looking for hidden meanings and possibilities. In the end, Alice made the decision for her. "Go for it! What have you got to lose?" Together, they composed a response and sent it.

"Hey, Alice, what are you going to do all summer long without me?" Lauren asked in a mocking tone, though the underlying truth festered just below the surface.

"Funny, I was thinking the same thing. What are you going to do without me?" The women laughed and hung up.

Again, apprehension twisted through Lauren's body. Was this the right thing for her family? Why was she so nervous at the prospect of a summer with her kids and husband? It made no sense... on the surface.

CHAPTER 12

Liza and Lauren agreed to meet in New York City, each planning to bring photos. It was one of those stunningly beautiful spring mornings, warm, and everything seemed to sparkle. Lauren took an early Metro-North train out of Poughkeepsie, arriving at Grand Central mid-morning. It gave her plenty of time to walk around the city before meeting Liza at 1 p.m. at a diner on 3rd Avenue, a few blocks below the train station.

The ride along the Hudson was relaxing, and Lauren gazed out the window, looking at the water and trying not to think about the peculiar behavior her kids had displayed of late. They'd been acting so far out of character for the past month or so, she didn't know where to begin or even how to wrap her brain around it.

David didn't notice a thing, but he was completely preoccupied by what was going on at work. She could probably paint the house blood red inside and out and he wouldn't notice. Whenever she brought up the subject, he said she was worrying about nothing, or she was being delusional. "Don't make problems when there are none," and, "You need to let them go, Mother Bear!" were two of his favorite phrases.

Satis, the child formerly known as Audrey, seemed so aloof—dark, almost. Her clothing and hairstyles were becoming more and more creative. Lauren couldn't stand this new look and felt her daughter was slipping down a dangerous slope. Daily, she forced herself to take a deep breath and remember how much her own mother had hated her leg-warmers-and-torn-sweatshirt look. Styles and fashion changed with every generation, and Lauren knew it was a rite of passage to hate your child's look or taste in music.

Lauren wasn't sure where she was going to get the strength to make it through this phase, but as "Daddy" pointed out all too frequently, his darling, perfect daughter always brought home exceptional grades. Did it matter that when she was home she barricaded herself in her room and barely acknowledged "Mother?" It was hard to argue David's logic, and he seemed blinded by her "Daddy's little girl" routine. Maybe she was envious and blowing it out of proportion.

Then there was Jason. Always gone. So many practices and meetings for this club or that activity. It seemed endless. His life was a whirlwind, and the only way Lauren knew he'd been home was by the level of liquid in the milk container. Again, she remembered when she was a junior in high school. Life was so full then, and she, too, had her first tastes of freedom. At least Jason seemed happy, unlike Satis and her best friend, Ra.

But Jason's grades had slipped—just the tiniest bit—and it worried her.

"Give it a rest, would ya?" David growled at her last night. "The kid has a million things going on, and his grades are still fine. He'll most likely get a full-ride scholarship from any number of schools. Do you need him to go to Yale?"

"David, you're not seeing clearly. You barely spend any time with the kids or me, even when you're home."

"So that's what this is, Lauren," David scoffed. "Everyone else has a life and you don't."

That hurt. Was it so unrealistic to expect family dinners like she'd had growing up? Maybe it was true. Maybe she did need to go back to work or get a hobby, as David had so harshly pointed out last night. It seemed hard to fathom that this was about her and not about her family's self-destruction.

"Grand Central Station, final stop."

As Lauren stepped onto the platform, all the self-doubt vanished. Here, back in her city, she became energized. The smells of the station, the exhaust fumes, the hum of anonymous people moving at a brisk pace… it transformed her. The suburban mom/wife persona was buried deep, and the youthful city girl was freed from the recesses of her mind. *I'm an idiot*, Lauren thought. *David is probably right; this is all in my head. And not being able to let go of the kids… I really don't have a life of my own.*

Lauren started down Park Avenue, headed toward 34th Street. From there, she would walk over to the New York Public Library. It was a great morning, and the idea of doing some people watching while sitting on the library steps between the lions seemed like the perfect thing to do before meeting this person with the cottage in Michigan.

As she sat munching a salty, street-vendor pretzel, the thought really sank in. She had no life of her own. For the past decade and a half, she'd been consumed with kid this or that. In the beginning, micromanaging occupies a huge part of a mother's job description, but the kids were doing fine and didn't need her hovering over them continuously. It was part of growing up. *So maybe it's my turn now.*

Lauren looked at her watch and headed up 5th Avenue, taking an indirect path to her meeting and enjoying the sights and smells of the city, completely lost in thought. She convinced herself that a family summer vacation was exactly what the doctor ordered. Then, in the fall, she would do some freelance work again or perhaps take a couple classes.

CHAPTER 13

Audrey and Ashley sat in Starbucks, each with triple venti lattes. They were feeling the caffeine rush and discussing what to do after they got their second drink. The fourteen-year-old girls were still youthful enough to create imaginary characters and play-act. Their current theme was Egyptian gods, and the caffeine buzz accented the all-powerful feeling that went along with the mood.

"Ra, we need headdresses to complete the look," Audrey commented, chugging the latte cooled with a bit of ice.

"Ahh, Great Goddess of Hunting, it would seem you have found new prey." Ashley spoke with great seriousness, as befit her position. "Do you have a suggestion for hunting grounds?"

"Yeah, let's bolt double-fisted and do the mall."

"Are you sure, Aud?"

"Speak to me as Satis! We must flood our bodies with the life-giving healing potions of the River Star-Nile." The girls melted into laughter and ordered four more lattes, one for each hand.

The two got off the bus in Poughkeepsie and walked toward Kmart. Filled with the so-called magical properties of the river Nile and jittery from the coffee, they were oblivious to the stares of the other shoppers. Dashing from one department to another, they "hunted" for the correct headdress.

Spying gold-toned headbands in the personal beauty section, the girls tried them on, laughing and complimenting each other at the regal look.

"Ra, I gotta pee bad!"

"Me, too!" Ashley said. "The bathroom is in the back of the store. Follow me."

They ran through the aisles, ricocheting off people without slowing down to acknowledge or apologize. This caught the attention of the store security staff, who, unbeknownst to the girls, were waiting for them outside the bathroom.

As they washed their hands, Audrey leaned over and whispered, "Let's steal the headbands."

"Are you serious?" Ashley was a bit unnerved at the suggestion. "What if we get caught?"

"Oh come on! Don't be chicken." Audrey kept her voice low. "We'll just keep them on and walk out of the store. Who's ever going to notice?"

Less than one hundred percent certain it was a good idea, but following in her friend's lead, Ashley went along with the plan. Having brushed their hair and looking as if they'd been wearing the headbands all day long, the girls strolled out of the bathroom and into the welcoming arms of store security.

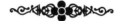

Ashley cried in the store manager's office while Audrey took the lead. She answered every question with complete confidence and a polished, polite tone.

"No, sir, we were not planning to steal the headbands. We tried them on and were heading to the checkout counter to pay for them," she explained. "You see, we were playing a game where we were pretending to be the Egyptian goddesses Ra and Satis." Audrey continued, using her obvious youth to her advantage.

"Where are your mothers?" the stern store manager asked.

Ashley was incapable of uttering a single word, so Audrey continued without batting an eye.

"My mom had to go to New York City for a few hours, so she dropped us and my older brother off here. He wanted to get pizza with a few of his friends, and we wanted to go shopping with the money our moms gave us." She continued, piling on lie after lie, completely confident she could talk her way out of the predicament. "I have a cell phone, and I said I would call him if anything happened. We're supposed to meet him at the pizza place in twenty minutes, so we went to the bathroom and were about to pay for the headbands."

The store manager remained silent as he studied the girls. Audrey didn't flinch, meeting his gaze with feigned innocence. He looked at Ashley, who could do nothing more than nod at him. Assuming she was scared but that the two were only guilty of being disruptive, he issued a stern warning.

"I believe you did not intend to steal the headbands; however, it is store policy not to bring merchandise into the restrooms."

"Oh my gosh!" Audrey blurted. "I didn't know. I'm so sorry, sir."

"Yes, well, there's the other matter of the two of you being disruptive in the store, running through the aisles and into our customers. We can't have that."

Audrey hung her head a bit and then looked up at him. "I'm very sorry, sir. I guess we got carried away with the game and weren't thinking. I promise we won't do it again. Really."

The store manager looked at the girls and deliberated for a minute longer before deciding to let them off the hook with a warning. He had no actual proof they were stealing the headbands, and police reports were time consuming.

"Okay, I'll let it go this time," he said. "I'll have security escort you out of the store, but I will keep your names on file. If you get into trouble here again, I will not be so lenient."

"Yes, sir, we understand. Thank you. And again, we are very sorry," Audrey said as Ashley nodded like a bobblehead doll.

The girls were escorted out of the store as promised. At first they walked slowly, nonchalantly, toward the far side of the mall where there was, indeed, a pizza shop.

When Audrey was certain they were in the clear, she exclaimed, "What a buffoon! I can't believe he bought all that. I have a craving for pizza. What do you say, Ra?"

CHAPTER 14

Lauren found the diner with ease and recognized Liza by her description. They introduced themselves and sat down in a booth, diving into the half-sour pickles placed on the table in front of them.

Lauren ordered a lox and egg scramble with a toasted plain bagel, her usual at any one of the hundreds of diners in Manhattan. Liza ordered the same. The busboy came by with coffee, and the two started in with the basic niceties. They quickly found a common ground from which to talk and were soon sharing intimate details of their lives as if they'd been lifelong friends separated by time.

When Liza asked why Lauren was looking for a summer vacation home, the tears and words just flowed. She hadn't realized how much she'd internalized her fears about her family and her marriage. At the end of the rant, covering everything she'd been thinking about for the past few weeks, Lauren sat back and took a breath.

All of a sudden it hit her: she'd dumped on a complete stranger nonstop for twenty minutes. Regaining her senses, she apologized profusely. "I don't know what just came over me! I'm so embarrassed." Lauren wiped the tears from her eyes. "I don't even know you, and here I just overwhelmed you with my own silly issues."

Liza took Lauren's hand in hers. Although she was younger than Lauren, her heart was touched by what Lauren had just shared with her.

"Please don't feel bad for telling me all that," Liza said. "First, you needed to get it off your chest before you exploded." Lauren chuckled but didn't remove her hand from the warm grasp of the woman across from her. "And, second, I completely get it."

Liza continued with her own tale about being the person who carried all the weight. How her brothers expected her to fix everything and contributed nothing. About missing her grandfather and her pressure to perform financially. "It's hard to be the responsible one in the family," Liza added. "Sometimes I just want to stop, walk away from it all, and let the pieces fall where they may... if only to see if any of the family notices." Liza paused to take a sip of coffee.

"But the problem with being the responsible one is that you can't help yourself. You are responsible—no matter what. It's innate, completely ingrained, and it will never be any other way. I'll bet you couldn't stop yourself if you tried," Liza added with a laugh.

The two women sat there for a moment, each lost in her own thoughts. The similarity of their feelings, despite their completely different situations, was astonishing. A bond was born at that diner, the kind of bond women often tend to develop. Each embraced the other's situation and was determined to help the other out, if possible.

Lauren agreed to rent the cottage for the summer season, sight unseen. Liza decided to drop the price to meet Lauren's budget. Although she wouldn't get the dues and extras completely covered with the agreement, she could come up to the cottage from time to time to visit her friends and get some sort of a summer vacation in. The house was more than big enough to accommodate Lauren's family, Liza, and a few guests, if needed.

Liza agreed to spend the first week of the rental in Charlevoix, introducing the family to the club members and showing them around. That way they would feel more at ease and really get the benefits the summer had to offer.

Liza didn't give a single thought to the more eccentric side of the club members. Like any family, everyone had their share of peculiarities. She didn't stop to consider how the party atmosphere might affect a family on the verge of falling apart.

Chapter 15

Karen was somewhere between fuming and panicked. She and Jason had been texting each other regularly since they'd parted company over a week ago. Jason kept saying he wanted to see her, but things kept coming up and the excuses were starting to wear thin.

She was deathly afraid he was the type of guy who would sleep with her and then ditch her. Or maybe he had a girlfriend... or a wife. At the same time, she missed him so badly it hurt. Her heart ached with longing and desire, she couldn't eat, and every time the phone rang or a text came through she pounced. Karen felt stupid for acting like a teenager.

On a Thursday night, almost two weeks from the last time Karen had been with Jason, he finally asked her out again. Of course she jumped at the chance and then cursed herself for being so easy. Dinner and a movie was his suggestion, casual, as if nothing was wrong. He didn't mention spending the night together or anything about the upcoming weekend.

In fact, now that she thought about it, she didn't really know much about Jason. He seemed secretive about certain things. Not in any overt way, but he often ducked questions or changed the subject back to things about her. It was flattering, and she was unable to recognize it when it happened, but in the end, when she lay alone at night thinking about him, she realized how little she actually knew.

Maybe it was simply an age thing. Maybe he was embarrassed to be in college while she'd already graduated. That had to be the reason for the secrecy. Jason was uncomfortable because he was still in school. Karen had to figure out a way to let him know she was okay with it, the age thing didn't matter. Besides, it was only a couple years. Worst case, he was twenty-one years old. If that was the problem, she needed to let him know four years wouldn't make much of a difference when they were thirty or forty. After all, Jason didn't know exactly how old she was either, and maybe he felt uncomfortable about being with an older woman.

Relieved now that she thought she'd figured out what he was hiding, she decided to find a way to make him more comfortable. She would lead the discussion at the appropriate time. So, with great anticipation, she picked out the sexiest sweater she could find—a black, fitted, angora that was soft against her skin and made her boobs look huge. *This man will not be able to resist my charms,* she thought. A little dab of perfume and she was out the door to meet her guy.

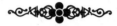

Jason had to lay low the entire week to calm his mom down. She'd flipped out on him when he came home from the weekend in the cabin. Granted, he'd pushed the limits, but he couldn't risk getting busted. There had to be some solution to this problem. At least his friends at school had calmed down, but they were riding him for being secretive, performing disappearing acts. Now Karen was starting to ask questions, too. That was all he needed. Why did people keep sticking their noses in his business? It was his life, and they should all just leave him alone.

Finally, he figured out a plan. His mom was away for the day, and Dad was stuck at work. If he left before they got home, he would only have to deal with the fallout when he got home late, assuming they caught him sneaking in. With any luck, he'd be able to get into the house without getting caught.

Audrey would probably catch him, but at this point he had so much dirt on her he could threaten back. She would back down fast, after the shit she pulled last week. If he busted her, she'd be grounded until the end of time.

Yeah, things were lined up pretty good. Maybe one of these days he could actually use Audrey, or whatever the hell she was calling herself these days, as an accomplice. Now that was a novel thought, something to consider later.

Jason threw on jeans, a T-shirt, and a sweater. At the last minute, he grabbed his backpack and sports bag. He could ditch them in the bushes and pick them up on his way home as an extra precaution to make whatever excuse he came up with seem reasonable. As he made his way out the door and jogged the half-mile to the bus stop, he thought about how much easier things would be when he got his driver's license next fall.

Jason got to the movie theater complex twenty minutes before he and Karen had planned to meet, so he wandered around a bit. Spying a small flower shop on the corner, he ducked in, figuring a flower or two might break the tension he'd felt from her. A rose implied too much; he needed something different, something with a touch of silliness to it. In the window display, there were some really cool flowers made of colorful pipe cleaners, created by local kids to support a cause he didn't care about. He picked out a multicolored daisy and hurried back to the theater.

Karen was waiting but didn't see him coming. Man, she was hot! Jason no longer had any interest in dinner and a movie, his mind turning to more carnal thoughts.

Jason snuck up behind her and wrapped the hand with the flower around Karen so she could see it. With the other arm, he pulled her into his body as tight as he could and whispered in her ear. "A flower for, without question, the most beautiful woman for as far as I can see." Jason kissed her neck, softly at first, then with a bit more intensity as Karen giggled and relaxed into his arms. Her body fit perfectly to his. Jason's desire for her became evident.

"I'm sorry, sir, but I'm meeting a friend here tonight, and while your offering is highly tempting, I'm afraid you'll have to take a number."

Jason turned Karen around. "I'm unwilling to take no for an answer," he said just before he kissed her deeply.

"Well, since you put it that way..." Karen wrapped her arms around his shoulders and kissed him back with equal intensity. The physical desire consumed them. Karen pulled away first.

Breathless, she asked if they could have dinner first, her treat this time. She'd already picked out a quiet Italian place near the movie theater and parked her car there in anticipation of his agreeing to her plan.

Jason agreed, hungrily kissed Karen again, and they started toward the restaurant. As always, Jason controlled the conversation, telling Karen she looked stunning and how much he'd missed her over the past two weeks. He didn't let her get a single question in.

Being a gentleman, he reached the door first to open it for Karen. As they were about to walk in, Jason ran headfirst into people he knew. The possibility had never occurred to him, and he was shocked into silence, stunned, not knowing what to do or say or how to cover his tracks.

"Jason, my boy, so good to see you." The man reached out to shake Jason's hand while clapping him on the shoulder.

"Dr. Thielman, Mrs. Thielman, nice to see you, too."

Stan Thielman was a friend of his parents, in his early seventies but still active in the community. His wife, Norma, looked from Jason to Karen and back but didn't say anything.

"Honey, look, it's Jason Breckenridge," Dr. Thielman said. "Why, we haven't seen you since you anchored the swim team relay that won the championship. You certainly have grown since then. Tell me, boy, do you still swim?"

The knot in Jason's stomach was enormous, and he could barely breathe. "Yes, sir, that was a few years ago. I play water polo now. It's good to see you, sir."

The Thielmans looked at Karen in anticipation of an introduction. Jason quickly recovered. "Oh, please excuse my manners. I didn't expect to bump into anyone here." He paused and tried his best to sound natural. "This is Karen Alderson, a friend of mine." Jason was positive everyone could hear his heart pounding. "We were just going to grab a quick bite before a movie."

"Oh well, then don't let us keep you, my boy. Do try the salmon special tonight. It was delicious, wasn't it, honey?" He didn't wait for his wife to answer. "And please give your parents our best when you see them. It's been far too long."

Jason shook hands with the older couple, as did Karen, and the two entered the restaurant without another word spoken until they were seated. Jason's heart was thumping a mile a minute, his mouth as dry as sandpaper. Thankfully, the busboy filled their water glasses right away, so Jason gulped half the glass while struggling to compose himself. He hoped Karen didn't notice his hand shaking.

As he drained his water glass, the waiter came up to the table to introduce himself, announce the specials, and ask if they wanted to order some wine. It seemed to Jason that the waiter gave him an especially long stare, and he decided now was not the time to push his luck.

"I'd just like some more water with lemon," he said. He asked Karen if that was okay with her and explained that he'd been dealing with a headache all day and just wanted to hydrate himself. Karen agreed, and the two decided to split a steamed artichoke and then have the salmon special for dinner.

Thankfully, the ordering was easy, and it gave him a few more minutes to regroup. Jason looked Karen in the eye and convincingly told her again how much he had missed her and how sorry he was for letting it go so long. Jason seemed sincere to Karen and she mistook his obvious distress as feelings of guilt for letting her down. She forgave him and let all of her misgivings go.

The rest of dinner flew by as the conversation sparkled between the two. Playful teasing, touching on current events and their musical tastes—the sort of magical evening new couples enjoy as they get to know each other. Karen and Jason were so wrapped up in their conversation that they barely noticed where they were or how the food tasted. By the time the check came, it was much too late to catch a movie.

Jason walked Karen to her car and leaned her against the side, pressing into her. The heat sizzled between them as they kissed with reckless abandon, grinding together, neither wanting to suspend the magic or stop the evening.

Jason pulled away first. "Oh my God, babe, you are driving me wild!" he groaned breathlessly.

"Good, then I'm succeeding." Karen pulled him into her again, rubbing his erection through his pants as he drove his hips against her hand.

"I need you! Now!"

It was not exactly what Karen had envisioned for the two of them, but she was also beyond the point of no return. Looking around the now-empty parking lot, she undid her jeans and pushed his hand between her legs. Once he felt how wet she was, it was too much. Jason demanded the keys to her car which she handed over quickly. Pushing her into the back seat, the two fumbled with their clothes until they were undressed enough for him to push inside her. It was over almost before it started.

Lying on top of her in the back seat, Jason whispered, "You drive me crazy, you are the most exciting girl I've ever known." They reassembled their clothes, and Jason ended the evening before she could invite him back to her place. He let her know he had an early day and asked if she was okay driving home by herself.

Later, in the shower, she had mixed emotions about the evening. Going at it in the backseat of her car felt odd. And he'd called her a girl. It all seemed so immature. Something was unsettling her, but she couldn't figure out what it was. The night went well, she enjoyed his company, and he certainly turned her on... but again, this nagging voice wouldn't go away.

With a good old-fashioned talking to, she told herself to stop overanalyzing things. It only serves to ruin things.

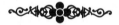

Jason watched Karen drive away as he walked back toward the movie theater. Once the coast was clear, he called Alec on his cell phone. "Dude, where are you? I need a ride bad."

"Jase, are you kidding me? It's late and I'm home."

"Seriously, man, I need a cover story, and it has to be a good one."

Alec dutifully picked his buddy up, and the two concocted a flat tire story for Jason's parents. Walking inside Jason's house together, they found his dad at the kitchen table. It was an easy sell.

CHAPTER 16

Another weekend with kids scattered. David and Lauren found themselves at home alone. They were on opposite ends of the house working on chores. Lauren had copious amounts of laundry piled on the bed ready to be folded and stuck in the kids' rooms. David was fixing something in the garage.

David could spend forever futzing around in his garage. Cleaning, organizing, fixing, painting... Who knows how he managed to kill so much time out there? It was as if the garage were his mistress and he her slave. The neighbors envied the pristine floors—you really could eat off them—and the pegboards with outlines of tools to show the less knowledgeable where to hang each item. Nothing out of place. Heaven forbid you borrow a tool and then put it back in the wrong location! Hell hath no fury like a man looking for his three-eighths-inch torque wrench.

As much as she teased and the neighbors envied, Lauren really did admire his ability to stay organized, and he could fix just about anything. They rarely had to hire a handyman, as David had this ability to take something apart, understand how it works, find the culprit, and replace it. This made him happy, so she steered clear. Particularly given the stress of his work situation.

After the mountain of laundry was finished, Lauren decided to lure her man out of his cave. They had much to discuss, and since the kids would be gone for the rest of the day, now was better than never.

Feeling playful and energized from her trip to the city, Lauren decided to try to recapture her youth. Digging through her dresser, she found a light blue silk teddy and matching tap pants—the ultimate in sexy waitress apparel.

Stopping in the kitchen, she made him a turkey sandwich and opened a beer. *This should get his attention!* She smiled at the thought. Thankfully, the garage door was closed to the outside as she entered the side door.

"David, I made you some lunch," she said playfully. His back was turned to her, so he didn't see the whole picture.

"Thanks, hon, just set it down. I'll get to it in a minute."

"David, it's hot now, and I wouldn't want you to miss out." Lauren tried to sound as mischievous as she could without ruining the effect.

David sighed. "Just one second, okay? I'll be right there." He never looked up. Lauren stood there for a minute, not knowing what to do and feeling foolish. The playful mood she was in drained away, only to be replaced with sadness and rejection.

Lauren's silence caught David's attention, and he turned around to find his rather shapely wife wearing slinky underwear and holding the lunch she'd prepared for him. Her lip quivered; he knew her well enough to know she was fighting tears.

"Lauren, what... ? I didn't know. I..." David's stammering didn't help the situation at all.

"What does it take for you to see me, David?" Lauren whispered as the tears streamed down her cheeks. "I don't know why I bother to try anymore."

David put down his latest project and walked over to her. "Lauren, sweetie, I'm sorry. I was preoccupied. Really. You look wonderful, and I do appreciate the lunch." He took the plate and beer from her and put it on a nearby counter.

Lauren just stood there, crying, and feeling like an ass. "David, you're always preoccupied with something or another. I feel as if I'm married to the house, not to a man. I'm a servant in my own home, and it hurts like hell."

David looked down at his feet, not knowing what to say. She was right in many ways; he just didn't want to admit it to her. David took her hand and led her over to his workbench, pulling her onto his lap as he sat down. He kissed her forehead and then each cheek—tender kisses that did nothing to stop the trickle of her tears. As he admired her nipples, he traced the outline of each with his fingertip and smiled as they hardened on command. Still no words were spoken. Lauren turned toward him and straddled his legs as she slipped her arms around his shoulders. David reached beneath her teddy, his fingers brushing across her warm skin. She quivered at his touch.

Pushing aside the crotch of her shorts, he reached inside her as she rocked instinctively against his hand. Standing slightly, he undid his own shorts and pulled them to his knees, pulling her on to him. Pressing his face between her breasts and keeping his hand between her legs they rocked together and in less than a minute both climaxed within seconds of each other.

David giggled a bit and kissed Lauren lightly on the lips. "Nice appetizer. Now what did you make for lunch?"

Lauren chuckled but felt empty inside. She straightened herself up and brought the sandwich to him while he pulled up his shorts. David took a huge bite of the turkey sandwich, offering Lauren a bite which she gratefully accepted.

After a pull on the beer, he paused, studying her. "I am one lucky guy. I have the best wife ever."

Lauren half-smiled. "And don't you forget it, buster." But her feelings did not match the words. She felt lonely. So much so, she suspected if she were in a room with 15,000 people she would feel the same way. Lonely.

After finishing the sandwich, the two sat on the bench in the garage, exchanging information on the week. One would be hard pressed to call it a conversation; it was more like a status report.

Lauren told David about Liza and the cottage in Michigan. She went over the amenities like a laundry list. She told him how much she liked Liza and that she would be there to introduce the family to the members of the club and show them around. David asked a single question about finances, and since it was priced within their budget, he simply said, "Sound's good. Let's do it."

David's news was a bit more startling. His furlough would begin June fifteenth and run through Labor Day. Because of his contract, he'd receive full pay and benefits. His staff was not as lucky; they would receive between fifty and sixty-five percent, depending on their position and years of service.

David told her he'd managed to negotiate that his whole staff would retain their jobs once the company started up again in September, but he expected some would have found other jobs by then, considering their talent level. His major concern was how much ground he would lose when they needed to ramp up for the next level of testing and development.

Lauren listened intently. She suggested to David that they host an early summer family party as a way of spreading good faith among his people. Perhaps if he brought the group together and reassured them the situation was temporary, then his staff might look at it as a summer opportunity to do something different and fun.

David thought it was a good idea. He kissed Lauren on the forehead and praised her for being so creative and caring.

Now that the plans were set, they moved on to implementation. They decided to wait until the beginning of June to tell the kids of the summer plans. It was late April, and they both felt it would be too much of a distraction when the kids needed to be focused on studying for finals. A month of not knowing wouldn't kill them.

Chapter 17

Audrey sat on the edge of the fountain near Town Center, bored to tears. She wanted something fun and exciting to do. Everything was so ordinary! She thought she was going to lose her mind. Jason had said he would take her to the baseball game but then ditched her as soon as they got to town.

He refused to tell her where he was going but threatened her with certain death if she said anything to anyone. Although she didn't exactly know what she wasn't supposed to tell, he'd found out about the shoplifting incident, and if he told their parents she was screwed. Audrey thought it was the perfect example of nuclear deterrence. Neither of them wanted to die, so they simultaneously threatened each other with disclosure. She must have been awake in history class that day.

She and Ashley had not seen each other much after they were busted. They'd had a scene at lunch one day, with Ashley insisting it had all been too scary and she didn't want to get into trouble again. *Wimp*, Audrey thought. *She really needs to grow up.*

Throwing her backpack over her shoulder, Audrey headed to the back of the park. It was where the stoner dudes usually hung out. She didn't know any of them personally, but maybe if she hung out she could score a beer or something.

It was early May and warm outside. She was fairly filled out for a fourteen-year-old and liked to use it to her advantage. She was wearing an old T-shirt that was a little too tight, so she figured if she took her bra off, she might meet some guy who would pay attention to her.

She approached the swing set where the older kids hung out. One of the guys was standing on a swing, seeing how high he could go without falling. With complete confidence, she walked up to the group of guys, the benefit of an older, highly competitive brother about to pay off in spades. "Betcha a beer I can go higher than your friend," she said. There was the expected laughter and eye rolling, but one of the guys, leaning against a tree to the side of the playground area, took her bet in a heartbeat.

"Look at this little girly girl who thinks she's so tough. I'll take that bet, girly."

He looked at a kid sitting on one of the other seats. "Russ, get off that swing so the girly girl can kick Brad's ass."

The boys burst into laughter, and Russ got off the swing with a mock bow. "It's all yours, girly."

Audrey sat on the swing first, and then she stood, pretending to be a bit unsteady. "Hey, girly, wanna make it double or nothin'?" the boy near the tree called out, eliciting more laughter.

On the other swing, Brad paid them no mind as he pumped away, the beat echoing through his headphones drowning out everything around him.

Audrey glanced at her challenger. *This is going to be fun.*

"What's the matter, girly, you chickening out?"

"You're on, double or nothing." Within a few pumps, Audrey had matched Brad's height. She listened as the boys on the ground urged him to go higher, but Brad already looked a bit green and unsteady.

A few more pumps and Audrey was flying as high as possible, to the point where the chain broke its tension as the seat of the swing paralleled the top crossbar. Brad saw this, sat down on the swing, and dragged his feet to slow himself. When he came to a complete stop, he staggered to the side of the swing set and puked.

The boys groaned and claimed to be grossed out, calling Brad a pussy for letting a girl show him up. Audrey, completely satisfied with the win, slowed the swing a bit, and when it reached a safe height, she jumped to the grassy area, landing in a crouched position. It was an Olympics-worthy dismount.

She brushed herself off, picked up her backpack, and walked over to the boy by the tree. He was cute in a stoner sort of way. His brown hair was shoulder length, and his eyes were a razor-sharp blue. "You owe me a beer, slacker," Audrey said to him.

The boy nodded toward a cooler, inviting her to help herself. Audrey had never tasted beer before, but she wasn't about to lose her nerve. She grabbed a can of Bud and popped it open, taking a swig as she'd seen other kids do. Her eyes watered and her throat burned, but the challenge was there and she wasn't going to lose.

She walked back over to the old oak and leaned against it. "You got a name, girly?"

"Bite me."

The boy looked her up and down and smiled. "Nice to meet you, Bite Me. I'm Matt." He laughed, and Audrey joined in with him.

"I'm Audrey."

They hung out for a bit, not really talking but bitching and teasing about one thing or another. Audrey was on her third beer when she saw Jason waiting at the fountain.

"I gotta go," she said, her words slurred. "My brother is waiting for me." Matt followed her glance toward the fountain and then looked back at her.

"Whatever you say, Audrey Breckenridge." She did a complete double take, looking from Matt to her brother and back again. Matt laughed a little harder. "Come back again sometime, girly." As she turned to go, Matt swatted her ass, and she couldn't help but squeal. He gave her a wink and sauntered over to his friends.

Audrey staggered over to her brother. "I don't feel so good."

"Jesus, Aud, have you been drinking?"

Audrey responded by puking at her brother's feet. Jason jumped out of the way just in time. The last thing he needed was to go home with a drunk little sister, both of them smelling like puke.

"Fuck, man, you're going to owe me big."

Audrey puked again.

Jason waited until he figured she had nothing left to throw up. Then he grabbed their backpacks, took her arm, and led her three blocks to the diner where Alec worked in the kitchen.

Jason walked her to the back door and parked her on a bench. He actually said "don't go anywhere," but from the looks of her he wasn't too worried about it.

He'd been with Karen for most of the day. It was the first time he'd gone to her place, and they had planned to go out. One thing led to another, and they ended up spending the entire day in bed, not that anyone was complaining.

He told Karen he couldn't stay late because he had a "family thing" he had to do. She asked a bunch of questions and he lied, saying his kid sister had a performance and he was expected to be there. It seemed to satisfy her curiosity, so he left it at that.

As he walked into the kitchen, Alec saw him and questioned why he'd come in through the back door. Jason headed to the slop sink, grabbed a stack of dish towels, and motioned out the door. Alec glanced out and rolled his eyes.

"Damn! These kids start younger and younger," Alec said. The boys burst into laughter, remembering a time not so long ago when the two of them had found themselves in a similar situation.

"Hand me the towels, man," Alec directed. "You call your peeps and tell them you're at the diner. I get off work in an hour and will drive you home. Say you're both studying or some shit. Maybe we can get the train wreck sobered up by then."

Jason called his parents who bought the lie—hook, line, and sinker.

Now that things were back in order, Jason turned his attention to his sister. He had enough practice at sobering up and wasn't too worried about this incident. He did, however, consider how useful the situation would be in terms of blackmail. It all fit together perfectly. Audrey would become a cover story for his relationship with Karen.

CHAPTER 18

Audrey and Jason were getting closer in an odd sort of way: each had dirt to hold over the other's head if they stepped too far out of line. But with this friendship of sorts came an understanding. They were able to share some of the secrets they'd been holding on to, relieving the pressure a bit. And with that truce, they helped each other avoid detection.

Their parents noticed the sudden bond and were pleased, thinking a closer relationship would be good for both of them. Lauren was lulled into complacency, assuming David had been correct after all: she'd been overreacting. She turned her attention to making plans. Not wanting to rock the boat, she continued to keep quiet about the upcoming summer's change of venue.

The month of May slipped by without any turmoil. David focused on the last-minute loose ends he needed to tie up before the shutdown. Lauren worked on plans for a Memorial Day pool party and cookout for David's staff in an effort to reassure them about David's commitment to keep all of them when the company reopened in the fall. David had convinced the company to issue retention bonuses in lieu of paychecks—a small advance now and then a more significant bonus six months after the company started up again. He planned to announce this at the party, hand out checks, and thank his staff for their efforts.

On the few times the whole family sat down together, their conversation was more a question-and-answer game than real communication. David, as patriarch, would ask questions, completely satisfied with "fine" or "good" offered up in response. Though sometimes the answers were followed by an equally shallow sentence of explanation, more often than not there was nothing more said. On the surface, everyone seemed content... busy, but content.

Eventually, Lauren relaxed and stopped looking for problems that didn't exist. She wanted nothing more than a simple, peaceful life. It was what she was accustomed to; it was the definition she'd been taught for the term "happy family."

Lauren's father served in Korea before she was born, but that was all she knew about it. He was a decorated veteran. He celebrated both Memorial and Veterans

Day by participating in parades with quiet dignity and pride. She knew he saw action and was wounded at some point, but he never talked about it. Neither did her mother.

What she didn't know was that her father had suffered significant trauma from the atrocities of war. He'd been a prisoner of war for long enough to affect him for the rest of his life. Survival became his life goal. When he returned, he was a significantly different person, and his young bride had to accept her new reality.

Lauren's father, once determined to make a name for himself, was now satisfied with complacency. He no longer aspired for anything but peace and quiet, and he'd passed this character trait on to his daughter. If everything seemed peaceful, then it was. Period. It was that simple.

Lauren became complacent in her own way: she became wife and mother, doing the best she could to keep her children content. It was the reason she'd never aspired to her own career or to lead any groups. She was the proverbial worker bee who did the tasks assigned to her with great care and attention to detail. Things ran smoothly in her volunteer positions, and that was exactly how she wanted her family to function. She trusted her children were telling the truth when Jason and Audrey said they'd stayed late at the library or coffee shop to study for finals.

The party went off without a hitch. The kids hung around to make an appearance and then went off to hang with friends for the weekend.

Lauren glowed with pride as her husband relaxed and socialized with his coworkers. David was in his element: happy, gregarious, generous, and funny. All the traits she'd fallen in love with years ago. Lauren looked and acted the part of the perfect wife. She refreshed everyone's drinks and made sure people were comfortable. She dressed the part, wearing a fitted floral sundress that flattered her figure and skin tone. Everything was perfect.

Throughout the evening, she would catch David's eye. He was happy as well; she could tell by his body language. The last of their guests had cleared out by 11 p.m. It was a clear, unusually warm night for late May. As Lauren picked up around the pool area, David strolled over to her and gently took the towels and empty glasses out of her arms, placing them on a nearby chaise.

Wrapping his arms around her, he whispered in her ear, "When was the last time I told you how amazing you are? Tonight was perfect. Thank you."

Lauren was at peace. She melted into her husband's embrace with tears of joy.

CHAPTER 19

Audrey ditched Jason at the diner. Matt and his friends had planned to go camping for the weekend at Lake Taconic, about an hour north of Millbrook. They had a van loaded, and at the last minute, Matt suggested Audrey join them. The group seemed comfortable with Audrey, and she was anything but bored when she hung out with them. Usually it consisted of drinking beer or something a little stronger and walking around town or sitting in a car listening to tunes.

Matt seemed to have taken an interest in her, which she didn't mind too much. He was cute. Audrey hadn't dated yet, so she was clueless when it came to relationships. The two of them were comfortable hanging out together. It was easy, and Audrey liked the feeling of acceptance.

The idea of going camping for the weekend seemed like fun. Jason wanted to go away for the weekend with his new girlfriend, so they'd concocted a plan. The cover story was simple: a club at school had a weekend trip planned. Jason agreed to act as chaperone, because he knew his parents had the big party that weekend. It worked so easily the two of them could not believe they hadn't thought of it sooner.

Without any fear or concern, they each simply went their own way with the tacit agreement of "don't ask, don't tell."

Audrey climbed into the van and wedged in the middle, her body pushed against Matt's. He put his arm around her as if she were his property for the weekend. Matt said a couple other carloads of people would meet them at the park.

By the time they found a spot and set up the campsite, it was getting dark. Someone started a campfire. Everyone was drinking beers and roasting hotdogs or eating chips. She overheard a group of girls talking about their friends' plans to drop acid, but since she really didn't know what that meant, she just smiled and nodded. Her goth look kept other girls at a distance. Audrey exuded an air of aloofness, more than anything else. She covered her insecurities with a gruff exterior. It was this challenging persona that attracted Matt to her in the first place. She was a curiosity, a play thing. He could tell she wasn't as experienced as she tried to portray. It became a game to him.

"Hey, Bite Me, you wanna smoke some weed with me?" He called her by her pet name as he had since the day they'd met. She wondered if he even remembered her real name.

But Matt knew exactly who she was. She was the great Jason Breckenridge's little sister. Matt was in Jason's class in school. When they were freshmen, Matt had wanted to be on the swim team. He tried out for the same events as Jason and came in second to him every time. The coach selected him for the team, but when it came to the individual events, he always lost to Jason. His own father, an abusive alcoholic, would look at the ribbons and in his drunken rants would blurt out, "Second place is the first loser."

After that year, Matt dropped out of swimming and practically everything else. He couldn't deal with his father's abuse, and he just didn't care. He and Jason never became friends; in fact, Jason was the embodiment of his anger. Not that any bad words were ever spoken. Matt's anger manifested itself in the form of perfect Jason Breckenridge. And now, here stood his kid sister, ripe for the taking.

Audrey played it cool and took the pipe from Matt. She had observed how he'd smoked it and tried to imitate the actions. Audrey pulled too much smoke into her lungs and fell to the ground in a coughing fit. She heard chuckling from those gathered around the campfire, and her face reddened with humiliation.

As she regained her composure, she downed half a beer to kill the burn and asked Matt to hand her the pipe. Matt, feeling a twinge of guilt, told her to take a smaller pull, hold it in her lungs as long as she could, and then let it out slowly. This time it worked much better. She felt as if her body was floating in slow motion. The stars were twinkling and everything seemed light.

She and Matt wandered down to the lake and continued to drink beer and get high for the rest of the night. When Audrey woke in the morning, she was lying on the beach with Matt spooning her. They were fully clothed, but she had no recollection of passing out.

As the other campers awoke, someone cooked passable scrambled eggs and bacon on the campfire, and one of the girls took Audrey to a park bathroom where they could get changed and wash up.

"Why does Matt call you Bite Me?" the girl asked. With a laugh, she told the girl the story, omitting the part where she puked for the rest of the afternoon.

"I'm Nancy," the girl said. "I hang out with Bill." Audrey was glad to have someone to talk to, though she wasn't exactly sure which of the guys was Bill. "So, are you like Matt's girlfriend or something?"

Audrey wasn't sure what to say, so she avoided the question with a shrug.

Nancy took that for a yes.

"He's cute," Nancy added in a nonchalant tone.

"I guess. My name's Audrey."

Nancy looked at Audrey for a second before responding. "I know. Everyone knows who you are."

Audrey was confused by the comment but didn't say anything. She changed into her bathing suit and a T-shirt, and the two of them walked back to the beach. Someone had brought a canoe, and there were an assortment of rafts and even a little sailboat. When she got within earshot, Matt called her to the water's edge.

He was knee-deep in the water, holding tight to the canoe. "Hop in," he said. It was more a command than a request, but she didn't care and climbed into the front. Matt pushed off and paddled away from shore. There was a tree-covered island in the middle of the lake, and he headed around toward the far side. Audrey relaxed and the two fell into a comfortable conversation about nothing in particular.

Matt found it easy to talk to Audrey. She didn't require much of him, just accepted him at his word. It was comfortable. He didn't have to work at it like with some of the other girls he'd dated. This Breckenridge chick was simple to be with.

He pulled up to the shore and hopped out. Audrey did the same. Matt tossed her a blanket which she spread out on the beach while he pulled the canoe further up onto the sand.

Matt produced his pipe and the two got stoned again. The conversation flowed smoothly, but they eventually quieted as the initial buzz mellowed. Matt pushed Audrey down on the blanket and kissed her. She was stiff at first but soon relaxed, thanks to the effects of the pot.

Without warning, Matt jumped up and climbed back into the canoe. "Pick up the crap and bring it over," he grumbled. Audrey had no idea what she'd done wrong. She worried she was a bad kisser and dutifully followed his instructions. They paddled back to the others in silence. Insecure about angering Matt and having no intention of showing it, Audrey adopted her gruff "whatever" attitude.

They rejoined the group, Matt going off with two of his buddies while she hung out with Nancy. The rest of the afternoon passed quickly, and by nightfall, the guys were passing out shots of a thick, sweet alcohol. Audrey hated the taste but enjoyed the warmth and buzz. She refused to feel anything.

Later that night, Matt walked up to her and sat down on a nearby log. He didn't say anything but handed her a pipe as truce. She relaxed as she smoked the weed. The smell of the smoke was different this time.

"What was that?" she asked.

"Hash." He struggled to his feet. "Let's go for a walk." Matt grabbed a blanket and a six-pack of beer, and the two headed away from the campfire.

"Sorry about before," Matt said once the others were no longer within earshot. Audrey said nothing, enjoying the buzz and not quite sure she could form words or thoughts anyway. "I freaked on you. Didn't mean to."

Audrey stopped walking and looked up at Matt. "No biggie. We're friends, right?"

"Yeah, right." His gut-laugh caught Audrey by surprise.

He spread the blanket on the ground and pulled her next to him. They lay there in silence, side by side, looking at the stars. Matt tucked himself in tight against Audrey's back and put his mouth to her neck, kissing and nibbling her with surprising tenderness. Reaching around, he cupped her breast with his hand and thrust his hips into her. She knew he had a boner, but the buzz took the edge off her nerves. She remained completely still, unsure of what to do. Soon, she heard deep breathing and knew Matt had fallen asleep.

The next morning, the campers moved slowly, packing up their belongings and heading to the cars. Nancy gave her a look that Audrey had no clue how to interpret.

When they got back to the diner in Millbrook, Matt and Audrey clambered out of the van and headed to the back to retrieve Audrey's backpack. As they stood behind the vehicle, Matt saw Jason looking out the diner's back window at them. He put one arm around Audrey, pulled her roughly into him, and kissed her hard, deep, possessing her.

When he'd had enough, Matt looked up at the window and made eye contact with Jason. "See ya later, Bite Me," Matt said loud enough for everyone in the van to hear.

Jason stared at his sister as she slid into the booth opposite him. He knew he should say something, but that would open up his weekend to questions. It was a risk he couldn't take.

So they said nothing and ordered breakfast.

CHAPTER 20

Lauren confirmed her family would all be home for dinner. She and David decided they would surprise the kids with the summer plans this evening. It was early June and the last day of school. There had been more grumbling than she expected; both Jason and Audrey had parties they wanted to go to.

Normally she would have shrugged it off and postponed until another night, but, filled with confidence from the party and excited about the summer plans, she told the children that she and their father had something important to tell them, and if they could just be home for dinner they could go out later.

Lauren spent the day marinating chicken and making a fresh mango salsa. As a gesture to introducing them to Northern Michigan, she baked a cherry pie. She had done research into the area, learning about the history and local lore. The cottage was near Traverse City, which was known for being "The Cherry Capitol of the World" and had a huge cherry festival each year. Well, she thought it sounded different, maybe it could be fun, though she could picture her family thinking her corny.

She told the family to be home by 5:30 for an early barbeque dinner. Lauren had just finished setting the outside table when she heard the doorbell ring. It was nearly 5 p.m. She wasn't expecting anyone.

❧⟡❀⟡❧

Karen had been crying for days. Once again, she and Jason had spent a great weekend together over Memorial Day. And, once again, he'd disappeared for the two weeks that followed.

She still knew next to nothing about him. Her instincts told her he was hiding something, but for the life of her, she couldn't figure it out. They'd been seeing each other for almost five months, and she'd never been invited to his home. They always met somewhere in public. Their sporadic weekends together were either at her place or the cabin. She'd driven them to Atlantic City once, but Jason didn't want to go to the clubs to dance or go drinking.

On the flip side, she was deeply in love with him. Their time together was magical. He was present—in the moment—and focused on her needs. Sexually, he was unstoppable. She also loved how playful he was at times. His youthful energy was infectious.

This week, for some unknown reason, she was overly emotional and feeling vulnerable. On her way home from work the other day she burst into tears without provocation.

Karen knew she had to get to the truth of the matter. Something was not quite right, and she wouldn't be truly happy until she found out what it was. A little bit of research on-line turned up an address in Millbrook. The listing provided only the first initial and last name, but it was her best shot. The thought crossed her mind that maybe Jason Breckenridge wasn't even his real name.

"Get ahold of yourself, girl," she muttered to herself as she drove through town to scope the place out. She was turning into a bona fide stalker. Thinking back, didn't they run into friends of his parents at that restaurant? The address could be his parents' place; he may not live there at all. He'd also mentioned his sister once.

But that was the whole point. It was *once*. He didn't share details about his life—not his school, not his work, not his family. Nothing. Karen took a deep breath. *What's the worst case scenario?* she wondered. *That he was living with another woman, and I was his affair. And, if that really was the issue, then wouldn't I want to fight for my man?*

Either way, she had to know. No more secrets. It was driving her insane. Karen gathered her courage, walked up to the front door of the home, and rang the doorbell. Her hands shook with each pounding beat of her heart, and she didn't trust her legs to keep her upright. She didn't know what to expect, but it definitely wasn't the pretty woman, just a few years her senior, who opened the door, dish towel in hand.

Karen's mouth went dry as the ugly truth hit her in an instant: she was the proverbial "other woman." Her peripheral vision darkened, and her knees buckled under her. She fell straight into Lauren's arms.

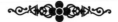

Lauren was a bit surprised when she saw the striking woman at her door. And when she toppled over into Lauren's arms, she didn't quite know what to do, but she couldn't just let the woman fall into a heap and slam the door in her face. Clearly she was in a great deal of distress.

Lauren struggled to get the woman into the house and settled her on the couch in the living room. The woman was shaking and sobbing; something had frightened her to her very core. Dashing into the kitchen, Lauren dampened a clean dishcloth and grabbed a bottle of water from the fridge.

"I would ask if you're okay, but clearly you're not." Lauren put the damp cloth behind the woman's neck and handed her the opened water bottle. "Here, take a sip. My name is Lauren Breckenridge." She paused to study the woman, who seemed to be in her late twenties. "Relax for a minute; take a breath. Can you tell me your name?"

The woman nodded. "Karen. Karen Alderson. I... I... Oh my God!" She sobbed, holding the towel to her face, spitting out a string of nonsensical words. But a few of them did come through loud and clear: affair, other woman, had to find out, didn't know. Lauren swallowed hard, a rock formed in her stomach, and she wanted to puke.

My God! Lauren thought, *David is having an affair with this young woman!* She had no idea how one handled this sort of situation, but her world came crashing down around her. Consumed by horror, shock, and disbelief, Lauren desperately wanted to believe this Karen person had the wrong house or was horribly mistaken somehow. But something resonated from deep inside her. There was no mistaking this woman's total heartbreak, and Lauren was perched on the edge of the abyss, ready to join her in utter ruin.

Fate has an extraordinary way of twisting the timing of events, and at that moment, as luck would have it, David strolled into the living room.

"Hon, I'm here. Are the kids back yet?"

Lauren came unglued. She picked up a piece of art glass and hurled it in David's direction. "You bastard! You son of a bitch! How dare you..." Lauren screamed at the top of her lungs. The sobs and terror filled her body as she launched herself across the room at her husband. "I trusted you! I believed in you!"

David deflected Lauren's swing and grabbed her, wrapping his arms around her in self-defense as her knees buckled. David looked at the crying woman on the couch, her splotchy face pinched tight in confusion. *What in the hell is going on here?* he wondered. *The Twilight Zone* was the only thing that came to mind.

He moved Lauren to the couch. "What in the hell are you talking about, Lauren? And who is this woman?"

"Don't you dare start lying to me, you bastard!" Lauren seethed with anger. "You cheated on me! For how long, David? For how long?" Lauren attempted to get back up off the couch, but David easily kept her sitting.

"There is some mistake. I don't even know this woman!" He glanced at Karen, hoping for help. "Would you please say something to my wife? Now!"

Lauren had to admit it; the woman on the other couch did look confused.

"Not him," Karen said. They were the only words she got out of her mouth before Jason walked in the front door with the nonchalant stride of a teenaged boy coming home for dinner. On time, for a change.

Jason stopped dead in his tracks the moment he saw Karen and his clearly-distraught mother. He locked eyes with his father. Time stood still as the three adults and one teenaged boy tried to comprehend the situation independently. Jason wanted to run, but that was not an option.

The next few seconds lasted an eternity. Karen looked at David, then over to Lauren, and finally to her lover. Stunned, she uttered a single, questioning word: "Jason?"

Jason's wide-eyed parents looked from Karen to their son as the shock slowly turned to recognition.

Jason, frozen, looked at Karen as tears pooled in his eyes. He had no idea what to say.

The next words broke the heavy silence and started time moving again. "Oh my God, Jason, what have you done?" his mother cried in an anguished whisper.

Jason bolted up the stairs to his room. Throwing himself on his bed, he sobbed into his pillow. With the flawed reasoning of a sixteen–year-old, Jason knew his life was over.

Chapter 21

Audrey didn't give a shit about her mother's plan for a family dinner. Whatever announcement she had to make probably wouldn't affect her in the least. School was over, and she wanted to make sure she was going to have a good summer. Ashley still wasn't talking to her, and the handful of other kids she hung out with from time to time had gone their separate ways.

Audrey headed to the park where she usually hooked up with Matt and his friends. Meeting up with them after school to drink or get stoned had become an unspoken habit. She would make this elaborate pretense of attending study groups or grabbing a burger with friends, and her mother bought it every time. She'd gotten good at acting straight at home—even when she was anything but.

Mostly, she liked smoking pot or hash with a few beers. The harder alcohol made it difficult for her to fake it at home. Still, she hadn't been caught. It was accepted that she and Matt were an item, although neither had verbalized it. Nancy told her Matt referred to Audrey as his girlfriend. At least he wasn't calling her Bite Me as frequently—only when he wanted to bust on her about something.

She'd finally figured out that Matt and David were in the same grade. Next year, he and his friends would be seniors, and she'd only be a sophomore. She didn't exactly know where she stood with the group, so she just accepted the status quo.

Tonight, the group was going to drive out into the country to an abandoned barn they knew about. The plan was to stay out all night. Her mother was screwing things up with the family dinner thing, and Audrey didn't want to deal. When she met Jason at the diner after school and told him what she was planning to do, Jason got pissed off. He didn't want to go home either, and now he'd have to cover for his sister. Yeah right. They quarreled and Audrey split, assuming he'd cover for her again.

"Whatever," she muttered. It was probably going to cost her big-time, but she couldn't risk starting the summer off on the wrong foot by missing out. Matt could hook up with someone else, and then where would she be?

The barn was way out in the middle of nowhere, accessible only by a dusty, dirt road. Grass grew tall between the rutted tire marks. It was a massive, old structure, deserted a long time ago. The lower part was open, occupied only by rusted tractor parts and a few stray tools. The stairs to the hayloft were rickety, but once upstairs, the loft was open and enormous. Hay was spread out across the floor, along with a collection of old, musty blankets. It was clear the barn was used as a party place, but what struck Audrey was how beautiful and peaceful it actually was. She loved the way the late-afternoon light filtered in through the dormers and mingled with the dusty, sweet smell of the hay.

While the others set up the keg and got ready to party, she walked to the far side of the loft just to soak up the atmosphere. She didn't hear Matt's friend, Brad, come up behind her.

"Pretty cool, huh?" Brad said. Audrey was surprised he was talking to her at all. He'd kept his distance from her since the day they met. He didn't even acknowledge her much when they all hung together.

"Yeah." Audrey wondered what he was up to. She didn't exactly trust him, but then there was no reason not to trust him, either. They sat down, their backs against a hay bale, and gazed out the open hay door to the empty fields beyond.

Brad handed her a bong, and she took a hit. They traded a couple times without saying much. The weed seemed different, stronger than what they usually smoked, but she liked the added tingly sensations. The world was awash in a rainbow of colors.

As the sun dipped below the horizon, Brad broke the silence. "So, you and Matt..."

Audrey turned to look at him and shrugged. "Yeah, I guess."

Brad sat there for a second longer and then leaned in to kiss her. He wasn't as gentle as Matt, but more forceful and intense. Not sure what to do, Audrey froze, not stopping him but not quite kissing him back, either. She didn't want to piss Brad off for fear he would say something to Matt. Brad took her hand and laid it on the zipper of his jeans. He placed his hand atop hers and pushed hard against the bulge that swelled beneath the taut fabric.

"Come on, babe, I know you want it."

Light-headed from the pot, Audrey didn't resist or pull back. In one smooth move, Brad unzipped his pants and freed his dick from his boxers. He wrapped her hand around it and pumped it up and down. Audrey tried to pull away, but Brad was much stronger. She found herself pinned between the massive hay bale and the wall. Brad kissed her harder, biting her lip, and continued to stroke himself with her hand in his.

"I know you want me, babe. You always have." Audrey tried to pull away again, but Brad slid his free hand to the back of her head and pulled hard on her hair.

Audrey gasped for air, relieved when he finally stopped kissing her. But her relief was short-lived. Instead of letting go of her, Brad pushed her head into his lap and shoved his penis into her mouth.

"Yeah, that's it. You go, girl." With his fists buried in her hair, he held her head in place and pounded his dick into her mouth. "That's it. Oh yeah! You like it, don't you? Wanna taste my cum, girly?" And with one last thrust, Brad groaned and filled Audrey's mouth with warm, salty fluid. Brad thrust a few more times and let her go. He stood, zipped up his jeans, and handed her a beer. "Yeah, you liked it." Then he turned and walked away.

Too stunned to move and trying hard not to vomit, Audrey rinsed her mouth with a swig of beer and spit out the foul-tasting liquid. A burst of laughter echoed from the other end of the barn. She closed her eyes, wanting to leave but unable to move. She wished more than anything that she was home.

Where was Matt? she wondered. *Why didn't he stop Brad? How could he let this happen?*

But the nightmare wasn't over. Soon a second and a third boy knelt before her, and the assault continued. There were more, too, but Audrey lost count of them. She didn't know their names. At some point they stopped bothering to kiss her or talk to her. They just used her to get off, one after the other, until she passed out.

Audrey woke with the sunrise, still slumped in the hay at the far end of the barn. Someone had thrown a scratchy, dirty blanket over her. Her head pounded, and she was overwhelmed by the desire to puke. The events of the night before played in her head like a fuzzy, out-of-focus dream.

She sat there for a few minutes, trying to clear her head. When she finally struggled to her feet and staggered outside, she noticed most of the other kids were gone. Only Nancy and one other girl remained. Audrey looked around, unsteady and confused.

"What... Where... ?" Audrey shook her head as if trying to clear her thoughts. Her face ached, and her tongue felt swollen. "Matt?"

Nancy handed her a bottle of water. "You okay?"

Audrey, still confused, nodded and looked away.

The girls picked up what remained of their things. Audrey climbed into the back seat of the Toyota hatchback and rode home in awkward silence.

It was still early when the girls pulled up in front of her house. Nancy looked at Audrey as she climbed out of the back.

"You gonna be okay?" she asked, her voice filled with concern. It was too little, too late. Audrey looked back at Nancy. She was still not totally clear about what had happened the night before. But she remembered enough... and none of it was good. She nodded and headed into the house. It was 6:15 a.m. Audrey hoped to get upstairs and into her room without anyone noticing. She desperately wanted to stand in a hot shower, to wash away the memories.

CHAPTER 22

At dawn, Lauren was curled in an overstuffed chair with a blanket draped over her legs. She watched as Karen slept on the living room couch and tried to process the events of the night before. The evening certainly wasn't the family dinner she had envisioned. As Audrey crept into the room, Lauren looked up at her fourteen-year-old daughter.

Audrey stopped dead in her tracks thinking she'd been busted but, honestly, not caring anymore. At second glance... *What the fuck?* There was a stranger sleeping on the couch. The room had been turned upside down, broken glass littered the floor, and her mother looked horrible.

Lauren took one look at her daughter and wondered if she knew her anymore. Tears rolled down Lauren's cheeks as they looked at each other in the awkward silence. Her mother's tears were more than Audrey could handle.

"Mommy!" she half-whispered as she dropped her backpack on the floor and hurried across the room, curling into the safety of her mother's arms. Lauren pulled a throw blanket over the two of them and stroked her daughter's head as they wept together. Audrey soon fell asleep, and the house stilled again.

Lauren looked around the room, surveying the wreckage, and was unable to comprehend what had gone wrong. Life had taken a sharp left turn, and apparently she hadn't noticed. As she held her sleeping daughter, Lauren was overwhelmed by confusion, sadness, anger, frustration, and guilt. Nothing made sense, and a deep, aching numbness consumed her, all feeling and thoughts replaced with a sort of low-frequency buzzing. Feeling chilled, she pulled the blanket closer and dozed off—a fitful sleep, if you could call it sleep at all.

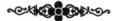

David awoke with a start. The house was quiet, and for a moment he wondered if it had all been a horrible, stress-filled dream. Lauren's side of the bed was empty.

Rolling out of bed, he threw on a sweatshirt and shorts. Peeking into the kids' rooms, he found Jason asleep in his clothes and Audrey's bed untouched. David knew the nightmare of last night was all too real.

As he tiptoed through the house, David found his wife and daughter asleep on the big chair. The woman who came to their door last night was asleep on the couch where he'd left her, covered by a blanket. There was so much upheaval from the night before it seemed people just ended up strewn across the house in heaps. He wondered how Audrey and his wife ended up asleep downstairs. Did he sleep through something?

David made a pot of coffee and considered some sort of food offering. Nobody had eaten dinner last night. Lauren had some frozen blueberry muffins, and he stuck them in the toaster oven to warm.

The gurgling coffeepot woke Lauren. She slipped away from Audrey, tucking the throw in tightly around her near-comatose daughter. She walked into the kitchen to find David, his back to her as he fiddled with the breakfast dishes. He stiffened as she wrapped her arms around him from behind and then relaxed and turned to his wife.

"I'm sorry I overreacted last night." Lauren tried not to cry, but it was wasted effort. "I don't know what came over me, and I'm really sorry for throwing the glass elephant at you."

David looked at his wife, his heart filled with love and sorrow. Not knowing what to say, he tried to make light of the situation. "Thankfully, you're a lousy shot, Mrs. Breckenridge." Neither of them laughed, but the dismal pall that had hung in the air between them seemed to lessen a bit.

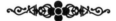

The night before, after Jason had fled to his room, Lauren, Karen, and David did their best to comprehend the situation. But tempers exploded and accusations flew—in addition to throw pillows and anything small within reach. There was nothing adult or reasonable about the things said. And when it became apparent to Lauren that Karen and her son were the culprits, she was reduced to calling the woman a whore and threatened to have her arrested.

David convinced Lauren to listen to what Karen had to say without interruption; the story she told them was horrifying. When Karen paused at what they hoped was the end of the story, Lauren sobbed. They were the heartfelt tears of a mother in total disbelief. Confused, Karen looked at David for an explanation.

"Karen, Jason is sixteen. He is finishing his junior year of high school," David said in a rather matter-of-fact tone.

Karen's face blanched. The full reality hit her hard. The situation was significantly worse than she ever anticipated. Suddenly, she was hit with a wave of nausea. Recognizing this, David helped her to the guest bathroom to give her some privacy.

Karen puked her guts up and then spent some time sitting on the floor, her back against the vanity. She thought back through their times together, looking for clues. In retrospect, there were signs, misunderstandings pointing to the truth, if she'd somehow been able to piece them all together.

Now she had to face the parents of a young man, a boy, really—parents who had the power and absolute right to have her arrested and prosecuted as a sexual offender. Karen's tears came again, as a new wave of dry heaves racked her exhausted body. She felt manipulated and powerless, but stupidity was no defense. Her life was probably ruined forever. In many ways, she wanted to call her own parents, but what would they say to her?

Finally, she stood up to view herself in the mirror. Her own ignorance stared her in the face and repulsed her. She splashed cold water on her face and ran her fingers through her hair, trying to regain her composure before walking back into the living room.

In the meantime, David crossed the room and sat in front of his wife. "It's not my fault!" Lauren said, preempting whatever her husband had planned to say.

"Lauren—"

"Shut up! Don't you dare say a word! You've had your head up your ass for months," Lauren continued, seething. "I do my best to keep everyone happy and the house running smoothly, while you use this place as your own personal hotel with a concierge sex service. In fact, you all use this place as a pit stop, not one of you taking a minute to be a family, and then when something goes slightly wrong, you look to me for answers or to fix it or to bail you out!" Lauren was ranting, her voice louder and louder as she continued. "I'm the only one in this house who gives a shit about anything!" She doubled over again as violent sobs overtook her.

David sat back, stunned. How did it get to this point? Was his wife really this angry with him, or was this a distraught mother's emotional—yet not unreasonable—reaction to an awful situation? David didn't blame his wife. Blame didn't solve anything. He wanted to get control of the situation and come up with a solution.

"Lauren…" he whispered as he rested his hand on her knee.

She pulled away in anger, staring out the window at the darkness.

David stood and went into the kitchen, pulling three bottles of cold water out of the fridge. It was well past one a.m. "Can we start from the top?" David spoke softly, and the three quietly contemplated the situation.

Karen broke the silence. "I'm sorry. Honestly. I didn't..." she whispered, faltering as she attempted to find the right words. Nothing would seem believable. "I didn't realize; I didn't know."

Lauren stared at the woman sitting across from her. "How is that possible?" she said, her voice as icy as her gaze. "Jason is just a boy!"

"Less boy than young man, Lauren," David said. "We both need to open our eyes and really look at our son. He's not little anymore."

"You are excusing this slut!" Lauren shouted.

Karen wanted to stand up for herself but had no valid defense. "She's right," Karen murmured. "I have no excuse, and I should have known better."

This admission seemed to diffuse Lauren a bit. For the first time, Lauren really looked at Karen, and she saw a young, heartbroken woman in complete turmoil and a great deal of pain. And then she understood. "You're in love with him?" But it was really more of a statement than an actual question. She knew the answer.

Karen hung her head and nodded, unable to say the words. Fresh tears fell from her eyes as she put her face into her hands.

David realized they all needed to calm down, rest a bit, and try to think clearly. They were getting nowhere, and the problem was certainly not going to solve itself in the next few hours. It was then he suggested they take a break and try to get some rest. Karen stood to leave and David rationally stopped her. "You can't drive, you need to stay here," she sat back down. "We can deal with this in the morning."

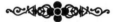

"I've made coffee and have some muffins defrosting. Maybe we can make sense of this situation and come to a sensible conclusion." David was treading lightly, nervous his words would unleash the anger which spewed from Lauren the night before. "I'll go wake Karen." David slipped into the next room before Lauren had a chance to respond.

Karen had already folded the blanket and was coming out of the guest bathroom as David entered. "Good, you're awake." Feeling awkward, he could only sputter, "There's coffee. We should talk."

David placed his hand on Audrey's shoulder "Punkin, you okay?"

Audrey nodded sleepily, not looking her father in the eye.

"Go upstairs and get some sleep. We can talk about what happened later."

Audrey stiffened. *How did he know?* "Dad, I'm fine. It's no big deal."

"Audrey, this... thing that happened with your brother affects us all. I can see you're upset, and it's better to talk about it. It will be okay. Now go get some sleep."

Audrey looked at her father with confusion and glanced over at the woman standing in the middle of the room. Whatever Jason did must have been huge, but she didn't give a shit. Without saying anything, she grabbed her backpack and went to her room, relieved to be alone, her fear of needing to explain what happened the night before alleviated.

"Miss Alderson, will you come with me into the kitchen?"

Karen swallowed hard and followed David without speaking. Lauren was sitting at the table and the two sat down with her. David poured her a cup without asking. The weight in the room seemed overwhelming.

"Where do you live?" Lauren broke the silence.

"Near Marist College. I work there." Karen fumbled for words, her discomfort visible. "I wasn't certain, but I thought perhaps Jason was a student." She paused. "I was getting the feeling he wasn't being honest with me. I know it doesn't excuse anything, I'm just saying." Her voice trailed off.

"You honestly expect us to believe you couldn't tell he was a boy?" Lauren's anger was barely controlled. "David, I think we should call the police. There are laws against this sort of thing."

"Lauren." David snapped. "Stop it. It seems pretty clear Jason's equally to blame, and do you really want this all over the news? Do you want our names splashed all over the local papers? Hell, this will make national news. Did you think about that? Did you think for even one minute about how it would affect my career?"

Lauren stared at David, her mouth agape. She was speechless.

"Ms. Alderson, Karen, surely you can see the damage this could cause. I'm sure you would agree with me there is a solution which doesn't splash our dirty laundry all over the headlines."

Karen nodded. She had no idea what this man was thinking. Was he looking for money? She had none. At this point, anything which kept her out of jail was a good option.

"I need you to leave this house with the promise you will never contact our son again. Now that you fully understand the situation, this should not be too difficult for you, correct?" David was all business. "It would be preferable if you were to move out of the area, but I don't know how I can force that to happen given your employment situation. Perhaps you could give it some consideration."

Karen nodded.

"Good, we are in agreement then." David stood. "I suggest you leave now, without saying anything to our son. My wife and I will take care of him. You need not concern yourself with anything to do with him from this point on."

Karen stood. Her knees were weak and she was in shock. This family had every right to call the police, and if it were up to the mother, Karen would be in handcuffs already. But somehow the father had taken control, and she was being escorted to the front door. No further words were spoken, and in minutes she was in her car, tears streaming down her face as she drove back to her apartment. Karen was devastated.

CHAPTER 23

With finals over, neither kid left the house, choosing instead to spend all of their time in their rooms. David spent most of his time at work finishing up the paperwork as his company shut down for the summer. Lauren prepared the family to leave for Charlevoix. It was decided they would drive in one car, taking the route through Canada and dividing the drive into two days.

As Lauren started working on the personal packing lists, it occurred to her that, in all the melee, they had yet to tell the children of the summer plans.

"Kids, David, dinner's ready, and I've got something I want to discuss with all of you," Lauren called out toward the living room.

Once everyone was seated and dinner served, Lauren took a deep breath, expecting her news to be greeted with an argument from the kids.

"As you know, your father's work is shutting down for the summer. We decided to take the opportunity to go away as a family, so we've rented a summer cottage in Northern Michigan, right on a lake, where you'll be able to swim, sail, even play tennis if you want. It's part of a club with other families and kids your ages to hang out with."

"Great. When do we leave?" Jason blurted out in a monotone.

Lauren did a double take. "Actually, day after tomorrow. I've made lists for you guys so you know what to pack."

Audrey held out her hand for the list and looked it over in silence. "Is there WiFi?" was her only question.

Lauren and David looked at each other quietly for a moment. "Cell service isn't great, but yes, there is WiFi at the house," Lauren said.

"What do you want us to pack our stuff in?" Jason asked.

"Your dad has pulled out some bags from the garage, and he's going to bring them to your rooms after dinner." Lauren paused. "Anything else?" she said in a tentative voice, expecting all hell to break loose.

"Nah," Jason said. "Getting out of here seems like a good idea."

Lauren looked at Audrey who was tight-lipped. She simply shrugged in apparent agreement, clearing her plate to the kitchen. "I'm gonna go start on this list. I'm not hungry."

Jason scarfed down his meal and followed in his sister's footsteps.

"Did that seem too easy to you?" Lauren was skeptical.

David looked at her, a sad smile on his face. "After the last few weeks, maybe the kids need a break just like we do. Jason's been through a lot."

"That really doesn't explain Audrey's reaction. Why isn't she having a fit about leaving her friends for the summer? In fact, don't you think she's been acting pretty weird?"

"Oh my God, Lauren! Are you really trying to make problems where they don't exist? Seriously? Now, because one of our kids didn't have a shit fit about something you think there's a problem? That's crazy."

David got up from the table in a huff, clearing his dishes into the sink. He headed to the garage to get the bags for the kids, leaving his wife sitting at the kitchen table, wondering what just happened.

Part 2

CHAPTER 24

Audrey stared out the window of the Escalade. The drive to Michigan seemed to take forever. Her parents kept pestering her with ridiculous questions and it was annoying. Glancing over at Jason, his earbuds stuck firmly in place, she rolled her eyes. His music was so loud it was irritating. She squirmed, pushing Jason's backpack into his leg.

"What?"

Audrey snapped at her brother. "Turn your damn music down. I don't want to listen to that crap."

"Kids, language" Audrey's mother chided from the front seat. "We're here and I want the two of you to behave."

The "cottage" Audrey's mother had been referring to was huge. It looked like some of the weathered beach mansions she'd seen in Rhode Island. Audrey had a hard time imaging what spending the summer here would be like. She just wanted to be left alone. Stepping out of the car, she watched her mother and some woman embrace and chat happily. She glanced over at Jason, who was casually standing at the bottom of the stairs.

"I'm Liza. You must be Audrey." The woman looked like she wanted a hug, so Audrey offered her hand to keep her at a distance. "I'm so glad you're here. Your mom has told me so much about you."

"Mmm, thanks."

Liza moved on to introduce herself to Jason and then addressed all of them. "I've got lunch set up on the back patio, and then I'll show you to your rooms."

David, Audrey, and Jason followed the women. The house was not what Audrey expected. The dark wood made the house seem cool but somehow comfortable.

Audrey answered the questions Liza directed at her. Her brother did the same. Her mother glared and seemed to be sending a message that she needed to be nicer.

After lunch, the woman addressed Audrey and Jason again. "Listen, I know you must be tired from the long drive. How about if I show you kids to your rooms so you can get settled?" Audrey refocused and started paying attention to what

Liza was saying. Finally, she could escape and be alone.

Liza told them what time to be downstairs. There was a beach picnic that night, and she would introduce them to the activities director. She felt bad, knowing they had been through a rough spring. Their sullen behavior said it all. Liza was optimistic that the pace of the summer would shake the negative thoughts out of them and put them on a better path.

Rejoining David and Lauren on the patio, Liza opened another bottle of wine and settled into the chair next to Lauren. The three fell into a relaxed conversation about club events and some of the people who lived there over the summer.

In the early evening Liza announced it was time to head down to the beach. She explained this was a weekly event for the residents of the club. The kids would be able to join others their age for burgers, and a movie would be shown on an inflatable screen at sunset. The counselors would be responsible for the kids so the adults could relax and enjoy themselves.

The group entered the beach area through a tunnel under a now-defunct railroad track.

"When we were kids, the trains still used the tracks—not for passengers as they did in the 1800s, but for hauling coal or rocks downstate. It was great fun to put pennies on the tracks and watch the trains flatten them. We would try to get the engineers to blow the train whistles. I'm sure it drove the adults nuts," Liza said.

The view from the beach was magnificent. Lake Charlevoix was much larger than Lauren expected; it seemed to go on for miles. In the early evening the lake was still alive with activity: a cluster of sailboats aimed for one general area, and a trio of water-skiers flashed past the end of a wooden dock. The smell of grilled chicken overwhelmed Lauren, and she realized she was quite hungry.

"Leave your shoes here," Liza said. "I'll take the kids over to the counselor and make introductions. The bar is open; help yourself. Oh, and don't worry, everyone is expecting you and will know who you are." She laughed and gave a wave.

The white sand felt soft and warm between her toes. David and Lauren watched warily as Liza took it upon herself to take charge of the kids as if they were her responsibility, but there didn't seem to be a moment to suggest another option.

Almost immediately, their attention was pulled back toward a group of adults when a female voice called out, "Oh hello, you two! You must be the Breckenridges!" Lauren focused on the petite woman in a floral sundress approaching them. "I'm Lindsay, Liza's best friend. Welcome. We must fill those empty hands of yours."

Lindsay led them to the bar and handed them margaritas. Lauren took a sip and grimaced, surprised at the strength.

"Oh, you'll get used to cocktail hour around here," Lindsay said with a smile. "Now let's introduce you to some people. It's David, right? Where is that errant husband of mine?"

Lindsay took David by the arm and led him over to a jovial group of men. They opened up the circle, making room for Lindsay and her guest. Lauren felt disconnected as Lindsay seemed to hold court, commanding the attention of everyone near. There was no question who was in charge. Lauren listened to the laughter, and from the looks of it, David was accepted into their crowd without hesitation.

A waiter came by with a tray of drinks, exchanging her empty glass for a full one. Lauren felt awkward standing there by herself, so she walked over to the playground area and sat down on one of the swings, rocking herself with her foot in the sand. The view was lovely and she enjoyed sipping her margarita, lost in thought.

All of a sudden, someone grabbed the ropes on both sides of her, and Lauren felt the swing being pulled backward. Her back was nestled against a man's chest, his arms securing her to the swing as he whispered softly into her neck, "I can't let a beautiful woman swing on her own."

Just as suddenly, he pushed her away and stepped back to watch her swing. Lauren caught her breath and let out a little squeal. The last few drops of her drink spilled, and she dropped the glass onto the sand.

"Oh dear! A gentleman always refreshes a lady's drink. Luckily, I brought a fresh one over for you."

"And you're a perfect gentleman?" Lauren responded, her tongue loosened by alcohol as she dragged her feet to slow the swing to a stop.

"Always. Richard Sawyer," he said with a grin as he handed over the margarita, "but everyone calls me Rick." He paused. "Okay, I get called Dickie a lot, too."

"Nice to meet you, Rick. I'm Lauren." She shook his hand. "And I don't have a nickname."

Rick smiled. "You probably will by the end of the summer. Do you come here often?"

"Me? No, I..." Lauren paused, flustered. "I was enjoying the view."

"So was I," Rick said as he gave Lauren a conspicuous once-over. He sat down on the swing next to Lauren, matching her gentle, gliding motion. "Swing much?"

Lauren looked at Rick, not sure how to respond. She wasn't sure if he was teasing or flirting.

"I can honestly say I haven't been on a swing for a very long time." Lauren tried not to laugh and fought to maintain her cool demeanor. She had to find something safe to talk about. "So can we eat soon? I'm getting hungry."

Rick chuckled. "What are you hungry for? Maybe I can help."

Lauren couldn't help herself. She turned beet-red and laughed. "You are a shameless flirt. I was trying to change the subject."

"I know. That's what made this so much fun. You're not as innocent as you pretend to be, and we both know it now." Rick locked eyes with Lauren. "Just so you know, my position on the club board is, in fact, Shameless Flirt, and it is my sworn duty to welcome all lovely renters to the club with insinuation and innuendo."

"Well, I'll be happy to write you a reference or, better still, a Yelp review. You've done a fabulous job of sweeping me off my feet."

"Ha! I see what you've done there. Well played, Mrs. Breckenridge. You and I will be great friends." Rick hopped off the swing, offering an arm to Lauren. "Now, you say you have this insatiable hunger which apparently only I can cure. May I lead you to some breasts with your name on them?"

As they approached the cabana, Liza called them over. "Lauren, Dickie, I have some seats over here. So glad the two of you found each other. My work here is done."

CHAPTER 25

Lauren awoke with a start. It was almost 10 a.m., and the house seemed dead quiet. Her head pounded from all the alcohol the night before. Getting home from the beach seemed fuzzy at best. Throwing on a robe, she went to the kitchen in search of coffee. After pouring a cup, she caught sight of a note on the table.

Good Morning! Hope your head is in one piece. Your hubby went golfing with some friends of mine, and I took the kids to crew so they can get signed up for activities. I'll meet you on the back porch for coffee. L.

Lauren couldn't process the information clearly, so she simply took her mug and, in a semi-comatose state, staggered toward the screened-in porch filled with wicker furniture and surrounded by birch trees. The last thing she expected was to run straight into a rather large man dressed in denim overalls and carrying a stack of newspapers.

Liza heard Lauren's scream and sprinted the last few hundred yards to the cottage. She discovered one of the groundskeepers in shock, trying to calm down a nearly hysterical woman clutching at her robe, a mug of hot coffee shattered at her feet.

"Lauren, it's okay. I'm here. I forgot to tell you about Frank. I'm so sorry." Liza looked at the caretaker. "Don't worry. This is Mrs. Breckenridge, my renter. I forgot to explain about what you do. I'll handle it. Are you okay?"

Frank nodded. "May I?" He gestured toward the door.

"Yes, of course. And really, everything will be fine. This is all my fault."

"Thank you. I'm sorry for scaring you, Miss." Frank nodded to Lauren before he slipped out the kitchen door.

"Watch your feet. You're not wearing shoes." Liza led Lauren to the porch and, after cleaning up the mess, came back with two steaming mugs of coffee.

"I put a shot of Kahlua in our coffee. I figured after that scare a little hair of the dog would be nice."

Lauren gratefully accepted the mug and took a gulp. It contained more than one shot, and her eyes opened wide. "Who the hell is Frank?"

Liza laughed. "Good morning to you, too."

"He scared the crap out of me."

"Yes, I can see that. He's always been a part of the club. I guess I forgot to tell you. Whoops." Liza gave Lauren a smile. "We have groundskeepers, and part of what they do is come into the house twice a day to make sure the fireplaces are laid so you can light a fire anytime you want. Frank also delivers the newspaper, sweeps the porch, and does any general maintenance that's needed."

"I was wearing a robe!" Lauren's voice went up an octave.

"Well, they usually come in when people are out and about. I'm sure he was just as shocked as you were. But even if you were home in your robe, they look the other way. I'm sure they get an eyeful, considering the goings-on at this inbred little club of ours, but they keep it quiet."

Lauren was about to ask what Liza meant by that statement, but Liza's phone rang before she had the chance. She wondered what there would be to keep quiet about. While Liza had an animated conversation about plans for the day, Lauren sipped her coffee. Her thoughts drifted to the interaction with Rick. It made her smile, and she wondered if she would run into him again.

"We're going to meet the girls in town for lunch." Liza's voice snapped Lauren back to reality.

"What? Oh, sure." In the back of her mind, Lauren wasn't sure if she was supposed to just leave the kids or touch base with David. It all seemed so haphazard.

An hour later, the two were driving in a Jeep heading across the Ironton Ferry toward town, while Liza described the surroundings and some of its history. Lauren was astonished by how antiquities like the ferry, well over a hundred years old, could still be such a functional part of day-to-day life.

As they drove into town, Lauren spotted an old castle on the right and asked Liza about it. "Oh, that's Castle Farms. When we were kids, we used to go to concerts there. We used to pack as many kids inside a station wagon as we could. We brought blankets and would lie under the stars getting stoned and listening to music. In fact—you're going to laugh at this—we used to drink Boone's Farm Strawberry Hill Wine. We thought we were so sophisticated."

Lauren looked at Liza and laughed. "I guess summertime equaled party time back then."

"Back then? Girl, this summer is going to loosen up some of those limbs of yours."

"What are you talking about?" Lauren chuckled.

"My dear, summer up north is one big endless playtime for adults. We work hard all year long. Even those who don't have a job, per se, work exceptionally hard on charity events. So by the time summer rolls around, we need to blow off some steam in a protected environment. Essentially, we're recharging."

"I think I got a pretty good idea last night."

"The beach picnic? That was nothing. Seriously, that wasn't even a party. That was just dinner on the beach, no big deal. There is a cocktail party at someone's cottage every night, and dinners at the club, and it's all fueled by alcohol." Liza was nonchalant. "I don't mean to make us sound like a bunch of alcoholics. Well, you'll see. It's like we're all still college kids, like we never grew up. And the thing is, it's been this way for generations."

Liza parked the Jeep in front of the Villager Pub and the two walked in, greeting Lindsay and Betsy, whom Lauren had met the night before. A surly bartender named Jessica came over and took the ladies' order: Pinot Blanc and a sun-dried tomato, pine nut, and basil pizza with Fontina cheese.

Bets held up her glass. "Let the gossip commence!"

Lauren expected to be left out, but the women were warm and included her in the conversation. By the end of lunch they had devoured the pizza and shared three bottles of wine. Lindsay looked at her watch and mentioned it was getting late. She grabbed the bill, counted out a bunch of twenties, and placed it on the bar. The woman all hugged each other before heading out into the bright sunlight.

Lauren was definitely buzzed when they climbed back into the Jeep. Liza seemed fine, so she didn't say anything about driving while intoxicated. Besides, it was a fun afternoon, and for the first time in what seemed like an eternity, she was relaxed.

Liza continued the driving tour, cruising past one of the other summer resorts on her way out of town. They drove past a marina, and Liza explained that Irish's was where most people kept their boats.

"Does everyone have a boat?" Lauren asked.

"Just about, but we all share." Liza went on to explain the variety of activities on Lake Charlevoix. When she was younger, they'd go waterskiing after dinner. The lake was like glass by 9 p.m., and since it stayed light until after ten during the height of summer, it was the absolute best time to go out.

"How old were you?"

"I don't know. We were allowed to take the ski boats out on our own by the time we were fourteen."

Lauren did some mental calculations. Would she ever let her kids take a boat out to go waterskiing at 10 o'clock at night? That seemed a bit much.

"I know what you're thinking," Liza said. They were back in line, waiting for the ferry. "In retrospect, I often think about what seemed like a total lack of supervision on the part of the adults."

Before Lauren could respond, Liza launched into her explanation. Honestly, it sounded more like a rationalization, but who was Lauren to criticize something she knew nothing about?

Liza continued. "Imagine never having to find a babysitter or not having to keep track of the endless schedule, events, or games. Plus, you didn't have to spend your summer in a car driving from one activity to another."

Lauren felt like she'd been struck by lightning. She got it. It really did take all the stress out of a mother's job.

"Actually, it sounds like heaven. A completely stress-free environment where kids and adults play together and separately." Lauren hadn't planned a "separate but together vacation." She'd hoped the family would spend time together after the turmoil of the spring. But the way Liza described everything, Lauren certainly could see the benefits.

David waved to them as they pulled into the driveway of the cottage. "Well, what do we have here?" David said as he walked to Lauren's side of the Jeep. "Excuse me, Liza, have you seen my wife anywhere? This beautiful, laughing woman bears little resemblance to the woman I drove to Michigan with or to the green lady I saw in my bed this morning!"

Lauren felt a twinge of irritation. David's comments felt mean-spirited, even though he was laughing. She glanced at Liza who also laughed, but the look on her face seemed hollow.

Chapter 26

Jason approached the cottage with some apprehension. Ever since the incident with Karen, his mother had been avoiding him, not looking at him directly. She didn't have much to say to him about anything, even when his grades tanked.

The way the past few weeks played out had been pretty bad. His mom had ended up crying and locking herself in her room for a couple days. She made it pretty clear she was pissed off at everyone for letting Karen off the hook.

Of course, they demanded he and Karen never see each other again. Jason was actually a little relieved. He wasn't in love with her, and Karen was becoming kind of intense. She was hot and the sex was awesome, but he never had feelings for her—not real ones, anyway. It was embarrassing to get caught.

Dad's lecture about "first love" was so awkward that Jason wanted to crawl out the window. And when Dad clapped him on the shoulder and called him a man, it was all Jason could do not to say something sarcastic. If ever there was a time when he wanted to melt into the walls and become invisible, this was it.

Karen wrote him a note, with permission from his parents. He brought it with him to Michigan but then decided to rip it up. He wanted to forget the whole thing ever happened. As the weeks passed, he cared less and less about what happened. With his new summer job, he had everything to look forward to. He just had to get the application signed by his parents and everything would be golden.

As Jason grabbed a soda from the fridge, he heard voices on the sitting porch and figured he might as well get it over with. His parents were talking to Liza, making arrangements for his mother to drive her to the airport in Traverse City. Audrey was sitting in the corner with her nose in a book.

"Hey," he said as he nodded in Audrey's direction. She returned the gesture. Her mood still seemed dark, more so than usual, and Jason wondered if she was lonely, missing her friends, or if something else was up. He couldn't shake the feeling something was wrong with her, but nobody seemed to be paying attention.

"Jase, the prodigal son, returns to the fold," his dad said a bit too loudly and put his hand on Jason's shoulder. "How was your day today?"

The conversation abruptly halted. All eyes were on him, so he figured now was his opportunity. Taking a deep breath, he decided to focus on his father, banking on the chip-off-the-old-block factor. He was pretty sure his mother would have something to say about it ruining the family vacation.

"Actually, Dad, I had an amazing day today. I was down at the beach helping out Mike, the head counselor. I guess one of the lifeguards quit or never showed up or something. I told him about my swim team stuff and lifeguarding over the past couple summers, and he offered me the job right there on the spot."

Lauren opened her mouth to reply, but David spoke right over her. "Jason, that's fantastic! When do you start?"

"David!" Lauren squealed.

Jason glanced at his mother out of the corner of his eye. As he guessed, she was not happy about the idea. Jason wanted this job badly; the idea of lounging around all summer with his parents seemed like hell. He preferred to be teaching swimming lessons to a bunch of kids and guarding a beach. Getting paid a decent amount of money to do it was icing on the cake. Hell, he would have volunteered to do it for free.

Jason felt a twinge of guilt when he ignored his mother's outburst. He kept his eyes on his father and responded. "Well, that's kind of the thing, Dad. I sort of started today. They just need you to sign this piece of paper and then it's official."

Jason pulled the application from his back pocket and handed it to his father, holding his breath. As he'd hoped, David, being an engineer, had a pen in his shirt pocket and signed the form in seconds.

"I think this is wonderful news, Jason. Of course I'll sign it. Why wouldn't we want you to get a job like this? Right, hon?" David handed the form back to his son.

"Thanks, Dad, you're the best. I really want to do this. It was great today. I even get paid extra if I teach private lessons. I'm going to run this up to the clubhouse now so they can get the paperwork done and I can work a shift tomorrow. See you in a bit." Jason hurried out the door before his mother could stop him.

"Isn't that fantastic news?" David said, beaming.

Lauren seethed. "Yes, it works so well into the plans for a family vacation—the word *family* meaning the four of us, doing things, together."

"Oh Lauren, you can't possibly be upset about this. He's a young man. He needs a job. There will be plenty of time for us to do things together. Liza, tell her this is a perfect opportunity."

Liza looked at the two of them and wondered how to extract herself from the awkward situation. Thinking on her feet, she tried her best to calm the nerves of her new friend.

"Actually, Lauren, much of what happens at the club is at the beach. We go there practically every day, and it's not like the lifeguards are in cages or anything. The reality is, it puts your son at the beach, on the end of the dock, every day. You can spend as much or as little time talking to him as you want to when you take your book to the beach. It's really not that bad."

Lauren relaxed a little; maybe she over reacted. "I just thought—"

"I know. You'll get used to life around here. It's really quite different." Liza paused, glancing at the nonexistent watch on her arm. "Would you look at the time? I do believe it's cocktail hour, and I have some icy-cold gin that's taking up space in the bar. Martini, anyone?"

Liza didn't wait for an answer and disappeared into the adjoining room.

Audrey sat quietly, watching the entire scene transpire. The precious Jason, who seemed to be able to get away with murder, just managed to get a job so he could skip out on this so-called family togetherness. *If he can get a job, so can I.*

Chapter 27

There were a handful of jobs listed in the Charlevoix Courier, but only one caught Audrey's eye—a part-time veterinarian assistant. It was close enough to the cottage for her to ride a bike there, and, best of all, she'd get to deal with animals instead of people. Perfect.

After a quick shower, Audrey threw on jeans and a T-shirt. Downstairs, her dad was sound asleep on the wicker couch. She didn't want to wake him, so she tiptoed out the door. It was a little past eight a.m. Audrey remembered how to get to the Ironton Ferry. From there she would ask for directions.

Spying a pair of Vespas tucked under the portico, Audrey guessed nobody would notice if she took one of them. She had never driven one before, but figured since she could ride a bike, she could deal with the scooter. She rolled it down the driveway and around the corner from the cottage, not wanting her dad to hear her start the motor.

Once out of earshot, she hopped on and started it up. At first she wobbled and almost fell off. The speed control was a little tricky to get the hang of, but soon she was relatively balanced and figured out how to brake and accelerate. It was fun.

Audrey found Dr. Hawkins' clinic easily. It was on the main highway as you headed toward town, a mile past the ferry landing. She parked in front of the clinic. There was nobody at the counter when she strolled inside.

"Hello! Anybody home?"

When no one answered, Audrey walked past the desk and down the hallway toward a back door, propped open with an office chair. She peeked outside and spotted a jean-clad black woman distributing food to a group of eager, kenneled dogs.

"Excuse me, I'm looking for Dr. Hawkins," Audrey called out.

The woman straightened and turned around. "Do you have an appointment? Where's your pet, honey?"

"No, wait. That's not what—"

"I'm busy right now. Office hours start at 1 p.m. Come back then." The woman turned her attention back to the hungry animals.

"I'm here about the job," Audrey blurted out. "Can I just talk to Dr. Hawkins? The ad said I should apply in person. Is he here?"

The woman smirked as she put down the food pail and brushed herself off. "How old are you, child?"

"Fourteen." Audrey sounded more confident than she felt.

"And what job do you want to apply for?"

"I'm here with my family for the summer. I don't want to just hang out on the beach all summer long, so I looked in the paper and saw the assistant job posted." Audrey had rehearsed the speech in her head during the ride over. "Oh, and I like animals."

"Do you now. Where's your mama?"

"At home."

"How did you get here?"

Audrey paused for a bit, wondering if this was going to get her into trouble. "I rode a scooter."

"Really? Hmmm..."

The woman studied the young girl again. She asked some basic questions: her name, where she was staying, and whether her parents knew she was there. Something made Audrey think she should be truthful about that last question, so she told the woman about her adventure with the scooter, sneaking it down the road and learning how to drive it.

"Well, I have to give you credit for being adventurous. You must be determined."

Audrey shrugged, not quite sure what to say.

"Put your backpack on the wooden bench over there," the woman said. "Then grab that bag of dog food and bring it over to the back cages."

Audrey followed her instructions, hopeful that the woman would let her talk to Dr. Hawkins once they were finished.

"It's heavy!" Audrey muttered as she struggled with the oversized bag of dog food.

"Yes, it is. You would have to lift bags like that if you worked here. Are you still interested in the job?"

"Yes, I am."

"Okay then, give me a hand feeding the dogs." The woman turned her back to Audrey and pulled the empty bowls from the cages. She instructed Audrey to rinse them and fill them with two scoops of the dry food. Audrey did what she was told, and they fell into a natural conversation.

She wanted to know what grade Audrey was in and about her family life. Audrey found the woman easy to talk to and soon opened up about her dad's job, the cottage they were renting, and even about the trouble Jason had gotten into that spring.

When the conversation turned to her own experiences, however, Audrey was not as forthcoming. She faltered and became awkward. The woman sensed a hurt and troubled girl beneath all the bravado and confidence. The mix of confidence and despair was compelling and reminded her of when she was young. She decided Audrey was in serious need of some guidance.

It took about an hour to finish the cages. Audrey followed the woman back inside the building. The woman poured two large glasses of ice water, and they drank in silence for a few minutes, the elder woman studying the child.

"So, do I get to talk to Dr. Hawkins about the job?" Audrey asked, breaking the awkward silence.

The woman across from her laughed. "Honey, you just did. My name is Dr. Claire Hawkins, but most folks around here just call me Claire."

Audrey blushed. "I... I'm so sorry. I didn't know."

"That's okay, sweetie, I kinda tricked ya." Claire looked at the girl for a good long minute. "And, if you want the job, it's yours."

Audrey was stunned, not quite understanding what had just happened. "Well, yeah! I mean, yes; yes, I actually do."

"Then consider yourself hired." Claire's smile was warm and genuine.

"Thanks, Dr. Hawkins. I really—"

"First off, call me Claire. And second, make me one promise." Audrey nodded, listening intently. "All I want you to do is try your hardest, and if you can't do something or you mess something up, just be honest with me. Everything else we can work on."

Audrey glowed. "Claire, that was two promises, and I agree to both of them."

Claire laughed. "I think you and I are going to work out just fine."

Claire handed Audrey a package of paperwork to fill out. "Do I have to get my parents' signature on them?" Audrey asked nervously.

Claire's instincts went on high alert. This girl really needed some help. "We can skip that for now. Your hours are Tuesday through Saturday from ten until three. Do you think you can handle that?"

"Absolutely! Thank you so much. See you Tuesday!" Audrey waved as she walked out the front door, the bell jingling after her. Stuffing the papers in her backpack, she rode back toward the ferry, giggling to herself and grinning from ear to ear. She got a job! All on her own.

There was a note on the kitchen table for her when she got home.

Sweetie,

Your dad, Liza, and I went to the softball game. Your dad is playing on the club team. Everyone needs to be back at the cottage and dressed formally for Sunday night dinner at the club at 6 p.m.

Love, Mom

Even better, Audrey thought. *I don't have to explain anything to anyone.* She headed up to her room, settled at the desk, and did her best to fill out the paperwork Claire had given her.

CHAPTER 28

The Breckenridge family and Liza walked to the clubhouse dressed in their finest for the formal Sunday night dinner, a tradition at the club for the past one hundred years. David and Jason sported jackets and ties. Liza and Lauren wore cocktail dresses.

Audrey had on a cotton skirt with a tank top. She didn't feel like she was dressed right at all. This was one of her nicest outfits, and all the girls at home dressed like this for parties. Once again she felt awkward, like she didn't fit in.

"You look like a dork," she hissed to her brother.

"Look who's talking, Cinderella," Jason replied.

"Behave," their father said as he turned to them. "Can we be nice, please? Just for one night."

As they entered the clubhouse, David was hailed by a few of the men he had been golfing with during the week and was quickly absorbed into their conversation. Jason and Audrey went to the Crew Clubroom where the kids their age hung out before dinner, a throwback to when kids were seen but not heard. The adults seemed to take every opportunity to separate themselves from the kids, and having them underfoot at a cocktail party was inconvenient.

"I'll go get us drinks," Liza said, touching Lauren on the arm. "Relax. I'll be back in a flash." Without waiting for a response, Liza headed toward the bar and disappeared in the crowd.

"My favorite swinger! How beautiful you look." Lauren felt a hand in the small of her back and blushed.

"I believe I met you at the swing set."

Rick grinned back and chuckled. "Why yes, I believe a long time ago, in our youth, you were swinging, slipped, and I was gallant enough to catch you before you fell to the ground."

"Funny, that's not quite the way I remember the story. Of course, my memory could have faded from the passage of time, but I could swear you pushed me off the swing, as boys tend to do." Lauren joked.

"If only to get the attention of an exceptionally beautiful girl. My immaturity must have outweighed my sensibilities." Rick and Lauren both laughed. "Allow me to correct my dreadful error in judgment."

"And how's that?" Lauren cocked her head but had a gleam in her eye.

"My dear, your hand is empty, devoid of drink. And, as luck would have it, I happen to find myself with two. It would be ungentlemanly not to share."

This time Lauren laughed. "That's right, and you are always the gentleman, or so you claim."

"Ask anyone. I've got references."

"Well, thank you for the drink, and thank you for rescuing me. Liza seems to be tied up over by the window."

"Doris Walsh and her husband. Liza is being interrogated about you, truth be told. A fact of life in a small club. Let's step outside on the porch where we can relax and talk." Rick guided Lauren through the screen doors toward a pair of rocking chairs. Lauren couldn't resist herself.

"You're determined to rock my world."

"I wouldn't have it any other way." Rick laughed. He was astonished at how comfortable he felt with Lauren. His plan of shameless flirting was obliterated with the discovery he genuinely enjoyed talking with her.

The two spent the rest of the cocktail hour talking about the history of the club and local area. Lauren seemed interested in discovering the area. Rick was surprised when she brought up Castle Farms, one of his favorite places. She quickly agreed to accompany him on a tour the following week. Rick couldn't remember the last time anyone was remotely interested in his history lessons, let alone willing to go on an excursion with him. His heart warmed with anticipation.

As the dinner bell rang, calling the members into the dining room, Lauren and Rick fell into step as if they were longtime companions. Liza watched them walk in ahead of her as she entered the dining room from the library. She did a double take. Her childhood friend Dickie was a consummate flirt, but there was something about his body language, about his relaxed stature, that alerted her to the fact that something was different about their budding friendship. Liza was getting on a plane for New York the next morning and wasn't sure if she would have the opportunity to get over to his table to speak with him during dinner. Perhaps she would get a chance when she came back in a couple of weeks for Venetian Weekend.

During dinner, the conversation with the Breckenridges covered some of the events they could look forward to, both on the club grounds and in town. Lauren was very interested in the Traverse City Cherry Festival beginning the following day since she was driving Liza to the airport. Liza explained most of the bigger events happen on the weekend, but there would be plenty to do on Monday if she wanted to wander around.

"That sounds like a plan. You should make a day of it. Maybe do some shopping while you're down there," David said. "I'm going fishing with one of the club elders. Apparently it's an honor to be invited out on the big lake with him."

Liza smiled. "Papa Doc. Yes, you must have impressed him. He doesn't offer invites to everyone; you need to be up early."

"That's what he said. We'll be out on the lake at sunrise."

With everyone's attention momentarily distracted, Lauren took the opportunity to scan the room and caught Rick's glance. Her heart skipped a beat. Lauren took a gulp of wine and quickly looked away. "Aud, would you like to come to Traverse City with me?" she sputtered, grasping for something to say, feeling as if she were a kid who'd been caught doing something wrong.

"No thanks, Mom. Not if you're going shopping. Totally not interested." Audrey held her breath.

"Oh, okay, sweetie. Is there anything you want me to pick up for you?"

"Actually, I could use some new jeans and T-shirts, but it's no big deal." Audrey tried to sound nonchalant, hoping her mother would go overboard, as usual, and she would have some new clothes to wear to work. "And probably a dress to wear to dinner here."

"Seriously? You're letting me shop for you? Since when has that happened?"

"Yeah, well, don't let it go to your head or anything. I just don't get the style they wear up here, and you like this sort of thing, so whatever. Knock yourself out."

Jason laughed. "I don't need anything, Mom. I'm living in swim trunks all summer long, just the way I like it."

Lauren risked another glance in Rick's direction only to see he was gone, and the table was being cleared by the wait staff. Her stomach sank just a little.

CHAPTER 29

Liza put her bags in the back of the Jeep. She planned to drive but made sure Lauren knew the landmarks to watch for on the way home from the airport.

"I wish you were staying for the summer," Lauren admitted. "I think I'd have more fun hanging out with you."

"Oh, I don't know about that. I think you're going to do just fine."

Lauren looked over at Liza to see if there was some sort of hidden meaning behind that comment. "Your friends seem nice."

"Yes, Betsy and Lindsay will keep you as occupied as you want to be, but I'm not sure that's who I'm talking about."

"What? Who are you talking about then?" Lauren gave her a quizzical look.

"Dickie."

"Who?"

"Oh, right." Liza smirked. "Rick Sawyer. Also one of my best friends since forever."

Lauren laughed. "He said some people called him Dickie. I guess he meant you."

"He meant everyone."

"He seems really nice," Lauren added quickly, her heart in her mouth. "In fact, he's going to take me on the tour of Castle Farms this week."

Liza did a double take. "Really?" She could barely contain her surprise. Here she was, about to warn Lauren about the flirtatious playboy who wreaked havoc on people's lives and couldn't be serious for a minute, and yet Lauren seemed to have discovered the other Dickie—the one Liza loved dearly. The one he hid from the entire world. Liza's Dickie was a smart, thoughtful, generous man who truly enjoyed history. He also passionately loved the small-town atmosphere of Northern Michigan.

The two spoke on random subjects for the remainder of the hour-long drive. Pulling into the commuter airport, Liza tossed Lauren the keys and pulled her bags out of the back.

Liza gave Lauren a warm hug. "Use the Jeep; it's yours for the summer. Just do me one favor."

"Anything."

"Be kind to Dickie's heart."

"What do you mean?"

"Just be careful. He's more sensitive than he seems. I don't want him to get hurt."

Those words stuck with Lauren as she shopped for Audrey. She had to admit to herself that she genuinely enjoyed the friendship she was forming with Rick. The flirtation was fun, but there seemed to be more depth to it. Lauren couldn't remember the last time she'd been in a position like this. College, perhaps. She wondered if she should be feeling guilty for enjoying Rick's company.

Stop it! It's a friendship. You're closer to Chams. Lost in thought, she'd finished shopping and headed back to the parking lot when she came to a pocket park overflowing with jubilant people, obviously part of the Cherry Festival.

The crowd, gathered around a massive booth, was cheering a college-age young man, the current participant in the cherry pit spitting contest. Lauren was drawn into the action and found herself enthralled by the enthusiasm. She was shocked by the distances people could spit a pit. Soon she was fully involved in the contest and cheering just as hard as the locals.

"I think you should sign up for a turn," a familiar voice behind her said.

Lauren jumped. Rick was suddenly standing by her side. She blushed, uncertain how long he'd been watching her.

"Oh, don't get shy on me now. You were having fun," Rick chided.

"Well, yeah." Lauren looked down at her shoes. "I admit it."

"Don't worry, I come every year."

The announcer called out, "Number 134, 1-3-4."

"That's me. Be right back." Rick squeezed his way through the crowd, turned in his ticket, and plucked a cherry out of the basket. He gave Lauren a mischievous smile before popping it in his mouth. Juice seeped from the corners of his mouth and down his chin. With the pit clean of any fruit, he stepped up to the line and spit as hard as he could, but his efforts didn't come close to some of the longest pits.

Lauren found herself cheering along with the crowd, applauding both his effort and form. The smile on his face was infectious as he made his way back to her side. "I've never come close to the pro pit spitters. I think they must practice in their basements all winter long." Lauren melted in laughter, and the two fell into step as they walked toward the picnic area.

"Are you hungry? The VFW's cherry-marinated barbeque chicken is delicious, one of the things I look forward to every summer."

"Show me the way! It sounds wonderful."

Rick took Lauren's bags from her, and they walked along Front Street toward Sunset Park. Rick regaled her with the history of the Cherry Festival and how Traverse City became known as the Cherry Capital of the World.

Lauren had to admit the chicken was delicious, and, surprisingly, she was not embarrassed to lick her fingers in front of Rick. The homebrewed cherry ale was not exactly to her liking but paired well with the chicken, so she ended up drinking the full sixteen-ounce cup. It went straight to her head.

"I really shouldn't drive back to the club right now."

"Oh good, I was hoping to extend the day. You're excellent company. I'm usually alone at these things."

"Why is that?" she asked as they walked toward the area of town where a band was setting up.

"I wish I knew. When we were kids, the counselors would bring the crew kids here on an excursion. I loved it. But as we got older, my friends just stopped wanting to come. When I got my license, I started coming by myself." Rick paused, looking toward the waterfront. "I do a lot of things by myself. People don't notice."

"Do you get lonely?"

"Lonely? Not in the sense you mean. I've met a ton of people. They've become my friends, too. It's strange, locals and club members don't tend to socialize with each other. So, because I disappear from time to time, I've ended up with an interesting reputation with the Lexington Club crowd. It makes me laugh."

"Why?"

"Well, they see me as this playboy, but really I'm the exact opposite." Rick paused and looked at Lauren carefully. "And now I will have to kill you; I've told you far too much about myself as it is."

Lauren laughed. "Yes, well, make sure you do it neatly. I would hate to think they'd find my mangled body somewhere. That would be horrible for the kids."

"But not the husband?"

"Oh, that was sneaky! You'll get no state secrets from me."

"You're a tough nut to crack, Mrs. Breckenridge, but I've got you under the lights. You'll buckle under the pressure. Nobody withstands my interrogation techniques.

"Is that so?"

"Well, it shall be from now on."

The two walked the length of the waterfront and back along Front Street until they got to Liza's Jeep.

"Are you sure you're okay to drive?" Rick asked.

"Yes, I'm fine now. You're kind to ask."

The two piled the shopping bags into the back of the Jeep and stood there looking at each other for a minute.

"Thanks again," Rick said as Lauren climbed into the car. She was surprised to see it was nearly eight p.m. She wasn't used to it staying light so late. She hoped the kids and David wouldn't be too upset with her. Even the thought of her family could not dampen the lightness she felt. Lauren smiled and headed for home.

Chapter 30

Audrey was focused on trying to come up with some sort of organized system for the client files. It was two hours before the clinic opened, and Claire was making house calls. Filing was clearly not something Claire considered a priority and Audrey wanted to surprise her.

The buzzer on the front door sounded, and when Audrey ignored it, it rang again. The second time she heard a desperate-sounding male voice call out for assistance. Audrey put down the files and darted to the front room.

"The doctor's not here. What do you want?"

"I tried to get the dog, but I couldn't!" he said breathlessly. "Can you help me?"

"Help you what? I don't know what you're talking about." Audrey was quickly becoming frustrated and a bit annoyed by the disruption.

"There's a dog running loose on the side of the road," the boy said, "and if somebody doesn't catch him, he's going to get hit by a car!"

Audrey sprang into action. She grabbed a leash and collar, along with a handful of treats. "Where's the dog?" The two rushed out the front door together.

"Just up the road. Not too far."

"Let's run!"

The boy took off down the road with Audrey at his heels. A minute later, she spotted the dog at the edge of the corn field. It was a small German shepherd, panicked and limping on its right front paw.

Audrey realized the boy was right: the dog was disoriented, and if it kept going, it would end up being hit by a car. Without hesitation, Audrey took action. She told the boy to be still and quiet. "I'm going into the field to get the dog. If anyone else stops, tell them I work for Dr. Hawkins and to wait by the road. Got me?"

"No problem."

Audrey crept toward the dog, making soft coaxing sounds. "Here, puppy. It's okay." Audrey repeated this over and over as she slowly approached the dog. The frightened animal stood still and growled, keeping a wary eye on Audrey.

It took a couple minutes, but soon she was beside the dog and had the leash on him. She was lost in the moment, completely unaware of Dr. Hawkins and another passerby who had stopped to help.

Once she had the dog under control and saw his name tag, she whispered, "Hello, Barney. Nice to meet you." The dog relaxed a bit, his growls replaced by whimpers.

Audrey examined his injured paw and saw a shard of glass sticking out of the pad. Looking up for the first time, Audrey saw Dr. Hawkins on the side of the road. Relieved, she picked up the dog and carried him over to Dr. Hawkins' truck.

"Nicely done, Audrey," Claire said.

"Thanks. It wasn't that big of a deal."

As Claire turned her attention to the dog, Audrey found herself facing the boy who had alerted her to the dog's dilemma in the first place. He was about her age and had the most amazing eyes. They were hazel with tiny flecks of gold that reflected the morning sunlight.

"You were awesome. I'm Dylan, by the way."

"Thanks." Audrey was completely tongue-tied.

"I can't believe you could just walk up to him like that. I've been trying to get him for at least half an hour." Dylan stood there for a minute. Audrey wasn't sure what to say. "How did you know how to do that?"

Audrey shrugged. "I don't know... I just kinda did."

"Dylan, this is Audrey. She's working for me this summer since Chrissie went downstate." Claire made the introductions official, and Audrey felt like an idiot. She hadn't even given him her name.

Dylan squirmed a bit. "Thanks, Dr. H. I guess I should be getting home now." Dylan paused, looking from Audrey to Claire and back again. "Would it be okay if I came to visit Barney?"

"Of course. Come in the morning around ten, before we have patients. Shall we go, Audrey? We have some owners to find." Claire nodded toward the back of the truck, where Barney was lying down inside one of the cages.

Audrey glanced at Dylan as she climbed into the truck. He was walking in the opposite direction, away from the animal hospital. He waved eagerly as they passed. Audrey blushed and pretended not to notice.

Chapter 31

A group of fourteen- and fifteen-year-old girls had taken residence at the end of the dock on the hours Jason had guard duty. And there was a surge of interest in individual lessons, especially for instruction in the butterfly, Jason's specialty. Mike, the lead counselor, teased him about his fan club, but Jason didn't think much of it. It was easy work.

On Friday afternoon, a girl dressed in tennis clothes walked out on the dock during his shift. She appeared to be about his age, but what Jason really noticed was how the muscles in her legs quivered and glistened in the sun. It was mesmerizing.

"You must be the Jason with his Argonauts everyone in the club is talking about," the girl said flippantly. Jason swallowed hard.

"Yes, and as captain of this ship, I may need to throw you overboard for talking smack."

"You wouldn't dare."

Jason stood and approached the girl, who immediately took off in a sprint down the dock. She was fast, clearly athletic, but Jason was faster; he caught up to her as they reached the sand. Grabbing at her waist and tossing her over his shoulder with ease, he sauntered to the water's edge.

"Okay, okay, you win. I give. Put me down!" The girl squealed.

Jason gently placed her on the sand. "Jason Breckenridge, lifeguard, at your service."

"You're a brute."

"Maybe, but I believe you started this."

"Nobody's ever caught up with me before."

"Lucky me. So, what's your name?"

"Morgan Stansfield. I play tennis."

"Well, since it's not Halloween, I kind of figured that." Jason overtly looked her up and down. "It's very nice to meet you. Please tell me you're here for a while."

Morgan blushed and averted her eyes. "Well, yeah, actually. I just finished a tournament in Newport Beach, and I have a two-week break before my next one."

"Well, Poseidon must be favoring me with good luck today, because I'm in the presence of a golden goddess."

Morgan stammered, stumbling over words and unable to form a rudimentary sentence. Jason laughed. "I guess I won that round." The two stood there looking at each other. Jason was the first to break the silence. "Listen, I've got another lesson this afternoon, but then one of the other lifeguards takes over and locks up. Do you want to grab something to eat later?"

"Like a date?"

"Sure, why not?"

"Well…" Morgan looked out at the lake, panicked. "I'm… well, my dad doesn't let me date."

"You're kidding."

"I've been focused on tennis practically my whole life. Next year I have an athletic scholarship at Stanford, and, as my dad says, I need to keep my eye on the ball."

"Like when you're playing tennis."

"Oh, he means in everything, anything that distracts from our goals. He says I can be a professional player, on the tour. He wants me to go to Stanford, play on their team and in tournaments then turn pro when I'm nineteen."

"Why so late?" Jason quipped. He was being sarcastic, not fully comprehending the seriousness of this girl's life plan and more than a little frustrated by her disinterest in him.

Morgan launched into an explanation, including details about needing to strengthen her emotional maturity. Her father felt players tended to burn out if they started out too young. As she mentioned the names of elite players she would have to contend with as part of the strategy, Jason stopped listening. He was captivated with how she used her hands to speak and how her eyes sparkled.

"Okay, so it's not a date. Would he be opposed to the two of us grabbing burgers at the Kids' Club after I lock up? That's just part of the standard club stuff, and we would just be running into each other. How's that?"

Morgan thought about it for a minute. Jason was really cute and she usually ate at the Kids' Club when she was home anyway. "I can't see how that would be breaking Dad's rules," Morgan said, her face flushing. With a smirk she added, "And you seem harmless enough."

"Oh, you're going to start that again?" Jason faked a lunge toward Morgan who jumped backward.

"You're going to have to work a little harder than that to catch me," she chided.

"I'm up for that challenge. See you soon," Jason called out as he walked out to the end of the dock. The rest of the afternoon sailed by, his mood euphoric at the prospect of seeing Morgan in a couple hours.

Chapter 32

The family seemed to settle into a predictable pattern of summer activities. Jason left the house early in the morning, spending the day at the beach where he seemed to hold court. Lauren had to admit the job agreed with him. Two weeks into their vacation and he was no longer gloomy or sulking. It was as if the whole incident with Karen had never happened. Lauren was happy to forget all about it.

David seemed relaxed and content. He spent all his time golfing with a group of men. There were so many courses, it seemed like they were always going to a different location. David was also on the club softball team, which took the interclub rivalries very seriously. They played league games twice a week in the evenings and held practices on the other days. When the family went to the beach picnics or club dinners, he was immediately drawn into conversation about one sporting competition or another. One of the club members was in hot pursuit, trying to draft David as "rail meat" for the Thirsty Thursday sailing regattas. David didn't know a thing about sailing, but Alec swore all he needed to do was sit there and be heavy.

Audrey disappeared in the mornings, too. She didn't say much at dinner, and every time Lauren brought it up to David, she was chastised for being overprotective and worried about nothing. The argument she used—she's fourteen—was his exact argument for letting it go. They were at an impasse.

Lauren had to admit she preferred this version of Audrey over the semi-goth version that appeared last spring. So, against her instinct, she tried to follow David's advice. Lauren remembered Liza's words, that the teens were supervised by the counselors and protected by the simple fact they spent their days on private property. Perhaps David was correct, and Audrey had made some friends and was just being a typical teenager.

Lauren was disappointed. Her grand vacation plans of family togetherness had disappeared, but since everyone was happy and enjoying themselves she decided to keep it to herself. For the most part, the family would come together at dinner time to trade stories of the daily events. After that they either retreated to their rooms for the remainder of the night or to a scheduled club event. It was certainly not what Lauren had envisioned, but somehow she wasn't unhappy.

The house phone rang, startling her. In this day and age of cell phones, when a phone attached to the wall rang it seemed so quaint. Lauren caught her breath. She hoped it was Rick.

But it was Lindsay, calling to invite her to a cocktail luncheon at the president's house starting at eleven thirty. The women of the club were going to discuss the selections of the summer book reading club—over a few bottles of champagne, of course.

Lauren declined politely but added she would love to be included in the book club. Today just wasn't a good day for her.

"I'm glad you turned them down," said a voice from the hallway.

Lauren nearly jumped out of her skin. "Does everyone just walk into each other's houses around here?" She sounded angrier than she felt, flashing back to running into the caretaker on her first day in the house.

"Well, actually, yes we do. Is that a problem?" Rick said sheepishly.

"It's completely disruptive and totally disrespectful. What if I were naked?" Lauren demanded.

"Well, then it would have been my lucky day." Rick disarmed her with a sexy smile.

"I'm serious."

"So am I." His voice deepened.

"Oh, you're being impossible. What do you want?" Lauren snapped. "Why are you here?"

Rick looked a little hurt. "I'm sorry. I've been walking into this house unannounced my whole life. I guess I really wasn't thinking. I mean, I wanted to surprise you, but I didn't mean to make you angry." He paused. "I'll go."

"No, don't do that." Lauren quickly recovered, reaching out to touch his arm. "I'm sorry, too. I overreacted."

"I'll accept your apology if you'll have lunch with me. Maybe we could go on a little excursion." Rick flashed a smile. "I mean, if you're not busy."

Lauren blushed. "I'm not busy. I didn't mean to lie to Lindsay, but I just don't feel like drinking lunch. Those ladies don't seem to stop."

"Don't worry, she didn't think twice about it. And to be truthful, you're right; they don't stop. They drink and gossip. Trust me, if you're looking for meaningful discussion about the books, you'll be disappointed. They might read the books, but the conversation amounts to 'did you like it?'"

Lauren laughed. "Oh Lord, I hope you're kidding."

"I wish I were," he said, eyeing her once over. "You look perfect. Are you ready to go?"

Lauren felt tinges of pink on her cheeks and caught her breath as the two headed out the kitchen door. For a moment she thought about leaving a note but then realized she would be home before the rest of her family, so there was no point in doing so.

"Wow! Your car is beautiful." Lauren admired the bright-red two-seater.

Rick grinned. "Thank you, I love her. She's a '62 Morgan. I've spent five years restoring her."

"You did this on your own?"

"Not completely. I had help with some of the body work, and then I had trouble getting the engine tuned just right. I have a shop where I tinker with things."

"I'm not so sure I would call this tinkering." Lauren sat back, enjoying the wind in her hair.

"Do you trust me? And are you up for an adventure?"

Lauren looked at Rick with caution. She was both excited and wary at once. As she held his eyes for a long moment, Lauren impulsively put herself into his charge. "Sure, why not? I'm game. Lead the way."

Rick smiled from ear to ear and accelerated the car a little harder than he would normally. Soon they were pulling into a marina parking lot with Rick waving to the security guard. "I'm taking you sailing."

"Really? I won't know what to do. I've never been sailing before."

"You haven't changed your mind have you?" Rick opened the passenger door, holding his hand out for Lauren.

"No, but I admit I'm a little nervous."

"I'll take care of everything. All you have to do is relax and enjoy." Rick held her hand as they walked down to a sleek black sailboat. Still holding tight, his free hand at the small of her back, Rick guided Lauren aboard the boat. "Welcome aboard the *Wataridori*. She's an Erickson 35, perfect for racing and cruising." Rick glowed.

"That name is unusual. What does it mean?"

"It's Japanese, actually. The name means *ferry*, and when you put it into the verb form, it means *wanderer*."

"You really picked a perfect name for it," Lauren said.

"How so?"

"You like to wander and explore. I mean, that's just you in a nutshell, right?"

Lauren watched as Rick moved from one end of the boat to the other. He released lines, took off the sail covers and stowed them below, and started up the engine. His movements were effortless, as if he had done this hundreds of times. When they were under way, he steered the boat out of the marina, waving to a group of people at the end of the jetty. Lauren was awestruck by his grace and ease of movement.

Rick reached out his hand. "Come here. I want you to stand over here." He took a step backward and she slid between him and the wheel. "Put your hands on the wheel and feel how the boat moves," he said into her ear. "You can feel the movement, can't you?"

Lauren nodded.

"Now look at the compass and keep steering in this exact direction. If we turn a few degrees, don't worry; just turn the wheel the tiniest bit, and the helm will come right back. Oh, and don't worry about me," he said with a laugh. "I'll be right back."

The next thing Lauren knew, Rick was scampering all over the boat raising sails and turning off the engine. Suddenly she could feel the boat lunge forward, and she got nervous.

"Rick?"

"Right here." He slipped in behind her. "Relax for a minute; you're sailing now." Rick turned the wheel a bit and the boat seemed to leap forward in the water. She felt her body press into his and it was heavenly. She didn't want to move.

Rick explained tacking and running downwind as he stood behind the wheel with Lauren in his arms. After an hour or so, he broke the spell, motioning for her to sit on one of the side benches as he expertly brought down the sails. When he pulled the boat into a slip, he called up to a dock hand and asked him to put her away.

Both of them had enormous smiles on their faces they walked back to the Morgan hand in hand. "I'm starving, and I know this great place where we can get burgers. How does that sound to you?"

"Perfect," Lauren said, but she wasn't really hungry. Honestly, lunch was the furthest thing on her mind.

Chapter 33

Audrey's favorite part of the job was exercising the dogs in the run. Dr. Hawkins had a soft spot for taking in dogs in need of homes; two of the dogs she'd taken in had served in combat. Audrey couldn't believe she was actually getting paid to throw tennis balls and play with them. They were so happy and grateful for the attention. It was the only time Audrey laughed and felt true joy. The residual feelings usually lasted for a few hours before the blackness of her world came crashing down again. But for the time she was tossing a tennis ball and romping with "her dogs," she felt light.

"Go long, Buster!" Audrey called out to one of the two German shepherds as she tossed a ball as far as she could. The two dogs barked and growled as they tussled on the far side of the pen over which one would have the honor of returning the ball to their human. Audrey laughed as she thumped the lone Rottweiler on his ribs for returning his ball. Suddenly the big dog left her side and ran to the door of the pen. "What's wrong, Roscoe?"

"Hey!" Dylan called out and waved to Audrey. He opened the run and greeted Roscoe who clearly knew him. Audrey froze. *How long had he been watching?* "You're really good with Dr. H's dogs. You looked like you were having fun."

"Yeah." Audrey's mood changed almost immediately. Now she was on guard, she felt like there was an intruder in her space.

"Dr. H lets me come here after school to play with the dogs. It's one of my favorite things to do." Dylan continued, oblivious to Audrey's obvious discomfort. He picked up a ball and tossed it for Roscoe who chased eagerly in its direction.

Dylan looked at Audrey, expecting her to respond. She was frustrated, annoyed that she couldn't just enjoy the dogs by herself. Roscoe dropped the ball at her feet, and she reluctantly picked it up, giving it a halfhearted toss.

"What are you doing here?

Dylan seemed caught off-guard by her abruptness. "I came to see how Barney was doing. Did you find his owner?"

"Oh, Barney. Right." Audrey was relieved. "Dr. Hawkins found them. They picked him up yesterday." She paused until the silence became awkward. "They were very happy to have him back... so, yeah."

"I guess we did a good thing," Dylan said.

"I guess." Audrey was not as cheerful. The two continued to throw balls for the dogs, but the joy Audrey had felt was gone. She was tense, nervous around this boy, wondering what he wanted and why he was still there. Her mood darkened and she wanted to leave.

Dylan seemed to ask one question after another. Audrey responded with short, terse answers. She didn't know how long she could deal with the small talk or why he kept pestering her. When Dylan asked Audrey how she felt about school, it was all too much. The question pushed her over the edge. "I fucking hate school, okay? Not that it's any of your business." Audrey pushed past Dylan and walked out of the pen. "I have to get back to work now."

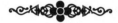

Claire saw the whole thing from her kitchen window. It was clear from his body language Dylan was crushed. She approached him as he started to leave the pen and lock it up.

"Try not to take it personally, Dylan. I think Audrey was hurt in her past and she hasn't dealt with it. I think she's very angry, but not at you or me. This has nothing to do with you."

"How do you know?"

"Oh, well, I've seen a lot of this. Sometimes when something really bad happens to a person they get stuck. And then little things remind them of that horrible moment. Then they're no longer reacting normally; they're reacting as if they were back in that horrible moment. I'm not certain, but I'm pretty sure that's what is happening to Audrey."

"So what do we do, Dr. H?"

"Well, that's the challenge, Dylan. We have to figure out what's wrong. But the important thing is not to give up. You like her, right?"

Dylan nodded, looking at his shoes. "She's really cool."

"I do, too. We need to give her time and some space. I think she'll come around. Now, run along. I'm going to have lunch with her and see if she'll talk to me."

"Thanks, Dr. H. I guess you're good with people, too."

"They're just two-footed animals, Dylan."

Claire Hawkins went in search of Audrey. She was impressed by Audrey's independence and hard work. In only two weeks, she had gotten into the rhythm of the office and seemed to manage it without much direction. She came in early, took care of the cages, played with the dogs before it got hot, and even made a significant dent in the filing backlog.

Claire had an inkling there was some dark truth Audrey was hiding. She'd tried to talk to Audrey a couple times over lunch, but whatever this girl was hiding wasn't going to slip out in casual conversation. Claire continued to nurture the relationship, hoping Audrey would begin to trust her.

"How were the dogs today?" Claire asked as she poured sun tea into tall glasses filled with ice.

"Oh, they were great. Pedro is getting more rambunctious. He's ready for his bandages to come off. At least that's how it seems to me. He wants to pull them off."

"Actually, his stitches can come out in the next day or two," Claire said. "Nice observation about canine behavior and moods. You have a talent for taking care of animals."

Audrey shifted uncomfortably in her seat and took a bite of the sandwich. Chewing was a great way to avoid a subject. Audrey didn't want to talk about herself. Claire usually respected her silence but not today.

"I'm serious, Audrey. You're young, but you have a real knack for this work. I've been impressed, and our clients are comfortable with you." Claire paused for effect and to allow her protégé time to swallow. "Many high schools have specialized programs for arts or sciences, and if you're interested, I think a medical magnate program would be appropriate for you. It could help you get into a veterinary program in college." Claire paused; Audrey said nothing. "Did you know they're actually harder to get into than med school?"

"Really? Why?"

"Well, for starters, there are less of them. Are you interested in veterinary medicine?" Claire asked.

Audrey looked up at Claire. She had to answer; the woman was waiting. "I don't know. I guess." She shrugged.

"Look, I don't mean to sound pushy. I care about you and want to help you, and if it's something you're remotely interested in..."

Audrey looked down at her plate, her lip quivering in spite of her efforts to control it. She didn't want Dr. Hawkins to notice. It was like she could see through her, and it made Audrey uncomfortable. But at the same time, she felt like she needed to be near Claire. It was very confusing.

"It doesn't matter," Audrey muttered.

"What do you mean it doesn't matter?" Claire realized she was treading on thin ice. The girl had to talk to someone. It was like gaining the trust of a wounded animal. Knowing how to balance moving with confidence and deference simultaneously was never easy. Slightly off kilter and the animal will spook and run.

All of a sudden Audrey burst out, "Why the fuck do you care?" She sprang to her feet, and her chair toppled backward. "You're not my mother, and even she doesn't give a shit." Tears of rage fell uncontrolled down Audrey's face. "Don't you get it? Nobody cares, including me, so just leave me alone!"

Claire watched in stunned silence as Audrey sprinted from the building. Her heart filled with sorrow as familiar memories flooded through her: shouting, pushed-over chairs, misunderstood feelings. Deep wounds opened and tears welled from the echoes of arguments long past. Claire knew she had to take action. She wasn't exactly sure where she would find Audrey but began the perfunctory step of putting the *Closed-on emergency call* sign in the window and making sure the phones were forwarded to the service. Locking the door and walking down the steps, she decided the logical thing to do would be to head toward the Ironton Ferry. If Audrey headed back to her summer home, that's where she'd be.

CHAPTER 34

Rick and Lauren ate lunch at The Landing, a quaint pub located near the Ironton Ferry. Rick ordered burgers for them both, and by the time they were served, she realized she was starving.

"Sailing and spending time out on the water will do that to you," Rick teased as he watched Lauren devour her lunch.

"You really seemed to know what you were doing. Doesn't it usually take a bunch of people to sail a boat?"

"When I race her, sure. But I also have her set up for single-handing. I love to be able to hop on the boat and go when the mood strikes me."

"Or when you want to impress the ladies," Lauren said. She had to admit to herself she was digging into his personal life to see if there were other women. She hated herself for wanting to know, but she couldn't stop herself either.

Rick smiled. "Oh, I've never taken any of my ladies, as you put it, out sailing." Taking a drink of his beer, he let Lauren sweat it out for a bit. "I suppose I shouldn't ruin my reputation like this, but I really don't have any ladies to speak of."

Lauren blushed, pushing the French fries around on her plate. She was secretly thrilled by this revelation. Looking up into his eyes, she said, "I find it very hard to believe no woman has captured your heart."

"Alas, it's true. My heart must be waiting for just the right person to come along, because I've never found anyone who captivated me." The words *like you* seemed to float, unsaid, between them.

They finished eating, and the intensity of the conversation made sitting there awkward, so Rick suggested they watch the ferry. As they walked to the landing, he told her all about the ferry's history. Lauren was surprised to learn how long it had been in continuous operation and laughed about it being in the Guinness Book of World Records. With something safe to talk about the momentary awkwardness dissipated.

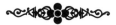

The line of cars at the ferry landing snaked down the street and around the corner. Claire located Audrey's scooter near the ramp as she pulled into the parking lot. The ferry was just unloading cars on the far side, so she knew she had five minutes to talk to her.

"Audrey, why did you run from me?" Claire asked when she was close enough to speak to the girl.

"Why did you follow me?"

"I wasn't going to let you run off like that."

"Why not? What do you care?" Audrey asked, angry and defensive.

"I do care, Audrey, I care a lot." Claire was trying to break down walls which seemed to have come out of nowhere. She realized she must have hit a nerve but didn't know what she'd said to cause so much hurt.

"You don't even know me."

"That may be true, but I like the part I do know." Claire was unwavering. "I want you to feel safe with me. You can tell me anything."

"That's not true. Adults judge kids my age. Nobody listens. It's like we don't exist."

"Audrey, I've opened my home and my work to you. I took a risk hiring you, and I've trusted you at every turn since. You know that. Don't you think you should trust me a little?"

"I don't know how." Audrey looked away as tears streaked down her cheeks.

The ferry had arrived, and Claire knew she was out of time. "Look, Audrey, I can tell you want to run again, and I'm not going to stop you, but think about this for a minute. You need to talk to someone. I'm willing to listen and I won't judge you, I promise."

As Audrey considered Claire's words there was a look of hope in her eyes. Suddenly a squeal of laughter echoed from the dock beside the ferry. Audrey looked up in time to see her mother snuggled close to Rick, his hands around her waist. She was smiling, laughing at whatever he whispered in her ear.

"Oh my God! Not you, too!" Audrey screamed. "I hate all of you!" Audrey cried as she hopped on the Vespa, spun the tires, and somehow managed to make the ferry just as the gates were closing.

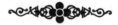

Neither Lauren nor Claire could react in time to get on the ferry.

Lauren was the first to regain her composure and approached the woman who had been with Audrey. "Who the hell are you, and what did you do to my daughter?"

"Excuse me? How dare you talk to me that way," Claire said. "I've done nothing but help that child. I believe she was reacting to you, because that sure as hell isn't her daddy." Claire glared at Rick.

"Ladies, ladies. Let's calm down here." Rick stepped between the women.

"Don't tell me to calm down, Dickie. This woman is making accusations about me." Claire made no effort to quell the anger surging through her.

"You know her?" Lauren said.

"Well, yeah. Claire, this is Lauren Breckenridge, and that girl you were talking to is her daughter, Audrey."

"Yes, I know. She works for me," Claire replied.

"Excuse me? What do you mean by 'works for you'?" Lauren's voice was still tempered with excitement. "And who the hell are you anyway?"

"Lauren, this is Dr. Claire Hawkins. She's our veterinarian," Rick explained.

"Well, she's out of her mind. My daughter does not work for a veterinarian."

"Actually, your daughter has worked for me since the beginning of the summer, and now I have a clue as to why she feels like nobody listens to her." Claire dug in her heels for a fight.

"Ladies, there is obviously a huge miscommunication that needs to be straightened out before we can move forward. Let's go inside and get some iced tea." He guided them toward the pub where he and Lauren had just had lunch.

Once they were seated and had ordered a round of iced teas, Rick turned to Claire. "How is it that Audrey came to work for you this summer, and did you realize her mother didn't know?"

Claire's explanation was simple, straightforward and rang of the truth. Lauren wanted to throw up. For the second time in less than six months, a stranger was telling her a story about an elaborate, secret life one of her children was leading. She could barely keep her head from exploding.

Chapter 35

Jason and Morgan were spending quite a bit of time together, and it was driving him crazy. Long showers just weren't cutting it. He couldn't stop thinking about her. Morgan was smart, funny, and sexy as hell when she walked. But the best part was he could just be himself around her, and she seemed to enjoy his company.

Walking back from the beach to Morgan's cottage, Jason couldn't take it any longer. "Morgan, we have to talk."

"What's wrong?" Morgan sounded panicked.

"Huh? Nothing. Wait…" When it dawned on Jason how his line must have sounded, he felt like an idiot. "Nothing bad, honest." Jason reached out and pulled at her hand so she was facing him. "You've got to know how much I like you." He took a step closer, not letting go of her arm. Morgan didn't pull away from him; this was a good sign. Jason slipped his arm around her waist and pulled her into him. Having her close felt so good.

Instinctively, Morgan reached up and rested her hands on Jason's shoulders, meeting his hungry gaze with one of her own. It was all the invitation he needed. Jason kissed Morgan softly at first, but the intensity quickly flamed.

"Morgan!" The booming voice brought them both back to reality in a hurry.

"Dad!"

"What do you think you're doing? And who is this boy?" Morgan's father was standing on the front porch of their house and he was furious.

"Dad, it's not what you think. This is Jason Breckenridge."

"The renter's kid? Morgan, it's exactly what I think! Is there more I should know about?"

"No!" Morgan glanced at Jason. "Well, not exactly. I like Jason. He's my friend."

"I thought we talked about this. Boys are a distraction you don't need. It will keep us from our goal." Morgan's father seemed to be in a world of his own. They listened to him lecture them about Morgan's path and her goals, about the need for absolute focus on their dreams in order to make them a reality.

"Daddy, please!"

"What?"

"Jason is different. He's not just a boy, and he's not distracting me." Morgan seemed to have her father's attention for the first time. Jason stood motionless, barely able to breathe. "We've been friends all summer long, and I won the last tournament, didn't I?" She didn't wait for an answer. "You need to let me grow up just a little bit, Dad. I'm seventeen years old, and I'm going to college next year. I'm allowed to have a boyfriend." Morgan defiantly slipped her hand into Jason's.

At this point, Jason fully understood the term *sweating bullets*. He was exhilarated that Morgan was standing up for herself, yet at the same time terrified of her father and what he might do. *Is having a girlfriend always so complicated?*

Morgan's dad was silent for a long time. Finally, he sighed and his shoulders dropped. "I don't have a choice in the matter, do I Aces?"

Morgan's voice softened, too. "No, Dad, you really don't."

"Jason, huh?" Morgan's father looked him up and down. "Well, your father seems to be a fine man. I've played a few rounds of golf with him this summer. Can I assume you're a chip off his block, if you know what I mean?"

Jason had no clue what he meant. "Yes, sir" was all he could think of to say.

"Well then, you better be good to my little Aces. I suppose you both should come inside. Your mother and I were about to have a cocktail; you can join us for a soda."

"Yes, sir." Jason squeezed Morgan's hand.

Morgan let go of Jason and launched into her father, throwing her arms around his neck. "Thanks, Dad. You're going to like Jason when you get to know him. I know it."

Jason wasn't sure what had just happened, but he was pretty sure the rest of his summer was looking up.

Jason followed Morgan and her dad into the house, secretly watching her leg muscles tighten under her short tennis skirt.

CHAPTER 36

Audrey was in her room when Lauren returned home after talking with Claire Hawkins. The initial shock of the situation was wearing off, and Lauren was trying to come to grips with all the new information about Audrey.

The enjoyment from the sailing adventure was gone, and her focus was on her daughter. Why did Audrey feel the need to lie? Claire mentioned she thought Audrey was dealing with some sort of trauma or anxiety issues, but Lauren dismissed the idea outright. Rick and Claire had no idea how difficult Audrey had been over the past six months, and this was just part of the big picture, a normal part of life with a hormonal fourteen-year-old girl.

To Lauren's credit, she knew Audrey had been keeping something from her this summer. Apparently it was this job. Lauren felt a little better, almost righteous, in her relief.

"Aud, honey, you need to sit up and talk to me." The girl didn't move. Lauren coaxed harder. "Come on. We're going to talk about this. You can't avoid it, and I'm not going away." Audrey sat up and glared at her mother who was perched at the end of the bed. Lauren wondered where all the anger was coming from.

"You want to tell me what's going on?"

Audrey simply shook her head.

"Okay, I'll start. I met Dr. Hawkins. I know about your job." Lauren softened her tone. "Sweetie, why didn't you tell me?"

"Because you would have said no."

"You don't know that. You didn't even give me a chance." Lauren fought hard to stay calm.

"You wanted this picture-perfect family vacation. So when golden boy got a job, I figured I could, too."

"Honey, Jason is hardly perfect."

"Yeah, right. He didn't even get into trouble for that whole thing with that lady," Audrey muttered.

"You have no idea what you're talking about." Lauren tried to keep her voice even, but the slightest mention of the incident tended to get her blood boiling.

"Well, it's not like anybody talks about shit around here. I have to figure everything out on my own, as usual."

"Watch your language. If you had questions you should've asked."

"Like you and Dad would have told me the truth. You would've handed me some sugarcoated pile of crap, and you know it."

"Audrey, I'm serious. Don't talk that way to me; I'm your mother."

"Really, Mom? Are you? What motherly things do you do with me? Do we go shopping and get our nails done together like all the other girls?"

Lauren took a deep breath. She didn't want to be baited into an argument with her daughter. Audrey knew exactly what to say when she wanted to hurt Lauren. Guilt crept into her heart and mind. They didn't do the so-called normal mother-daughter things Lauren had looked forward to since Audrey was born. "Can we stay focused for a minute? You got a job without permission and you've been lying about it. That is the real issue."

"Whatever."

"Look, I'm trying not to get angry about this, so don't push me. Dr. Hawkins said you happen to be really good at your job. She said you could have a career as a veterinarian. I'm trying to weigh that positive news against your lies and come to some sort of middle ground."

"Wait, you mean I can keep the job?" Audrey perked up.

"Well, yes, but you're missing—"

Audrey launched herself into Lauren's arms, "Oh Mom, thank you so much. I was afraid you and Dad were going to say no. I'm sorry. I promise I'll never lie to you again. I swear."

Lauren felt the relief in her daughter's body and decided the rest of the discussion wasn't worth it. It seemed like Audrey was genuinely sorry for lying, and there was no actual harm done. Lauren believed she would be honest from now on.

Dr. Hawkins seemed nice enough. Rick had told her some compelling things: Claire was a decorated veteran from the Iraq war, respected in the community, and a genuinely good person. Rick reassured Lauren that Audrey was in good hands. Lauren needed to relax. She trusted Rick completely.

"Okay, we'll put this behind us. Let's just tell Dad you got a job. We don't have to go into all the details. He'll be surprised and proud of you. It's not exactly the summer I planned, but it's turning out pretty good."

As Lauren left the room, she failed to notice how quickly the light left Audrey's eyes.

CHAPTER 37

By mid-July, the whole town was buzzing with Venetian Week activities. Tourists packed the hotels to overflowing, T-shirt and fudge shops were bustling, and the town shut down to focus on festival activities. The week culminated with two fireworks shows, a lighted boat parade, and a street carnival.

The Lexington Club had its own celebrations, including a tennis tournament where everyone dressed in garb from the turn of the century. Instead of the normal Sunday buffet dinner, the chefs prepared a lobster dinner on the lawn in front of the clubhouse.

Liza would never miss this weekend. It would have been easy enough for her to stay in a cottage owned by one of her friends, but she was happy the Breckenridge family welcomed her back to her own home. She genuinely liked Lauren and knew the two of them would remain friends long after the rental was over.

Liza was driving through town on her way to the cottage when she saw her friend walking down Bridge Street.

"Dickie!" Liza called out after she parked the rental car.

Rick cringed and took a deep breath. He loved Liza, but he'd been trying to outgrow the nickname since he was eleven.

"Hello, beautiful! You're a sight for sore eyes, but do you think you could refer to me by my grown-up name?"

Liza hugged Rick with the warmth of a lifelong friend. "And ruin the fun of watching you cringe? Not a chance."

Rick squeezed her ass with both hands. "Well, then, I get liberties. And you haven't been to the gym this week."

Liza shoved Rick away. "You're horrid, Richard!"

Giggling, they strolled into Kilwins for handmade ice cream and then walked along the docks toward the Beaver Island Ferry slip. Liza grilled Rick about the summer happenings to date.

"How are my renters doing?"

"Oh, they're great. Lovely people," Rick replied.

Liza heard something in his voice and questioned his choice of words. "Lovely? What does that mean?"

"What are you talking about?" Rick barely hid the lump in his throat.

Liza stopped in her tracks. "I've known you my entire life, Dickie, or Rick, or whatever you want me to call you." Liza hissed. "You're up to something. I hear it in your voice. Spill it. Now!"

Rick focused on his melting ice cream. He was unsure if he should tell Liza the truth or try to keep his feelings a secret. Feelings he knew he shouldn't have. Feelings he wasn't sure were even returned. How could he tell his best friend he'd fallen in love with Lauren—a very married woman, no less. Given his track record, he doubted Liza would even believe him.

"Have you lost your mind?" Rick sputtered. "The son is working at the beach and seems to be getting along with Morgan. I just found out the girl started working for Claire Hawkins, who apparently thinks she has a talent. And the husband has totally fit in. He worked his way into the golfing-softball crowd."

"And Lauren?"

"What about Lauren?"

"You two seemed pretty chummy before I left."

"What do you want me to say, Liza? We're friends. That's it." Rick held his breath while Liza eyed him for what seemed like an eternity.

"Okay. I'm sorry. I guess I'm seeing conspiracy theories everywhere. It's been tough at work this summer. I need a vacation."

Rick put his arm around his closest friend and the two fell into step together. "I guess you do, so make the most of the weekend and chill out." He took a bite of her butter pecan. "I still prefer peppermint. I wish you could stay for the finish of the Chicago-Mac sailboat race next week. I have rooms at The Grand again."

Liza relaxed. She really was home, with nothing to do but enjoy the weekend. "Are you racing?"

"Just serious spectating this year. I'm hoping to get some company to go with me this year. It gets old going alone."

"Dickie, if I know you, you'll be alone for maybe ten minutes. I'm sure you'll sweep some cute thing off her feet in no time."

"So you think."

"So I know."

CHAPTER 38

The Lexington Club put on a show for the Founder's Tournament held on Venetian Weekend each year. The entire membership, including the competitors, dressed in turn-of-the-century garb and limited their play to the club's eight clay courts. When President Harvey Winslow announced Richard Sawyer and Lauren Breckinridge as one of the doubles teams, Rick was at Lauren's elbow in a flash. "It's a conspiracy. I paid him off in Scotch." Lauren giggled, not sure if she should believe him.

Liza looked on with interest. She wasn't sure how to read their body language. Something was up, but she didn't sense the heat of a raging affair. Whatever was going on was subtle, almost tender. Was it possible they were unaware they had feelings for each other?

David was paired with one of the elder club matrons. Lauren watched as he entertained her, charm oozing from every pore. Upon seeing his wife standing with Rick, David walked over to greet the two of them.

"I understand the two of you are paired today." David leaned toward Rick and whispered, "Watch out, she has a mean backhand. I usually get it right before I'm sent to the doghouse."

Rick smiled halfheartedly as the color drained from Lauren's face. She wondered how he could say such inappropriate and hurtful things without realizing their full impact.

"Oh look, I see our match has been called." Rick took Lauren by the elbow. "We're up on court seven. Best of luck in your match, David." He steered her quickly toward the stairs. The two were quiet as they made their way to the court.

They were pitted against Edith and Allen Baxter, the reigning club champions, and lost their set to the experienced doubles pair in no time flat.

When the match was over, Rick guided Lauren straight for the champagne punch. She would have preferred water, but none seemed available. As usual, the alcohol went straight to her head.

"So, I was thinking, since you enjoyed sailing so much..." Rick fumbled for words. "The finish to the Chicago-Mac is extraordinary. I get invited to corporate events, and if you're interested, we could go watch the finish. I get rooms at the Grand Hotel every year. Now that I think of it, The Grand is a place you wouldn't want to miss. It would be up one day and back the next."

Lauren wasn't sure what Rick was asking; the words were distorted, her heart hammering. All she could focus on was the possibility of an overnight trip with Rick.

"I'd love to go. It sounds like fun." She had no clue how she'd get away, but she'd figure out the details later.

The rest of the afternoon was a blur, spent drinking champagne and eating finger sandwiches. Eventually everyone ended up at the beach for the first night of fireworks. Lauren truly felt as if she hadn't a care in the world as she relaxed and let the day unfold around her.

CHAPTER 39

Audrey was about to lock the front door when two panicked women rushed in, one carrying a medium-sized terrier.

She tried to get them to fill out the forms, but they insisted on seeing Dr. Hawkins right away. Sensing the urgency and guessing Claire would not turn the women away, she did her best to reassure them and took them to a treatment room. Once they were settled, she went to the back to get Claire.

After greeting the Stovell sisters and doing an exam, Claire pulled Audrey out of the room to discuss the situation. "Puddles is in serious condition. She has a bowel obstruction and needs emergency surgery or she's not going to make it. There's no time to get her to the surgery center in Petoskey or to get a surgical assistant here. I'll need you to be my assistant. Do you think you can follow my instructions to the letter while I'm performing the surgery?"

"I don't know. Is there any other choice?" Audrey was nervous. This seemed like too much responsibility. She didn't want to let Claire down or let Puddles die.

"I'll be very clear with my instructions. I'm confident you can do this. Just trust yourself a little bit and follow my lead. It's Puddles' only chance."

"Okay, I'll try."

Claire explained the situation to the Stovell sisters and excused herself to prep the surgical room. The women cried and fawned over the ailing dog. Audrey did her best to calm them and herself.

"Dr. Hawkins is an amazing vet. She'll be able to help Puddles. Would you like me to hold her while we wait?"

The sisters were grateful for the help and handed the distressed, semiconscious dog to Audrey, who instinctively stroked her ears and talked to her in a low, soothing voice. Puddles relaxed in Audrey's arms. It seemed to calm the Stovell sisters as well.

Claire reappeared in ten minutes. "I have everything set up. Audrey, please bring Puddles back. Ladies, I'll send Audrey out as soon as we get past the major part of the surgery."

Audrey followed Claire into the surgical room. At first she was tense, but soon her curiosity overcame her fears. Audrey followed Claire's instructions, moving lights, handing her instruments, or holding a retractor. Audrey acclimated to her new role quickly, and Claire saw more of the natural talent in her young surgical assistant.

When Claire finished most of the surgery and began closing the dog up, she sent Audrey out with good news. Puddles would recover nicely. The Stovell sisters were certainly relieved to know their dog would live and shared their appreciation.

Later, Claire poured a cup of water from the cooler in the front room and sat down on the couch. "What a day!" she said, drinking half the cup at once. Audrey sat in silence on the arm of the overstuffed chair across the room.

"What did you think?" Claire asked. All Audrey could do was shrug. She was emotionally exhausted, but her mind was going at ninety miles an hour.

"Well, I'll tell you what I think," Claire said, her tone businesslike. "You were great. That wasn't easy, and most kids couldn't have handled what you did." She paused. "I'm proud of you and impressed."

"Thanks. I liked it."

"Good," Claire said as she eyed her young helper. "If you want to, you can come with me to the surgery center one of these days to watch how we really do surgery. You might like it. Now hit the road; it's late. I'll clean up."

"Are you sure? I don't mind staying."

"I've got it. You've already put in a ton of extra time today. See you tomorrow."

Audrey was distracted by the day's events and hadn't really paid attention to the time. As she pulled into the driveway, she realized she'd missed the children's dinner, and the adults were sitting on the porch having drinks.

She was starving, so she slipped into the kitchen through the back door and found cold cuts to make a sandwich. Later, when she heard people on the stairs looking for her, she pretended to be asleep. She didn't feel like talking about her day to anyone. The deception worked like a charm.

Chapter 40

Jason sat by the flag pole watching Morgan play in the tennis tournament. He had the day off, so he wasn't required to be at the beach. Morgan was the only teen allowed to play in the event, thanks to her skill level.

Jason was mesmerized as Morgan floated over the court, graceful and achingly beautiful. His desire for her was overwhelming. Morgan's skills far exceeded her partner's but were not enough to carry them past the quarterfinals, so by late afternoon she was part of the spectating crowd. Spying Jason, she slipped away from her dad to join him.

"Thank God! Someone to talk to," she said as she sat on the grass next to Jason.

"Hi!" Jason squeaked. "You're amazing."

Morgan gave Jason a quizzical look. "You okay?"

Embarrassed, Jason popped up and looked around. "I'm thirsty. Hang on; I'll get us something to drink." He soon returned with two red Solo cups filled with champagne punch. He had already downed half a glass and refilled his cup while nobody was looking. He needed something to calm his nerves.

Jason handed the cup to Morgan who took a sip, coughed, and almost spit it out. "Are you kidding me? You got the punch?"

"Sure," Jason countered. Seeing her face, he quickly added, "They were out of lemonade and I'm thirsty."

Morgan stared at him for a moment then took another hesitant sip. "My dad will kill me."

Jason held his cup up to hers. "Cheers! I'm not planning on telling him, are you?" Jason took a big gulp. Morgan eyed him warily but joined him nonetheless.

The alcohol relaxed Jason, their banter once again coming easily. Jason felt flushed, warm from the punch. His nerves were a thing of the past.

The finals match was in full swing, so he was able to refill the cups without being noticed. He brought sandwiches with the third refill, and they lay on the grass talking, hidden from view by a massive oak tree.

"You were so beautiful on the court today," Jason said, his tongue loosened by the alcohol. He reached out and brushed the strands of hair out of her face. "So beautiful."

"You watched me play? Wait, you think I'm pretty?" Morgan asked, stunned. "Nobody has ever said that to me before."

"So pretty I couldn't stop watching." He continued to play with her hair. "I want to kiss you." Jason leaned forward, the champagne fully in charge, desire pulsing through him.

Morgan was shocked but wanted to be kissed. She had been protected by her father her whole life. Boys had never been in the picture. Morgan finally felt like a normal teenage girl. Every inch tingled and all self-control was gone. At first their kisses were soft and hesitant, but soon they were carried away, lying side by side on the grass, oblivious to the adults forty feet away.

Nobody noticed; nobody cared. Jason and Morgan were locked in pure teen passion fueled by alcohol, kissing with abandon. The applause marking the end of the match broke the spell, and they scrambled to their feet. Morgan stumbled into Jason's arms as she tried to regain her footing.

"Oh my God, I think I'm drunk." Morgan squealed.

"Shhhh," Jason said, "don't announce it. We have to get out of here."

"Yes, but where? We can't go to the beach now."

"That lady who owns the cottage is staying with us this weekend, so our house is full," Jason said.

"My cottage is full, too. Wait! I know! Let's get the keys to the boat. My dad isn't planning to go out on the boat for the fireworks this year, so we can go there."

Jason agreed and the two stumbled hand in hand to the boathouse. The keys to the boat were kept on a hook just inside the door. It was going to be dark soon, and Morgan suggested they drive the boat to Depot Beach for a better view of the fireworks.

"Your dad lets you take the boat out?" Jason wondered out loud.

"I know how to drive the boat. Besides, it's just going to sit here. What's the harm?" After clearing the breakwater, Morgan guided the boat, picked up speed, and headed out into open water.

Jason went below deck to check out the cabin. He had never been in a boat this size before. The refrigerator was fully stocked, so he grabbed two beers in hopes of continuing the mood from earlier and went back on deck. Morgan found a place to stop and shut down the engine.

"Um... don't we need to anchor or something?"

"Not really. We do this all the time. The boat doesn't drift much." Morgan sat down on the bench seat along the stern of the boat. "We won't get lost, either." She laughed. Jason handed her an open beer and sat down next to her.

Morgan grabbed the second round of beers before the fireworks started, and Jason wrapped his arms around her, pulling her close as they watched the show. Maybe it was the alcohol affecting him, but he was surprised how comfortable he felt with this girl.

The fireworks show was extraordinary, with spectacular combinations and new exotic rockets. By the end of the show, he felt happier than he had in a long time.

"I think we need to get the boat back," Morgan grumbled. "I'm getting sleepy."

"I could stay here with you forever, but you're probably right about the boat." Jason was feeling the alcohol, but his pride didn't allow him to admit how much.

Motoring back across the lake only took ten minutes. Morgan didn't go fast, and finding the general direction was easy. It was when they got to the part of the lake where the club was located that the situation became complicated. They traveled up and down the shoreline three times, looking for the entrance to the docks and boathouse.

"I don't understand! The entrance is just gone," Morgan said, her words slurred. "I can't do this anymore."

"Well, I don't know how to drive the boat, so I can't exactly take over. What if we tie it to the swimming raft and wait for a bit?"

"That seems like a good idea," Morgan replied.

Jason got the line off the stern and sat on the edge of the boat while Morgan pulled up to the raft. She bumped it hard, and Jason fell into the water.

"Oh my gosh! Are you okay?"

"Fine, just wet." Jason laughed, pulling himself onto the raft. He tied the boat to a cleat the best he could.

Stepping onto the boat, he asked if they had a towel on board. Morgan went into the cabin and returned with a small towel and a comforter. She tossed the towel to Jason. "Take your shirt and shorts off and get dry. I won't look."

"There are easier ways to get my clothes off. You didn't have to toss me into the water."

"I swear it was an accident!" Morgan squealed.

"Sure. I believe you. Really, I do." Jason mocked her with a gleam in his eye. Soon the two were lying on the bench, the comforter wrapped tight around them. Jason warmed up quickly. "If I didn't know better, I'd say you planned the whole thing," he whispered.

"You're the one who got me drunk, you know."

"Then shouldn't it be the other way around? Shouldn't you be naked under the covers?"

Morgan laughed. "I guess I just beat you at your own game."

"I call foul. You're not following the rules, and you have way too much clothing on."

"Well, I wouldn't want to be accused of cheating." Morgan flirted back, slipping out of her dress.

Jason wasted no time pulling her close to him. "Now this is nice," Jason murmured.

The two drifted off to sleep, not noticing the boat rubbing up against the raft. Morgan had forgotten to put bumpers out to protect the boat from the edge of the dock.

The next morning, Mike, the head lifeguard, swam out to the boat, which had come loose from the platform. "Holy shit! Did the two of you spend the night here?" he said as he boarded the boat. "Jason, man, you gotta get up! Your first lesson is in ten minutes."

Jason opened his eyes, the sun blinding him. "Aww shit."

Morgan groaned. "Everything is spinning. I don't feel so hot."

"Did you guys get drunk?" Mike asked.

"Yeah, kinda," Jason answered. "Hey man, you got extra swim trunks?"

"Sure, in the shed."

"Good! I'm swimming to shore to get them." Jason stood up, covering himself with the towel. "Nothing happened, okay? I fell into the water. My wet shit is around here somewhere."

Jason dove into the water, swam to shore, and sprinted to the shack. He found the shorts, a towel, and a T-shirt. After getting dressed, he ran back down the dock as if it were a normal day at the beach. Dropping the towel and T-shirt at the end of the dock, he swam back out to the swim raft where the boat and a hung-over girl were waiting. Suddenly, Jason didn't feel so hot either.

Morgan was sitting in her underwear, her head in her hands. Mike had gotten her a bucket from down below, just in case.

"Jase, you've got a problem here," Mike said as Jason scrambled onto the boat.

"Thanks for pointing out the obvious. I really appreciate it."

"Hey, don't get pissy with me."

"Sorry, man. I'm in over my head. The Arbruster girls are going to be here any second. I have no idea what to do with this boat, and Morgan is in no condition to drive it."

The two looked at the girl, who was now nearly passed out on a deck chair. Mike considered the situation. "First things first: get Morgan back in her dress. I'll get the dinghy, and you can row her to shore. Prop her up in a beach chair while you do your lesson, and I'll get the boat back to its slip. Then I can take over for you while you get the poor kid home."

"You think that'll work?"

"Sure. This is the weekend when there's a lot of collateral damage," Mike replied. "With any luck, nobody will notice."

As Mike eased the boat away from the raft, Jason noticed a black streak on the side of the boat. He was pretty sure they were screwed but focused on getting Morgan home. She looked rather green.

By nine thirty, the Arbrusters' lesson was over, and Jason got Morgan home. He helped her put on a T-shirt and get into bed. He glanced down the hallway; the coast was clear. Somehow, Jason managed to slip down the stairs and out the front door without anyone noticing. As he walked back to the beach, he was overcome with nausea and puked in a bush in someone's front lawn.

CHAPTER 41

Lauren convinced Audrey to go into Charlevoix with her on Sunday morning for a mother-daughter day. The Venetian Festival was winding down, and Lauren wanted to take advantage of the discounts in the shops. Audrey decided to tag along since she had nothing better to do.

The two set out early with the plan to have breakfast at one of the diners before continuing down Bridge Street with all its touristy stores. Audrey's mood was flat. Lauren was relieved; at least they weren't arguing for a change.

Lauren asked Audrey about the job. The conversation flowed without drama. Audrey was answering questions about her duties and telling stories about some of the animals and clients they treated. Lauren was impressed by how much her daughter seemed to have learned about the practice. Audrey obviously respected Dr. Hawkins a great deal. Lauren found herself more relaxed about Audrey's work situation. It had turned out to be a good idea after all.

As the two left a store near the amphitheater across from East Park, they heard a band warming up. Lauren nudged Audrey. "Would you like to go listen to the music?"

Audrey shrugged. "I guess."

They crossed the street and headed to the amphitheater, where the band was playing 70s rock and roll. Audrey felt awkward sitting with her mother, who was enjoying the music and people watching. A burst of laughter from a group of teens dancing near them caught their attention. The girls, dressed in shorts and bathing suit tops, were flirting with the boys. The joyous laughter made Audrey squirm with discomfort.

"Mom, are you sure you want to stay?"

Lauren missed the subtle clue. "Sure, this is fun. I'm fine, honey."

Audrey sulked. Her mother could be so dense sometimes.

A boy called out, "Audrey! Hey! I can't believe you're here." Lauren looked up at the young man, and then glanced at her daughter, who did not respond with the same level of enthusiasm.

The boy approached them, looking expectantly at Audrey and then her mother. Audrey barely acknowledged him and didn't make introductions.

"Hi! You must be Mrs. Breckenridge. I'm Dylan. I met your daughter at Dr. Hawkins' office."

"It's nice to meet you," Lauren replied eagerly. "Audrey really seems to enjoy her job there."

"Oh, you should see her. She's amazing with the dogs," Dylan gushed. It was clear to Lauren this boy had a crush on her daughter. Finally, some normal teenage behavior she could understand.

"I'm pleased to hear that, Dylan. I met Dr. Hawkins the other day. She seems quite nice."

"Dr. H is really cool. I sometimes help out with the dogs, too. They need a ton of exercise, and Dr. H lets me play with them."

"I'm sure she appreciates your help. Are you here with your friends?" Lauren tried to make small talk, hoping Audrey would take over the conversation.

"Yeah, those are some kids I go to school with," Dylan said with a nod toward the group of rowdy teens.

Lauren considered the situation for a moment. "You know, Audrey, if you want to join them, I would be fine sitting here by myself. We could meet in an hour or so." She glanced at Audrey.

Audrey turned pale and her body stiffened. "That would be totally cool with my friends, Audrey," Dylan said enthusiastically, jumping at the chance to be with her. "They would like getting to know you."

"Mom, no!" Audrey jumped to her feet. "This is stupid, and if you don't take me home right now, I'm going to walk or call Dad or something."

Audrey stormed away, disappearing into the crowd, leaving the two of them staring after her.

"I'm sorry, Dylan. I don't know what came over her just now," Lauren stammered, embarrassed by her daughter's behavior.

"It's okay, Mrs. Breckenridge. Dr. H. explained the whole thing to me." Dylan spoke calmly, but it was clear he was disappointed by Audrey's reaction.

"She did?"

"Yeah, she said there was something Audrey was having a hard time dealing with, and we need to give her space. Whatever happened to her was pretty bad, and she sometimes just overreacts to situations normal people are cool with. Dr. H. said the best thing to do was just be her friend. Eventually whatever it was would come out, and then we could help her get over the bad stuff."

"Really? She said all that?"

"Yeah. Audrey flips out at work a lot. But now that I understand, I just give her space. She's really cool." Dylan paused, trying to see where Audrey had gone. "It's hard to see her get all upset though."

"Yes it is, Dylan. And you are obviously a good friend. I appreciate that more than you know."

Lauren said good-bye to Dylan and made her way back to the car. Audrey was waiting for her. She put the bags in the back and the two headed toward home. It was Lauren who finally broke the awkward silence.

"Aud, is there something you need to talk about?" Lauren asked gingerly, not knowing how to handle the outburst.

Audrey was silent. She simply looked out the passenger window.

Lauren reached out and squeezed her daughter's hand. "I'm here for you, whatever it is."

Lauren did not see the single tear fall from her daughter's eye as she watched the scenery pass.

CHAPTER 42

Pregnant? Pregnant! This can't be happening. Lauren crumpled the note in her lap.

She sat at the antique correspondence desk, looking over a packet of mail forwarded to them from home—mostly bills, notices about school, and a handwritten envelope addressed to her. *Karen has some fucking nerve.*

Lauren uncrumpled the letter to read it one more time, but the words didn't change: pregnant; keeping the baby; letting us know; didn't expect anything. Lauren wadded the paper and threw it across the room. "How about a jail cell? Would you like that?" she yelled.

She was glad nobody was home. What was she supposed to do with this information? Act as if everything was fine? Tell Jason and ruin his life? Tell David and ruin the summer? Lauren started crying. The summer had been fine so far, and now everything was coming back to haunt them. It wasn't fair! This woman broke the law. David convinced her to let the whole thing go because of what Jason would have to go through if they did anything about it. But it didn't go away as he'd said it would. Now what?

Lauren thought about burning the letter in the fireplace and pretending she never got it, but there would probably be another one. This was an impossible situation.

"Hey, Lauren, you here?" The voice startled her.

What? Oh shit! Rick. She'd completely forgotten he was coming over to talk about going to Mackinac Island for the Chicago-Mac. Lauren tried unsuccessfully to wipe the tears from her face as Rick entered the main room. *Why the hell do people around here just walk into each other's homes like they own them?*

"There you are. I... Hey, what's wrong?" Rick crossed the room in two steps and took her elbow, his voice filled with concern. "Come here. Sit down." Rick guided Lauren to the couch, pulled a handkerchief from his pocket, and dabbed at the tears still glistening on her cheeks. "Seriously, tell me why you're crying."

Lauren shook her head; she couldn't find her voice to start. "I can't" was all she could whisper before the sobs escaped her.

Rick pulled her to his shoulder and let her cry. His heart melted for this woman. Whatever was wrong shook Lauren to her core, and it had an effect on him as well. His eyes filled with tears for her, and he was determined to fix whatever was wrong. "Tell me. I'll make it better, I promise."

"You can't," Lauren said, struggling to compose herself. She felt both embarrassed and strangely comforted by Rick's calm demeanor. He didn't shy away from her emotional outburst; in fact, the opposite was true. Rick was encouraging her to express herself. This was not something Lauren was accustomed to. Emotional outbursts were to be smothered, silenced, not encouraged.

"Try me," Rick said. "Give me the highlights. Whatever it is can't be all that bad, can it?"

Lauren took a deep breath. "My son had an affair with a much older woman. I just got this letter. She's pregnant. I have no idea how to deal with this... what I'm supposed to do."

"You mean Jason? He's sixteen, right? How old is the woman?"

"She's in her mid-twenties, maybe almost thirty."

Rick sat there, stunned. He wasn't sure what to say. Many thoughts crossed his mind, but one thing was certain: a mother had the absolute right to be horrified by the situation.

"Lauren, I'm sorry. This is a mess, isn't it?"

"Yes, it really is." Lauren leaned back against the couch cushions. "I have no clue what to do, Rick. I really don't."

"Yes, I can see that. Let me get you something to drink. It certainly won't hurt and might actually help you relax."

Lauren nodded, amazed. Rick seemed to understand and showed no sign of being judgmental. Maybe she did have someone to talk to who could help her make some sense of the situation. Maybe he would see a solution she'd overlooked.

Lauren gratefully accepted the glass of chardonnay he handed her and downed half of it before she knew what hit her. Rick encouraged her to tell the whole story, and by the time she finished, they were halfway through the second bottle of wine. Lauren was relieved to get the shame of her son's affair off her chest.

"Lauren, the first thing you need to do is stop blaming yourself. You've done nothing wrong," Rick said as he placed his hand on her knee.

"How can you say that? It's my son who's been screwing that whore!" Lauren said exactly what she was thinking as the alcohol loosened her tongue.

"My point exactly. Lemme tell you something, man to man." He leaned in close, his lips near her ear.

Lauren laughed. "Except I'm not a man."

"See? You're laughing." Rick chuckled. "Minor detail. Anyway, you know what I mean. Every sixteen-year-old boy on the planet wants to get laid by an older woman." Rick poured the rest of the wine into Lauren's glass. "It's in our nature."

"Excuse me?"

"It's true." Rick held up his hands. "Don't shoot the messenger. At that age, a stiff breeze will give you wood, and getting laid is a life obsession."

"This is my son we're talking about!" Lauren squealed and giggled all at once.

Rick went to the bar and returned with a third bottle of wine.

"It's like a dog chasing a car," he said. "What on earth will the dog do if he catches the car? But if a high school boy catches a woman who is willing to show him the ropes, he may not know what he's doing at first, but he's willing to learn."

Lauren fell into a fit of laughter. The alcohol and Rick's company made her forget, for just a second, the disaster now in her lap. Instead, they were just two people laughing over drinks in a cottage in Northern Michigan. The tears were long gone, replaced by warmth and security. It was easy to feel close to this man.

Lauren looked up suddenly to find Liza and David standing in the doorway. The unexpected appearance of people caught Lauren and Rick by surprise, like two teenagers caught red-handed.

David was the first to speak. "What are we celebrating?"

"Celebrating? Now that's really funny, David," Lauren replied. "The answer to your question... I guess we're celebrating how fucking unpredictable life is." Lauren's happy mood evaporated into dark anger. She jumped up, turned on her heels, and stormed out of the room.

After her exit, David and Liza looked at Rick, expecting some sort of an explanation. The three wine bottles were hard to miss.

Rick answered the question on everyone's mind. "Lauren received some upsetting news in the mail today. My timing was such I became caught up in the whirlwind." He nodded toward the wine bottles.

"What news?" David asked.

"I think your wife should be the one to answer that question, but she's quite upset. I tried as best I could to lift her spirits, but it obviously didn't last."

"I'm confused. Has someone died?" David asked.

"Oh no, nothing like that." Rick tried to smooth the man's ruffled feathers. "She was really upset when I got here—crying, in fact." Rick's brain was swirling from the wine, and he was desperate to get out of the spotlight. "I'm not sure I even got the whole story. I just tried to cheer her up a bit."

"Well, I appreciate your efforts and concern." David awkwardly reached out to shake Rick's hand.

Liza wasn't buying it for one second. She knew Rick too well. They had gotten ten percent of the story, all facts accurate, not a single lie, but nowhere near the real truth. Rick avoided Liza's eyes as he shook David's hand.

Liza took the opportunity to jump in. "Listen, I'll go talk to Lauren. You know, girl talk." She gave Rick a look and headed toward the bedroom without waiting for a response.

David perked up, visibly relieved that he'd escaped dealing with a drunk and angry wife. "Oh, thank you," David called after Liza. "I fail miserably in the girl-talk department," he said to Rick as he gathered up the empty wine bottles. "It looks like quite the little party."

"Yes, I seem to have lost my head and drank too much," Rick added.

"That happens up here daily, or so it seems."

"I should be heading back to my cottage," Rick said, struggling to find some sort of graceful way to extricate himself from the situation. "I hope all of this blows over quickly."

"Yes, I do hope you're right. Thanks again."

CHAPTER 43

"Oh my God, Lauren!" Liza wrapped her arms around the tearful woman. "I don't blame you one bit."

The two sat on the bed with a box of tissues between them. The second time through the story was a little easier than the first. Of course, Liza knew about the affair, so catching her up only took a few minutes.

"I honestly don't know what to do," Lauren lamented. "It's like I've been punched in the gut and reality is worse than my imagination." She was sobering up faster than she cared to, the feelings of pain and despair washing over her again.

"To be honest, I don't know what I would do in your position," said the younger woman. "But my grandfather would tell me to break the problem down into little steps, and take it one step at a time." Liza paused, pulling back from Lauren. "I know it sounds cliché, but believe it or not, it works."

"What can I do from here?" Lauren felt powerless. Her overwhelming desire to press charges against Karen returned with a vengeance. This woman had violated her son, and she needed to pay for her crime, despite what David said.

"There's nothing you can do about this situation right now, so why let that hateful woman ruin your summer? Deal with her in the fall when you return to New York. She'll still be pregnant; nothing will have changed."

"She really is despicable. I can't understand why David won't see her for what she is."

"Probably because he's not a mother. Who knows, but David's assessment of her doesn't change the situation, does it?"

"What do you mean?" Lauren looked at Liza, grabbed a tissue from the box and blew her nose.

"This woman is awful and she has broken the law. That is the truth of the matter. Right?"

Lauren agreed.

"Okay, so why let her control your life? Don't wreck your lives because some woman was—at best—stupid. You control the timeline, not her." Liza could tell

Lauren was not quite following her lead. "Lauren, don't do anything now; just try to enjoy the time you have left and forget about it until you go home to New York. Then call the police if you want to, or confront her, or do nothing if you prefer. But make your decision after your summer vacation. Don't ruin everything because of her."

"I see what you're saying. Why should I mess up our lives even more?"

"That's right! Why should you?" Liza repeated.

"If I tell either Jason or David, their summer will be ruined. I can't imagine what this will do to Jason."

"Exactly!"

"I need to keep this secret from my family until we get home. I can't let this woman control our lives." Lauren worked hard to convince herself that hiding the news was the best thing for all of them. "In fact, maybe when we get home, I should just deal with her myself. Certainly David's plan didn't seem to work very well, did it?"

"Exactly. That's something you can decide later. In the meantime, you put a lot into this family vacation. Don't let some unstable woman ruin it for you."

"Finally, something that makes sense." Lauren hugged her friend. "I'm so glad you're here. I don't know what I would have done without you." Lauren smiled, relieved. "Only one thing... how am I going to explain tonight to David?"

"I'll tell David you had upsetting news from a girlfriend, and then I'll pretend I didn't know the players." Liza gave her friend a conspiring grin. "He won't press me."

"You're brilliant!"

"You relax and try to get some sleep. I'll smooth everything over downstairs. Tomorrow's another day. We can grab some breakfast before you run me to the airport." Obviously it was not the time to ask questions about the electricity she saw between Lauren and Rick.

"I wish you could stay for the rest of the summer," Lauren said.

"Me too, my friend; me too." Liza tiptoed from the room, hoping Lauren's head wouldn't hurt too badly in the morning. Rick, on the other hand, deserved a sledgehammer-pounding hangover. What was he thinking? Liza fully intended to head up to his cottage and rip into him.

Liza found David reading the newspaper by the fire. He had cleaned up the evidence of the alcohol binge and was perfectly willing to buy Liza's tale without hesitation. Liza wondered why he ignored the obvious. How could someone be so self-absorbed that he didn't see the clues dangled right under his nose? Liza excused herself for the evening, telling David she was heading to a friend's house before heading back to New York in the morning.

CHAPTER 44

"Are you out of your mind, Dickie?" Liza ranted. She stormed into his cottage and found him on a sleeping porch, lying on his bed.

"Liza, I've had too much to drink. I can't deal with this now."

"Tough shit. A little late for that now, buddy. What the hell is going on between you and Lauren Breckenridge?"

"You're not going to believe me when I tell you, so why not just make something up and go away?" Rick rolled over, his head spinning.

"Nice. Except I'm not going away, and you're going to tell me the truth." Liza fumed and plopped down on Rick's bed, leaning against the footboard. "I can't believe I just found you tanked, consoling my renter. That's a new low, even for you."

"It's not like that, Liza."

"Then you better tell me how it is."

Rick propped himself up against the headboard and faced his childhood best friend. She was visibly angry with him, and he couldn't blame her. Sometimes he wondered why he didn't just keep to himself and stay out of trouble.

"Liza, I'm in love with her."

"Oh bullshit." Liza rolled her eyes and gave him a kick.

"Are you going to give me a chance to explain or not?"

"Wait, you're serious?"

"Yeah, I think I am. I've never felt like this before, and I mean never."

Liza appraised her friend. "But what makes you think you're in love with her? How is this one different?"

"Well, that's just it; it's completely different. We talk about stuff, we laugh. When I'm with her, I can relax and just be myself. Like I am with you. I don't have to pretend to be something I'm not, and she accepts me for who I am."

Liza squirmed on the bed. "So... you're friends. Have you had sex with her?"

"Not even a kiss." Rick held up his hand. "I swear."

"You're kidding." Liza was astonished. "You?"

"See? I knew you wouldn't believe me." Rick fell back onto his pillow and groaned. "Iz, I've got it bad. I can't sleep. I think about her all the time. I find stupid ways to be near her. Get this—I invited her to the Chicago-Mac."

"What? Dickie, she's married!"

"And this is a problem. Her husband is a great big giant ass, if you ask me." Rick pouted. "He treats her like shit."

"Said every person having an affair since the dawn of mankind," Liza pointed out. "Tell me, how many people with really great spouses have affairs? It's a lame excuse."

"Now there's the thing—we are not having an affair, not even close." Rick defended himself. "Nothing sexual whatsoever. Maybe some flirting but I'm telling you, I flirt more with the little old ladies in the club than I do with her. How do I say this? I'm not myself when I'm with her, but I'm exactly myself."

"Oh Lord, you do have it bad." Liza laughed.

"This is what I'm saying. I've actually fallen in love with Lauren."

"You want to tell me what you plan to do about this?"

"I wish I knew, Liza. I'm clueless, and it's eating me up inside. Hell, I don't even know if she likes me."

"You sound like you're in high school. Do you want me to pass her a note in Study Hall?" Liza teased her friend.

"Thanks. I really appreciate your help here. I'll remind you of this when you fall in love."

"This isn't about me, Dickie. And I'm not out playing around with married men, am I? You got yourself into a mess, and I don't know how you're going to get yourself out of it, but you've got to stay away from her. She's had a really rough ride this spring, and throwing this at her really wouldn't be fair. It's the last thing she needs." Liza got off the bed and headed for the door.

"Liza, did you ever think maybe it's exactly what she needs—some love, friendship, and respect?"

"Dickie, your heart is in the right place, but she isn't a project; she's a person with feelings. Her family is going through a lot, and they don't need anything else to add more confusion. Just stay away from them, okay?"

"You've always known better than me, Liza, ever since we were kids. Are you going to boss me around when we're eighty years old, too?

"Go to sleep, Dickie. You'll feel better in the morning."

Liza closed the door behind her. She was concerned with this latest development but hoped her friend would remain a gentleman. She was afraid if he actually made a pass at Lauren, in her current state, she would give in to the temptation and revel in the moments of pure escapism rather than face the difficulties of her own life. And how could Lauren guide her son when the example she would be setting was just as wrong? Liza felt partially responsible for the mess between Lauren and Dickie, but she wasn't sure if she could prevent the relationship from moving forward.

CHAPTER 45

On Tuesday after Venetian Weekend, Jason was in the middle of his last group lesson of the day when he spied Morgan heading toward the dock. He gave her a quick wave while continuing to focus on the kids' breathing exercises. By noon, the nannies were back on the beach, ready to take their charges home for lunch.

Jason did not have lifeguard duty on Tuesday afternoons, so after his lessons he was free for the remainder of the day. Walking to the end of the dock, he plopped in the beach chair next to Morgan. "How are you feeling?"

"Better today. Yesterday I could barely move."

"I know. I checked in at your house. They said you had the flu." Jason chuckled.

"It didn't occur to anyone that I was hung over. Thanks for not saying anything."

"Me? Never. I do have to admit, though, this place was... well... quiet without you."

Morgan did a double take, not sure what Jason was saying. "Quiet? I'm loud?"

Jason laughed. "You're going to make me say it, aren't you? Okay... I've missed you. Better?"

Morgan blushed. "Oh, I didn't mean to..."

"Yeah you did. You just wanted to hear it. And now I've said it." Jason enjoyed having the upper hand; plus, Morgan looked cute when she was flustered. Visions of Morgan in her panties flashed through his brain. It was all he could think about, but he wasn't sure how to get into a situation where they would be alone again. "So, are you hungry or anything? I could use some lunch."

"I guess I could try to eat something. I haven't eaten anything since Saturday."

Jason started thinking about it. His house was cleared out for a few hours. Maybe it was a perfect opportunity. "Why don't we head over to my place? Mom's got sandwich stuff in the fridge." Jason held his breath, hoping Morgan would agree. At least he would be alone with her, a good first step.

"Are you sure she wouldn't mind?"

"Nah, it's fine. In fact, nobody's home right now. We'll have the place to ourselves for a couple hours at least." Jason tried to sound as casual as possible, but he was a bundle of nerves, hoping Morgan wouldn't see through his plan and back out. She was hypersensitive her dad would catch her doing something.

Morgan agreed and Jason's heart skipped a beat. He was thankful for the sweatshirt in his lap; it hid his true intentions. Morgan suggested she meet him at the cottage in half an hour. He ached with anticipation as he watched her walk away. Waiting for his replacement seemed to take an eternity.

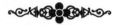

"Jase, you here?" Morgan called from the kitchen stairs.

"Yeah, come on in."

"What's for lunch? I'm starved."

"Lunch?" Food was literally the last thing on Jason's mind.

"Remember? Food, lunch, the sandwiches you promised?" Morgan teased him, wondering where his brain had wandered off to. "You didn't eat without me, did you?"

"No, of course not. I was distracted, sorry. Mom's got some turkey or tuna salad. Which do you want?"

"Turkey is good." Morgan responded eagerly. Jason made two sandwiches and suggested they take them into the living room where they could put on Netflix and chill.

"Wow, you have Internet in this house? Most of the cottages don't have it. A lot don't even have TVs."

"Actually, it's on my laptop, but it's better than nothing."

Jason sat down on the floor in front of the couch and placed his laptop on the coffee table. When Morgan put her plate on the table, Jason grabbed her wrist and tugged her onto his lap.

"This is an awkward position for lunch," Morgan said.

"I can think of a few more positions I'd like to put you in." Jason growled as he kissed her neck. Morgan caught her breath. She was not used to someone being so aggressive with her. She didn't want him to stop, but maybe he needed to slow down a little.

"Kiss me," he whispered, hungry for much more than a turkey sandwich.

Morgan kissed him softly at first. He pulled her head toward him and kissed her with intensifying passion. Morgan resisted but felt her body suggesting otherwise. Jason's urges had taken control, and he reached under her shirt. She gasped as his hand brushed over her breast. Then he reached behind her back and unhooked her bra.

Taking her gasp as a positive sign, Jason pushed Morgan onto her back and lay on top of her. He lifted her knee so he could push himself against her. Morgan felt how hard he was, and she trembled as fear swept through her.

"Jason, I've never—"

"It's okay. I'll show you." Jason reached down toward her shorts. "I want you so bad."

Out of nowhere, Lauren's voice called out from the kitchen. "Jason, are you home? You left a mess." Scrambling, the two sat up, and Jason helped Morgan pull her shirt down. They jumped on opposite sides of the couch, pulling their sandwich plates into their laps just as Jason's mom came into the living room.

"Mom! You're home!"

"Yes, I decided to come home early. Oh, I see you have company." Lauren looked from Jason to Morgan and back again, waiting for an introduction.

Jason swallowed hard. "Oh, sorry, I didn't expect you. Mom, this is my girlfriend, Morgan." He was stumbling, not sure what to say.

Morgan sat there frozen, afraid to move and wondering what just happened. "Hi, Mrs. Breckenridge" was all she could manage.

Lauren had the feeling she had interrupted something, but there was no evidence of any wrongdoing. "Sorry. I didn't mean to interrupt your lunch. I'll leave you alone. Jason, clean up the kitchen when you're done eating."

"Yes, mom. I won't forget."

Lauren headed toward her bedroom, leaving the teens by themselves.

"Jase, I should probably go," Morgan said as she put her plate down on the table and stood up.

"Are you okay? You don't have to leave."

"I'm fine. Everything is fine. I just... I don't know. Your mom's home; it's awkward," Morgan said. "I'll see you tomorrow, okay?"

Jason nodded. Morgan said everything was fine, but somehow he felt like she wasn't telling him the complete truth. *What went wrong?* he wondered.

CHAPTER 46

Audrey eyed her mother and Dr. Hawkins nervously. The two were sitting at the kitchen table in the break room. Lauren had supposedly decided to drop in to visit her daughter at work, and the two women were chatting amicably while Audrey exercised the dogs in the run.

"I'm really glad you came in to discuss this. I wasn't sure, after our first meeting, if I should reach out to you," Claire said, pouring hot tea into their cups. "Dylan is correct about what he's told you. He's a great kid with a really good heart."

"In certain situations Audrey freezes up, and sometimes, out of the blue, she'll have a burst of anger." Lauren looked horrified. "Oh, please don't take it the wrong way. It's never been with clients or with the animals. Her work here has been extraordinary." Claire reassured her. "The outbursts seem to have very specific triggers; I just haven't figured out what they are yet."

Lauren had now been witness to the same thing and had to admit that it seemed odd. "Honestly, don't you think she's just a rebellious fourteen-year-old girl? I wonder if my daughter isn't lost in the shuffle somewhere. She's been fighting me more and more this spring, but I can't say why. Our family had some issues with her older brother, and since then she has just shut down." Lauren took a sip of tea and thought about the spring and how Audrey behaved. "They had been getting closer, and I assumed she was reacting to his situation, but now I'm not so sure."

"What do you think it could be?"

"I'm really not sure, to be honest," Lauren said softly. "I know she had a falling-out with a girl she's been friends with since second or third grade. I thought it was odd, truthfully." Lauren was scrambling for ideas, but even as she articulated this possibility it didn't seem likely. The timing was off.

"I suppose it could be something like that, but in my experience, Audrey's reaction seems as if it came from something more traumatic. It's as if she's reliving something, and her base fight-or-flight instinct is kicking in. Is that possible?" Claire asked, genuinely concerned for the girl.

"With the spring we've had, I would believe anything," Lauren quipped. "I'm sorry. I shouldn't be snide like that. Truthfully, though, we've had a rough time."

Lauren was about to explain some of the details, thanks to the willing ear of Dr. Hawkins, when Dylan and his parents appeared in the break room. Dylan introduced his parents to Lauren. He seemed genuinely excited she was visiting the practice today.

"I made my parents stop. Our church group is going on a rafting trip on the Jordan River this Saturday, and I thought I'd see if Audrey wanted to come with us. It's really a ton of fun." Dylan was animated, excited about both the trip and including Audrey.

"Hang on a second; I'll call her in." Claire stood and walked toward the back door. "The Jordan River is great, and she might really enjoy it."

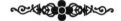

Audrey froze as she walked through the door, not expecting anyone but her mother and Dr. Hawkins. Dylan immediately introduced his parents and started babbling about the river trip. Audrey's chest tightened, and the room seemed to close in around her.

Suddenly everyone seemed to be talking at once, insisting she go tubing on the river trip. She had no interest in going anywhere with Dylan or anyone else. Audrey backed against the door, unable to catch her breath. The room seemed to shrink as her vision blurred, darkening around the edges.

The voices seemed to envelop her and increased in volume until all she heard was screeching and screaming. Terrified, Audrey batted them away, afraid they were going to hurt her. She knew her mother was there, but somehow she couldn't reach her for help. Crying out, Audrey crumpled to the floor and curled into a ball. The room went black.

Audrey was lying on a stretcher with paramedics standing over her. She had an oxygen mask on and an IV in her arm. Looking around, she realized she was about to be loaded into an ambulance. Audrey took off the oxygen mask. "Mom?" she called out in fear.

"Well, hello. Look who's back. Your mom is right here," a woman's voice echoed from somewhere above.

Lauren was by her side in a flash. "It's okay, sweetie, you're safe now. Stay calm. I won't leave you." Lauren tried to sound composed for her daughter, but, truthfully, she was terrified. The last fifteen minutes could have been fifteen hours. Watching her daughter panic and lash out with no provocation scared everyone.

Dylan had jumped into action. Responding to Claire's instructions, he'd called 9-1-1 as soon as Audrey's attack began. Claire had instructed the adults to back away from Audrey, giving her room to breathe but Lauren didn't listen and ended up in the line of fire, her face badly scratched. At that moment it was clear to everyone in the room Audrey was dealing with some intensely dark demons.

Once the ambulance pulled away, Claire offered to drive Lauren to the hospital. On the way, she'd told Lauren she knew the perfect person who could help Audrey work through her issues.

"How could it get so bad?" a shaken Lauren asked, though the question was really rhetorical more than anything else.

"If anyone's going to figure it out, I'd put my faith in Erin. I've seen her work miracles." Claire put her hand on Lauren's. "We'll get her through this."

CHAPTER 47

"David, the doctors say she had some sort of panic or anxiety attack." Lauren was agitated, pacing in the living room. She and Audrey had gotten home from the hospital an hour ago and Audrey was in her room. The ER nurses said the medicines should keep her calm overnight, but she would be groggy. "They think she needs to see a therapist or attend a support group."

"Did they say why this happened?" David was concerned but unconvinced.

"That's the whole point. The therapy would uncover the source of the problem. I think something happened to her last spring, and we missed it because of this whole Jason fiasco." Lauren's voice was raised; she was angry. Mad at herself, mad at David, mad at their situation. "I had a long talk with Claire Hawkins today, and she completely agrees with me. She knows a person for us to contact."

"What could she possibly know about our situation?"

"David, you're not listening... again." Lauren was exasperated. "Why am I even bothering to try to talk to you about this? You never listen! You just dismiss what I have to say, because it doesn't fit the picture in your head."

"Hey, now that isn't fair. I'm listening to you. I just don't happen to agree with you."

"I suppose, in your infinite wisdom, you think you know better than the medical professionals, too? David, you weren't there. You didn't see what happened to her, so for once just shut up about this. You are wrong." Lauren was on a roll. She'd kept her feelings bottled up for far too long, and she was starting to erupt.

"Lauren, you've had a tough day. I think you need to calm down. You're starting to sound a little crazy."

"Now I'm sounding crazy! What do you know? You're barely involved with this family. I have to take care of everything." Lauren glared at her husband. "Do you even care what's going on? I'm sick of the endless secrets. Every time I turn around it's another fucking lie!" Lauren was on a roll, so oblivious to her surroundings that she didn't notice Jason and Morgan standing in the doorway.

Audrey heard her mother's voice and came stumbling downstairs. "Mom?

Why are you yelling at Dad?"

Lauren didn't miss a beat and gestured toward Audrey. "Did you know your daughter's job started with a lie? She rode the Vespa to the vet's office every day without telling anyone, and I caught her. I told you something was going on, but you didn't believe me; instead, you completely disappeared, so I had to deal with everything myself."

"Everything? What 'everything' are you talking about?" David said.

"Everyone in this so-called family is so busy running off in every direction that once again I'm left alone with the dirt!" Lauren yelled.

"Lauren, you've totally lost it. You've got to calm down."

"Shut up, David. You don't understand. You weren't here when I got the letter from that whore, Karen, telling me she was pregnant. I had to deal with that one on my own."

Now it was Jason's turn. "What? What did you just say, Mom?"

Lauren spun around at the sound of Jason's voice. "Well, I guess the cat's out of the bag now. Jason, that bitch you were screwing sent me a lovely note. And David, this whole plan of not calling the police backfired, because she's pregnant and planning on keeping the baby. Our sixteen-year-old son is going to be a daddy. And I get to be a grandma."

Morgan gasped. She looked up at Jason, her eyes brimming with tears and a multitude of questions. Jason was frozen, staring at his mother, uncertain what to say. Morgan burst into tears and sprinted from the house. When Jason turned to follow her, his mother's angry voice stopped him in his tracks.

"Don't you dare move, any of you! I'm not dealing with this bullshit on my own. I trusted all of you, and each of you lied to me, betraying my trust at every turn. Well, it's going to stop right here."

Audrey had heard enough. She refused to listen to her mother's bullshit a moment longer. "So are you going to admit your affair with that Rick guy, or are you just going to blame us for shit?"

Lauren took two steps toward her daughter and slapped her hard across the face. "You have no idea what you're talking about, and don't you dare talk to me in that manner!" Audrey crumpled to the ground, stunned and sobbing.

"Lauren, stop!" David grabbed his wife's arm and pulled her closer to him. "You are totally out of control."

"Yes, and that's all you've ever cared about—being in control, looking like the perfect family. Well we're not."

"And you're the biggest liar of them all, Mom," Audrey said. "Dad's not the one who wants things perfect; you are. You don't listen to anything. What makes you think Jason and I are going to talk to you about a damn thing, when you only care about grades or sports?" Audrey glared at her parents as tears streamed down her cheeks. "We aren't going to come to you for shit."

"Aud…" Jason knew his sister was about to step over the line.

"What?" she snapped back at him. "It's true! She just wants a pretty family postcard, not a real family."

When no one responded, Audrey was more than willing to fill the silence. "Does anyone even notice shit in this family? Our so-called mother didn't. What does it take? I get drugged and raped by my shitty boyfriend and half my fucking class, and you all treat me like my ice cream just fell off the cone. No big deal. Whatever it is, she'll get over it."

Lauren gasped, falling to her knees next to her daughter. "Audrey! Is that true?"

"Yeah, whatever. Go take care of your precious boy and his baby, Grandma." Audrey hissed as she sobbed uncontrollably.

"Oh my God! What is wrong with us?" Lauren cried.

Audrey was the first to speak. "Well, I can tell you one thing: I'm not going back to that school, and you can't make me. I refuse. I don't ever want to see those people again."

David wiped tears from his eyes, crossed the room and pulled Audrey into his arms. "Honey, I'm sorry. I've let you down. I should have seen these things, but I was too wrapped up in my own worries." David kissed Audrey's head and held her close. "I can't fix everything, but I can fix some things. I promise I'll get us back on track."

Jason sank to the floor and put his head on his knees. His life was over.

Chapter 48

Lauren helped Audrey back into her room. With the drugs still in her system, she fell asleep fairly quickly. Lauren could hear the muted voices of David and Jason from down the hall. She watched her girl sleep and could only imagine what had taken place last spring. Lauren wanted to run away. She didn't want to deal with the repercussions of any of the issues. She was tired of the struggle. She was tired of pretending to be strong when all she wanted to do was cry. It was all too much. Out of the corner of her eye, she saw David appear in the doorway.

"Is she asleep?"

"Yes. Don't stay long. She needs to rest." Lauren pushed past David and hurried from the room. He joined Lauren in their bedroom a few minutes later.

"Why didn't you tell me about the letter and the pregnancy?"

"Because I didn't want to ruin your perfect little vacation. Besides, you didn't exactly handle it well the first time we had to deal with Karen. You said we should just drop the whole thing and it would go away." Lauren fumed. "It didn't exactly go away, did it?"

"I thought we were together on that decision. Now it's my fault?" David tried to stay calm, keeping his voice low so Jason wouldn't overhear them.

"You talked me into it. I wanted her arrested, remember?"

"I'm sorry. Apparently I made the wrong decision. But we're still a team, right?"

"Are we?" Lauren made no effort to hide her bitterness.

"Okay, we haven't been acting like it, but the fact remains we are one." He paused, but his wife refused to look at him. "Lauren, we need to get on the same page in order to have a chance. Look, I need to ask you something." David took a deep breath, crossed the room and sat down on a chair.

"What's that?"

"I can't believe I have to ask this," he muttered half under his breath. "Are you having an affair with Rick?"

Lauren stared at David for quite a while without saying anything.

"I never left this marriage, David. You did. I've been in the same place since the day we got married, since the kids were born. At some point, you left. I just don't know when it was."

"Lauren?" David implored.

"What? It's the truth. When was the last time I was anything more than member of your staff? Or maybe an object. That's not teamwork; it's ownership." Lauren swatted away the tears that threatened to fall. "I'm tired, David, so damn tired of all of this. But if you need to have an answer, it's no; I have not come close to having sex with Rick. We're friends. But, damn it, the truth is, I needed a friend because I was lonely, David."

"I love you. You know that."

"Do I know that, really?" Lauren sighed. "Maybe in the same way you love a favorite toy, but when was the last time you saw me as a person? A woman? Where is that love?

David was stunned. She was right. "Look, I don't have all the answers, but I'm not giving up on us."

Lauren sat on the bed without responding. At that moment she wasn't sure if she loved David or if she was interested in continuing the marriage. The thought surprised her. She remembered how she felt when she was sailing with Rick but tried to put it out of her mind. Running away wouldn't solve her other problems; she still had to deal with her kids.

"What's next?" David asked. "I don't know where to start."

Lauren just shook her head. "I don't know, David. Maybe you should go to New York to find out what Karen wants. In the meantime, I can get Audrey started in some therapy. We can talk after that."

"That sounds reasonable. I'll take care of this Lauren. I promise."

CHAPTER 49

Lauren was relieved David would be out of town for at least two days. The questions she had about their relationship were overwhelming, and she wanted to put them out of her mind.

Lauren needed to focus on the children. Once again, they were crumbling in front of her. Both were shut in their rooms, neither one talking to her. Lauren wondered why mothers suffered emotional abuse at the hands of their children. As she drank a second cup of coffee, she wondered which problem to tackle first. Both issues seemed like nightmares and she honestly didn't know where she would get the strength to deal with either kid. She decided to start with Jason.

Lauren tapped on the door. "Jase, you awake?" she asked as she eased open the door. Jason was lying facedown on his pillow. Lauren paused. Her little boy looked more like a man, and she wondered when that happened. She crossed the room and sat on the edge of the bed.

"Honey, we need to talk."

"About what?" Jason snarled.

"Jason stop," Lauren whispered to her son.

"Oh, you mean you want to talk about how I knocked up some bitch, and now your life is ruined."

Lauren recoiled. Maybe she'd underestimated how Jason felt about this whole issue. "Come on, that's not fair," Lauren said. "I came here to talk to you, not get into an argument."

"There's nothing to talk about."

"That's not true. Now sit up and talk to me."

Jason rolled over and pulled his knees up to his chest. "So?"

Lauren decided to try a different approach. "So... when you walked in last night you were holding hands with that cute tennis player."

"Morgan."

"Right. Are you dating her now?"

"We're not having sex, if that's what you're worried about." Jason's anger bubbled just below the surface.

"I admit I'm relieved to know that, but it wasn't what I was asking."

"Mom, my life is over. What difference does it make if we talk?" Jason sighed. "It changes nothing."

"Jason, your dad will take care of Karen somehow. What she did was wrong, and you are not responsible." Lauren tried to sound more confident than she actually felt.

"You're talking about Karen? I don't give a shit about her," Jason said. "I was talking about Morgan. She heard the whole thing, and now she's never going to talk to me again."

Lauren was stunned. "Morgan? How can you be thinking about her when your ex-girlfriend says she's pregnant?"

"Mom, Karen wasn't my girlfriend. We hung out for a couple months and always used protection. Besides, she's crazy. She's probably lying about the baby to get near me."

"What are you saying, Jason?"

"Mom, I basically stopped seeing her three weeks before she showed up at our house. She was texting me all the time. I couldn't deal with her; she was totally nuts. It's not like I was in love with her. God, this is totally awkward... but it was, you know, just sex."

Lauren was astonished. Jason's explanation seemed so simple. Lauren wanted to believe him.

"Wait. Then why are you so upset?"

"Because of Morgan. I like her. It's the first time I've ever really felt comfortable with a girl. And now it's ruined by some bullshit story. Sorry, Mom, but it's true."

Lauren didn't correct his language; she sided with her son. "Jason, if this is true, it will be fixed. Your dad will get to the bottom of it, and then you can go to Morgan with the truth." Lauren paused, but Jason didn't look convinced. "Jase, the truth usually comes out on top. Morgan will recognize it and get over this mess if she cares about you. I promise."

"How do you know?" Jason grumbled but he was clearly listening.

"Because I was a seventeen-year-old girl once." Lauren tried to recollect the raw feelings of being a teenager. "It's hard, but it does get better. Now get up. You have work to do."

Lauren left the room, closing the door behind her. It had not gone the way she'd expected, but somehow she felt better about the whole thing. She considered calling David to tell him what she'd found out, but decided to talk to Audrey first.

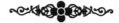

Lauren made Audrey her favorite coffee with vanilla and cinnamon. Perhaps it would help soothe her frayed nerves. Lauren put the coffee on the nightstand and opened the curtains. It was nearly noon, and the sunlight poured into the room.

Audrey sat up to take a sip. "Thanks," she grunted.

Lauren curled up in a wicker chair by the bay window. "This is one of the nicest rooms in the whole house. I love the view."

Audrey looked at her mother but said nothing. Lauren knew this wasn't going to be easy.

"Sweetie, this is complicated. We have a lot to talk about. But I need you to know I love you very much."

"Are you going to punish me?"

"Of course not. How could you ask that?" Lauren was lost; it felt like anything she had to say was going to come out all wrong. "Do you want to tell me what happened?"

"Not really."

The silence between them was uncomfortable. Lauren took a deep breath. She needed patience, and it was not something she had a great deal of at the moment. "Okay, how about if I start. I'm not having an affair with Rick."

"I saw you with him," Audrey said.

"And sometimes we see things which can be misinterpreted. Rick and I are friends; I won't deny that. But he's younger than me by at least ten years, and what you saw was him preventing me from falling on the rocks. I would never cheat on your dad."

"It didn't look like that."

"That's right. Things are not always as they appear. You made an incorrect assumption."

"Sorry."

Lauren marveled at how many syllables could be packed into that word, completely changing its meaning. She decided not to take the bait. "There's no need to be sorry; it was an honest mistake. My main concern is why you didn't ask me about it first. Why don't you talk to me anymore?"

"Mom..."

"No, Audrey. A lot has happened, and we're going to talk about it. How about you start by telling me when this whole mess happened." Lauren couldn't bring herself to say the word *rape* in reference to her daughter.

"You know the night that woman came over?" Audrey looked down at the bed, not making eye contact with her mother. "Then."

The whole ugly scene flashed through Lauren's mind. She remembered Audrey coming into the room early in the morning. Lauren pictured her crying and curled up in her lap. How had she missed that before? It was certainly not normal behavior. In retrospect, it was as plain as day.

"Shit," Lauren mumbled. "I'm sorry. I don't know what to say. I should have seen how upset you were, but I was caught up in the drama of that night." Lauren paused. "That's no excuse. I feel terrible." Guilt overwhelmed Lauren as she put her arms around her young daughter.

"I'm not going back to that high school, Mom. I can't," Audrey said with a whimper.

"We need to get you help, emotional support. You've been dealing with this on your own far too long. We will face this issue."

"How, Mom? You can't make it go away. I've tried."

"Honey, the situation won't go away, but you will learn how to handle your feelings, and that will make everything so much better. I can promise you that."

"I don't see how. I couldn't deal with stupid kids my age, so I got the job at Dr. Hawkins'. And then there was Dylan. I helped him save a dog, and he was perfectly nice, but I froze. It was like I was back in the barn with those kids I thought were my friends." Audrey sobbed, unable to continue.

"You can tell me, honey. Go on."

"I can't. I can't talk about it, Mom. Not to you."

"I understand. We need to find a person you feel safe with. Dr. Hawkins and the hospital gave me the name of a therapist. I put a call in to her this morning."

"Dr. Hawkins said I could talk to her, but I kind of blew it."

"Somehow I doubt that, but what did you do?"

"Well, I kinda got angry with her. She's been so nice to me, and I snapped at her. I really like her, Mom." Audrey finally sounded a bit more like herself.

"She seems nice and very understanding. Would you like to go back to work for the few weeks we have left up here?"

"Can I?" Audrey sounded hopeful.

"My guess is Dr. Hawkins would be happy to have you when you're feeling up to it. She's very worried about you. She called here this morning to check on you and wants an update this afternoon."

Audrey nodded and yawned. Lauren saw how vulnerable her daughter looked.

She wondered why she had not recognized this until now. "How about if you try to get some more sleep. I'll check on you a little later and bring you a sandwich. Then tomorrow we can go see Dr. Hawkins if you're up for it."

"Thanks, Mom." Audrey climbed under the blanket. Lauren watched as her daughter fell asleep. She looked so peaceful. Lauren could only imagine the horrors she had faced.

Lauren silently wiped away her tears. She didn't want Audrey to know she was crying. She blamed Karen for all of this. If she hadn't come to the house, Lauren would have recognized the pain her daughter was in and things would have been completely different. Who knows how events would have played out if that loathsome woman had not shown up on their doorstep.

Chapter 50

David sat opposite Karen in the same pizza place where she and Jason had first met.

"Thank you for coming," David said. Karen's face seemed puffy and pale, perhaps due to her pregnancy. "This can't be easy for you." David could not image how she and Jason had crossed paths in the first place. They seemed on two different emotional levels.

Karen studied the man opposite her. He was an older version of Jason, and the contrast made Jason seem even younger. Her stomach churned. "It's not... Easy, that is. I wasn't sure what to expect."

"Well, it would seem the situation has become complicated, and I wanted to discuss it with you—sooner rather than later."

"I'm not sure what there is to discuss, really. And isn't this something I should be talking to your wife about?"

"Yes, well, about that." David grimaced. "Your letter was not well received by Lauren, and whatever your intended goal, I'm quite sure you missed the mark."

Karen stared at David. "I didn't have an intended goal."

"Which is one of the things I need to find out, don't I?" David sighed. This meeting was already going badly. "I don't want to be adversarial with you; I just want to talk honestly. Is that okay with you?"

"I'm sorry. I didn't know what to think when I got your call." The pizza arrived, and David served Karen a slice.

"Karen, my son is sixteen. You're what, twenty-five?"

"Twenty-six."

"My apologies. Twenty-six. You had a relationship of some sort with my son, and now you find yourself pregnant. Is that correct?"

"Yes, it is." The thought was depressing enough. Karen didn't like hearing it out of the mouth of a stranger.

David took a deep breath and forged ahead. "Are you under medical care? That is, has this been confirmed by a doctor? It's not that I don't trust you; I have to ask."

"I understand and yes; yes to both questions." Karen's voice was flat.

David sighed. "I hate asking this... but are you sure my son is the father?"

Karen gritted her teeth. "I'll try not to take offense to that question, but yes, I'm quite sure the baby is your son's."

"I'm sorry. I had to ask, given the circumstances." David wondered how he could gain this woman's trust so she would open up to him. "I'm upsetting you. Maybe we should back up a bit. Why don't you tell me your side. How did this begin?" David tried to sound encouraging.

Karen nodded. As David ate a slice of pizza she unveiled how she met a flirtatious young man on a random night out with friends.

David interrupted. "Didn't you wonder about his age?"

"They were drinking beer. It didn't occur to me that they had fake IDs." As the story unfolded, she explained how she'd been lonely, having been cheated on by her last boyfriend. Jason seemed gentle, sweet, and willing to listen. He was genuinely nice, and it was refreshing.

By the time she finished her story, David was reeling. It was obvious that Jason had deceived them about his weekends away and overnight visits. They'd had quite a few dates, and their relationship had been intensely physical. It had also gone on far longer than he'd anticipated. It was clear from the way this woman was telling the story that she had not yet fully accepted the fact that Jason was still a boy. It was also clear she was in love with him.

"How far along are you?"

"The last time we were... together... was the only time we didn't use protection." Karen avoided David's eyes. "It was a few weeks before I came to your house. I guess that makes it close to three months."

"But you're not certain?"

"No, not exactly. I've been so shocked and confused." Karen tried hard not to cry. "You can't imagine what I've been through."

"Tell me. I want to understand," David said gently.

"I can't."

"Please trust me. I'm not the enemy. I want to help you." The words came out of David's mouth before he really had a chance to think about what he was saying. He wanted to try to understand what this woman was thinking.

Karen sighed. She had no one to talk to, no one to confide in. Maybe if she explained her situation a resolution would become obvious.

"I was falling in love with Jason. Or maybe I was already in love with him. There was something about his attentiveness that made me feel alive and full of energy.

But deep down I knew something was wrong. Honestly, I thought it was another girl. At the end, I was going crazy with jealousy." Tears streamed down Karen's cheeks; it was clear to David her heart was broken. Maybe they had misjudged her.

"I actually thought your wife was Jason's wife when she answered the door. I made so many bad assumptions. I wish I could take everything back," she whispered. "And now I'm pregnant and in love with someone who never really existed. After that awful day, I became very depressed. I didn't realize I missed my period. By the time I went to the doctor and they told me I was pregnant, I honestly couldn't remember the date of my last period. I didn't believe it at first, but I heard the heartbeat during an ultrasound. I knew I couldn't abort this baby."

David's heart did a flip. This poor woman—girl, really—was alone... and carrying his grandchild. "Karen, you don't need to do this by yourself," he blurted out. "That's my grandchild you're carrying. I'll help you."

Karen looked at David, stunned. David was shocked that he'd said it, too, but he meant every word. "Look, there are so many things wrong with this, but that baby is innocent. Maybe if I'd been a better father we wouldn't be having this conversation, but we are, so let me do the right thing now."

Karen could only nod. "The financial part will be tricky, but I'll figure out a way to get money to you to pay for your medical expenses. As for the rest, there is email. We'll be back in New York in a couple weeks. I can arrange to see you on occasion so you're not so alone. My wife and Jason can never know about this, but I'll do what I can. Will that help?"

Karen stared at the man sitting opposite her. A great weight was lifted from her shoulders, and suddenly she was famished. "It's not what I expected, not at all, but I feel better. In fact, I suddenly feel like eating for the first time in weeks." Karen's smile was genuine.

David smiled back. "Well, you do have two to feed," he said as he served her another slice of pizza.

CHAPTER 51

Lauren walked along Hemmingway Point. This part of the shoreline of Lake Charlevoix seemed remote. It was rocky and scattered with pine trees, a far cry from the manicured lawns and beach of the Lexington Club. Rick said he would meet her there in half an hour. Lauren decided to head out early so she could collect her thoughts.

With two weeks left in their vacation, life was suddenly filled with upheaval and uncertainty. David's quick turnaround was only two days, and he would be back from New York in four hours or so. He'd called from the Chicago airport to tell her he'd run into someone from the club who would give him a ride to the cottage, so there was no need for Lauren to drive to Traverse City to get him. She appreciated the breathing room.

Both Audrey and Jason went to work, giving Lauren a few hours to herself. She took a chance and called Rick to see if he wanted to go for a walk. Lauren wasn't sure if she was looking for a momentary escape from her troubles or if she needed someone to talk to. In either case, the thought of spending a couple hours with Rick bolstered her mood.

Lost in thought, she stopped to admire the wildflowers growing amidst the rocks along the shore.

"Queen Anne's Lace." Rick's familiar voice echoed from behind her. "Related to the carrot, believe it or not."

"Ahh, Rickly's Believe It or Not. I love that game."

Rick laughed. "I see what you did there. Cute. Well, regardless, it's one of my favorite flowers, even if it grows wild."

The two fell into step, listening to the crunch of the rocks beneath their feet. It had only been four days since he last saw Lauren but it felt like an eternity. He had so many questions for her about the situation with her son, but he didn't want to pry. It was hard to know where to draw the line in their relationship.

He also was having a hard time controlling his emotions now that he'd articulated his feelings to Liza. It was almost as if the cork was out of the bottle and it wouldn't go back in, no matter what he tried to do. He'd tried sailing the day before—his usual means of escape—but it hadn't worked. He'd pictured Lauren sailing with him, his arms around her, and it made his desire for her irrepressible.

Lauren was so deeply distracted by her own issues that she didn't notice the unusual silence between them. She was comforted by his presence; just being near him calmed her somehow. It was soothing being with Rick.

Without warning, Rick stopped walking and grabbed Lauren's forearm, pulling her around to face him. He looked at her, his eyes brimming with emotion. In one quick motion, he slipped his arm behind her back, pulled her body into his, and kissed her. Lauren responded by wrapping her arms around his neck and pressing back with equal passion.

Rick pulled away from the kiss but didn't let go of her. "Lauren, I... I couldn't help myself."

Lauren was filled with mixed emotions. She wanted to stay in Rick's arms but felt the weight of her wedding band on her finger. The two hugged tighter, Lauren's head on Rick's shoulder.

"Rick, I can't. I'm married."

"I know. I'm sorry; I shouldn't have kissed you."

"We're friends, right?" Lauren sputtered, still trying to deny her feelings for Rick.

"Are you saying you don't have feelings for me?" Rick said, his stomach clenched in fear.

"No, no I'm not saying that at all. I... I don't know what I feel." Lauren hesitated and looked up at him. "Rick, the past two days have been overwhelming, between the thing with Jason and now Audrey."

"What's going on with Audrey?" Rick held Lauren at arm's length for a second, his eyes filled with genuine concern. His compassion dissolved her defenses, and Lauren once again found herself enveloped in Rick's embrace, the warmth and protection of his body providing the strength and safety she so desperately needed.

Without answering his question, Lauren reached up and kissed Rick, her lips soft against his, the complexity of their relationship expressed in the tender moment of understanding. Lauren needed the momentary break from reality. Having to rehash everything would obliterate the gentle purity of the moment.

Against her will, Lauren forced herself away from Rick. "I can't do this, Rick. My husband will be home any minute, and I need to deal with all the crap going on."

"Can I help?" Rick's heart was pounding in his chest. He longed to hold on to this woman and never let her go.

"Yes and no." Lauren looked out at two passing sailboats as she tried to organize her thoughts. "I need to deal with David and the kids. But knowing you're here makes me feel so much better."

"So where does that leave us?"

"I don't know. Let me get things settled with the kids. I feel something; I just don't know what. You're very important to me, but it's all so confusing. Please, just give me a few days."

"I'm not going anywhere. Let's head back to the club, and you can tell me about Audrey on the way." Rick took her hand and the two walked back toward the cottages while Lauren shared the truth of her situation.

As they reached the cottage, Rick kissed her on the cheek and let her know he was only a phone call away.

Chapter 52

"Hon, give me fifteen minutes to shower and get changed, and then we can go over what I found out when I spoke with Karen. Is that okay?" David asked as he gave Lauren a peck on the forehead. He didn't wait for an answer and headed toward the bedroom.

The shower was a diversion; David had to formulate his game plan. If he told his wife the truth about Karen, she wouldn't listen to him. Karen was credible, in his opinion. He'd felt her pain, and he believed her story. The truth would turn a precarious situation into an ugly argument. He desperately wanted to avoid more conflict. David wanted peace. He wanted life to return to normal.

Lauren was waiting for him in the kitchen. She'd poured two glasses of iced tea and made sandwiches for lunch.

"Thanks. I didn't grab anything to eat before getting on the plane this morning," David said as he took a seat at the table. "What have I missed around here?"

David listened to Lauren as she went over everything she knew. She detailed Audrey's issues and shared information about the support group recommended to them. She also described Jason's perspective regarding his relationship with Karen. It was a lot to take in all at once, and the part about Jason made David particularly uncomfortable. Karen's story was significantly different.

When Lauren finished, she urged him on with a nod. "So, what happened when you met with Karen?"

David sighed. "This is hard. That's a lot to take in. How are you handling all this?"

"Me?" Lauren scoffed. "It's almost irrelevant. I'll be fine once we get the issues with the kids handled."

"Okay, we can talk about the kids first, but your feelings are not immaterial to me. We can set your feelings aside for now. Jason or Audrey first?"

It seemed to Lauren like David was dealing with an engineering issue rather than a personal one. She was beginning to wonder if he had any feelings at all.

"Well, you spoke to Karen."

"For the most part, her story is the same as Jason's, with the caveat being her story is from a woman's perspective."

"What does that mean?" Lauren snapped.

"Simply that she was far more emotional. There were lots of tears." David took his time, trying to tell Lauren enough so it seemed truthful without getting her all worked up again.

Lauren looked surprised. "She was in love with him?"

"I believe so. I also believe she was unaware of his actual age," David said, trying his best not to take sides. If he sounded like he was defending Karen, his wife's rage would surface again. "The bottom line is; the main details are the same."

"What about the baby?"

David hesitated a split second. "She said she had a miscarriage."

"So she lied about the pregnancy?"

"Whether we believe she was pregnant or not is irrelevant. The fact is we don't have to worry about a baby now. That's all that really matters, Lauren." David held his breath. Having Lauren buy this lie was crucial to moving forward. He needed to make everyone believe the problem had gone away. A miscarriage seemed the easiest explanation.

She sat there in silence for a few moments. "Do you believe her, David?"

"Honestly, Lauren, it's hard to know exactly what to believe. But we have to make a choice. Frankly, I don't think Jason is ready to be a father." David felt a little guilty but decided this was the best solution for their family. Once he made up his mind there was no turning back.

"I don't feel like I know the whole truth." David could hear the uncertainty in Lauren's voice.

"And we're never going to. That's something we're going to have to accept." David pressed on. "I talked to Karen; she believes her truth. She wasn't lying; that much I know. You talked to Jason. You're his mother. Was he lying?"

"No, he wasn't."

"We're caught. We have two different perspectives: Jason, who is almost seventeen and not yet a man, and a woman who didn't recognize that fact. Yes, we have to question her judgment, but how do we know who's 'right' here?"

"I didn't think about it that way. But how could she look at our boy and think she was dating a man her own age? What was she thinking?"

"The only thing to do is move forward with what we know. We no longer need to worry about a baby." David hoped the issue would be put to rest. He would figure out a way to support Karen and her baby without his family knowing, but for now he needed to protect them from further damage.

"Okay, so now can we focus on the more immediate and pressing issue?" Lauren said.

"What do you mean?"

"I'm talking about Audrey. I'm at a total loss to comprehend what happened or how to handle the situation. And in addition to everything else, she's refusing to go back to her high school."

"That's unfortunate."

Lauren looked at David, questioning his choice of words. *Unfortunate?* That seemed a bit cold and void of emotion. "We have an appointment with a counselor at the hospital in the morning. I'm driving her, but Audrey insists on talking with the counselor alone. I think we should respect her need for privacy. I don't think she wants either of us to hear the details."

"God, I don't know if I want to know the details, truthfully."

"I'm not sure we should avoid the truth. It seems like an awful lot for a young girl to deal with on her own."

"She's a strong girl, Lauren. And she's got to grow up eventually. Besides, like you said, she's not going to be on her own; she's going to a support group."

"Well, we'll see what happens tomorrow." Lauren put their plates in the sink and headed out of the room.

"Wait! Can we talk about us?" Lauren paused in the doorway as David continued with what was obviously a well-rehearsed speech. "Lauren, we need to put us first. I think we went wrong when we stopped being a couple and became parents."

Lauren started to interject but David cut her off. "Hear me out first. Please?" She didn't stop him.

"I think we got our priorities out of line. When we were young and new together, everything was about us—what we did, when we did it—as a couple. We were happy. Do you remember?" Lauren nodded. "When we had kids and got busy dealing with them, that feeling eroded. We stopped taking care of us. We need to come back together and prioritize our relationship. I still love you; I've never stopped. I just want that feeling back."

David's impassioned plea made complete sense, but Lauren wondered if it was too late. She didn't know if she could feel the way she used to feel about him.

"What makes you think we can go back to how it was?" Lauren asked.

"We can if we try. I know I've been a jerk. I focused on everything except what was right in front of me the whole time. You're beautiful, an amazing wife; you always have been. I took you for granted as I built my career. Give me a chance to make it up to you somehow. I'm going to try my hardest. I promise."

"I don't know, David. I guess we'll just see what happens, take it one day at a time. It's not like I'm in any hurry to leave."

Chapter 53

Lauren and Audrey drove toward the Charlevoix County Hospital. Audrey stared out the window at Round Lake Harbor as they made their way through town. Lauren could only imagine what she must be feeling.

"You okay, sweetie?" Lauren asked, trying to sound cheerful despite the pall that had settled between them.

"I'm fine, Mom."

"You don't have to do this alone. I'm willing to come inside," Lauren said as she pulled the Jeep into the parking lot.

"I know. I think I'll be more comfortable if I don't know anyone." It sounded stupid the minute she said it.

As the two approached the hospital's front doors, they were greeted by a young woman with bright blue hair styled in a pixie cut. She wore army pants and a black T-shirt and couldn't have been more than twenty-five years old.

"Are you Mrs. Breckenridge?" she asked with a bright smile. Lauren confirmed. "Then you must be Audrey. I'm Erin." She took Audrey's hand and squeezed it. "I know you've felt alone and powerless, but not anymore! I promise that, in time, you'll be strong again, but from this minute on, you will never be alone."

The cheerful young woman turned to Lauren. "We'll take it from here. I'll work with Audrey individually first, and then I'll bring her into the group. We'll do this for the first few sessions until she feels she only needs group. As I said on the phone, we meet three times a week for the first phase. It's an intense schedule, but I've found it really helps to kick this thing to the curb quickly, particularly when the woman is so young. Since this is our first session, please come back in two and a half hours. You might bring Audrey some lunch when you come back. She'll say she's not hungry, but I bet she'll change her mind. They usually do. Okay?"

Lauren nodded. She was spellbound as she watched Erin lead Audrey through the doors of the hospital. This young spitfire simply took over the situation, managing both Lauren and Audrey at once. There was no question who was in charge, nor was there any question about doing exactly as she instructed.

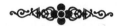

Audrey looked around Erin's office. It looked more like a lounge. The couches and chairs were worn and mismatched, but the collection still looked like it belonged together, almost as if it had been decorated that way on purpose. The room was warm, inviting, and comfortable. Audrey was able to relax in the space.

Erin gestured for Audrey to sit in one of two armchairs in front of a massive picture window that offered a stunning view through the treetops to Lake Michigan in the distance.

"I'm not what you expected," Erin said.

"Not really."

"I get that a lot. I guess when people hear *social worker* and *group therapy,* they automatically picture someone older and, you know, formal."

Audrey tried to hide her smile. "Exactly."

"Well, fuck it. This is me, and I'm good at what I do." Erin looked at Audrey with intensity, but for some reason the eye contact didn't make Audrey feel uncomfortable, in fact, if anything it made her feel more comfortable with Erin. "When you feel comfortable, you can tell me what happened to you, but it's not required." Audrey relaxed a little as Erin laid out her expectations. "I don't believe in wallowing in the past. Shit happened; it sucked. We deal with it and move on. I'm not saying that in a cold, callus way. Many people in our position end up being victims their entire lives, and that gives all the power to the assholes who committed the crime. I don't believe in that, and this is what I'm going to teach you."

"You were... ?" Audrey couldn't finish the sentence.

"In your position? Hell yeah. I was sixteen. It was my mother's boyfriend. How fucked up is that? He raped me—more than once—and my mother didn't believe me. She was a drunk and sided with him. When I was seventeen, I ran away from home. We lived in Florida at the time, and I knew I had a grandmother in Portland so I went to find her. I'm one of the lucky ones."

"How were you lucky?"

"My grandmother was cool. She made me finish high school and encouraged me to go to college. She helped me see I was strong. Because of her, I ended up on this path. I got my Master's degree and now I help other girls. You see, when you're abused like we were, it's so easy to become trapped, to always see yourself as a victim. Your entire life can be ruined because of a bad person."

"But what if it was your fault?" Audrey whispered.

"That's what they want you to believe. That is their power over you. But Audrey, listen to me, it's never your fault. Never. Nobody has the right to do anything to you unless you're willing. It's that simple. Girls need to know this. When you get it, it's empowering."

Audrey wasn't sure what to say. It all seemed to make sense, but, at the same time, it didn't seem to apply to her life. Erin sensed her uncertainty. "This will make sense to you soon enough. Let's get your forms filled out, and then you will meet the other people in our group. You don't have to talk today if you don't want to. Just listen, get to know everyone. It's totally cool. Each one of them has been exactly where you are today."

Erin handed Audrey a package of forms and left her alone to fill them out. As she wrote, it struck Audrey that, for the first time in months, she felt hopeful. She genuinely liked Erin and trusted her completely. Audrey couldn't remember the last time she'd felt so comfortable.

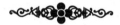

Lauren was surprised to see Erin and Audrey laughing when they walked out of the building. Audrey gave Erin a hug before getting into the car, and the two waved good-bye as Lauren pulled away from the parking lot.

"I brought you a tuna salad sandwich and water. It's in the cooler at your feet."

"Thanks, Mom. I'm actually pretty hungry."

"Erin seems nice," Lauren said cautiously as Audrey munched on her sandwich.

"She's actually pretty great. She's smart and funny. I like her."

"Good. So, the session went well then?"

"Yeah. I'm going to talk to Dr. Hawkins about moving my hours a little. That way I can ride the Vespa into town for group and go to work after. I mean… if that's okay with you."

"I think that's a great plan. I'm sure Dr. Hawkins will approve."

Lauren glanced at her daughter and smiled. Audrey seemed more relaxed than she'd been in weeks.

CHAPTER 54

Jason sat alone at the end of the dock with a stolen six-pack of beer. It was dinner time, the beach cleared out hours ago. Earlier in the day he'd stopped by Morgan's house to try to talk to her. He desperately wanted to explain his side of the situation, but she was ignoring his texts and calls. The housekeeper told him she was in Long Island with her father for a tennis tournament. His heart sank. Not knowing when she would return, he feared he might never have an opportunity to talk to her again. The beer helped to numb his pain.

"Hey, Jason!" a chipper voice called out from behind him. "You shouldn't be sitting all by yourself. Where's the fun in that?"

Jason looked up to find the perky fifteen-year-old redhead with big tits whom he'd been giving swimming lessons to all summer long, "Oh, hey Kylie." She was wearing cutoffs and a bathing suit top. Jason wondered why he hadn't noticed how hot her body was before now.

"If you want, I'll join you." Without waiting for an invitation, the girl sat down close enough to Jason so that their arms were practically touching. "You don't seem like you're in a good mood."

"I'm not, really."

"Oh." Kylie was quiet for a minute while the two watched a water-skier pass the end of the dock. "It's because your girlfriend left the club, isn't it?"

"What? Yeah, Morgan left town." Jason grunted. At this point he should be used to the fact that everyone in the club knew everyone else's business. He didn't care.

"I know how to make you feel better." Kylie crawled behind him and got to her knees. She rubbed his shoulders as he finished his beer and popped open the fifth can. He took a long swig and leaned into her massage.

Kylie sat down behind him and hooked her legs around his body. Massaging his back with one hand, she deftly removed her bathing suit top and pressed her breasts against him.

"What are you doing?" he said, groaning, unable to hide his surprise.

"Doesn't it feel good?" She leaned harder into his back and reached around to rub his chest.

Jason moaned in response. Between his current mood, the beer, and his raging hormones, Jason was no longer in control of the situation. Kylie was on a mission. She knew exactly what she wanted, and she was determined to take advantage of the situation.

"Just go with it," Kylie whispered, lowering her hand to his bulge and rubbing hard. "I'll make you feel better."

"You're driving me crazy." Jason gasped.

"Well, don't just sit there; feel free to join in at any time." Kylie laughed, arching her back and rubbing her breasts against his back.

It was more than Jason could bear. He turned around and rolled on top of Kylie, his hands and mouth exploring every inch of exposed skin. Kylie wriggled out of her shorts and wrapped her legs around Jason's hips. Breathlessly, he pulled his trunks down to his knees and pushed into her as hard as he could until the two of them could no longer move, fully satisfied.

"I knew I could get you to fuck me this summer," Kylie whispered.

"What? What are you talking about?"

"Don't play innocent. All the girls have been trying to get you to do them, but you only wanted Miss Priss Morgan. I told them I could get your attention."

Jason was still lying on top of Kylie as she confessed her intentions. He felt himself starting to get hard again. "You wanted to get fucked by me? You really want to get fucked?" Jason got on his knees and flipped Kylie over on her belly. Lifting her hips to him he thrust into her with great force.

Kylie gasped, squealing with delight.

"You shoulda said something sooner, 'cause with a hot bod like yours, I'm good to go."

CHAPTER 55

"Karen? It's David Breckenridge." David stood in the parking lot of the golf club talking on his cell phone. He had just wrapped up a round of golf with three of the club members and had a few moments of privacy before he headed back to the cottage for dinner with Lauren and the kids.

"Oh, hi. I wasn't expecting you to call."

"I wanted to see how you're feeling and to find out about your doctor's appointment."

"Really?"

"Yes. I was serious when I said I wanted to be part of this. I may not be able to go to the appointments with you, but we can talk, can't we?"

Karen wasn't sure what to say. She wondered if there was some other reason for his sudden interest. She was the one who'd alerted the family in the first place, but this wasn't the reaction she'd expected.

"Are you there?" David asked.

"Yes, I'm here. Sorry. You caught me off guard. I don't know how to take your interest."

"Take it at face value. I'm not hiding some ulterior motive. In fact, starting next week you'll see automatic deposits into your checking account from a company called NanoTech. It's not an error. You're now on the payroll as a consultant. You'll receive two thousand a month to use for baby expenses. You'll also be put on the company insurance plan. It covers everything, including deductibles, so you won't have any medical expenses."

"David, I don't know what to say."

"How about you start with telling me about the doctor's appointment?" David said.

Karen could almost hear his tender smile.

CHAPTER 56

Audrey looked around the room at the five other girls in the group. They seemed completely normal to her. None of them appeared to feel as awkward as she felt. When it was their turn, they just told their stories and said what was on their minds.

"After the first time, my mother's boyfriend threatened to hurt me if I told anyone. So whenever he and my mom got drunk, she would pass out. Then he would come into my room, and that's when it would happen." Mia was speaking as the rest of the group listened in rapt silence.

"Can you tell us what happened?" Erin said. "It's not easy saying the words, but they are just words. Remember, this room is filled with shared understanding and support. Our goal is to turn this person's cruel behavior into words. That way, we'll have more control over our reaction to the hurt and humiliation. Words don't hurt; actions do."

Audrey listened to Mia struggle with the rest of her story. Her stomach knotted as she empathized with the pretty seventeen-year-old girl who'd been repeatedly raped. Mia had endured further humiliation when her mom threw her out of the house, believing she'd enticed the man into having sex with her. Mia now lived in a teen shelter. She'd dropped out of high school and was working at a diner to support herself.

Erin squeezed Mia's hand. "You're doing great. Allowing yourself to have feelings is part of the healing journey we're all on together. Thank you for trusting us. It means a lot to me." Erin looked around the room. "Who feels like talking next?"

It was Audrey's third session, and to her great surprise, Erin had not pressured her to speak at all. She'd said she could sit there until she was ready, and it really seemed like she meant it.

"I think I'm ready, Erin." Audrey's voice faltered.

Erin crossed the room and sat down on the floor next to Audrey. "We're all grateful for your trust in us. We know it's not easy to begin. Where do you want to start?" Erin spoke softly but with confidence.

"Well, I guess the whole thing was fucked up from the beginning. I met this guy when I was bored. I'd had a fight with my best friend, and I was lonely. I didn't even think he was cute or anything; he was just there. I didn't know Matt hated my brother, Jason, because he always beat him in every sport they played together. So I guess Matt decided to get even. He got me drunk and stoned. I don't even know all the different kinds of drugs I smoked. In the beginning he tried to use me for sex, but things got weird. What I found out later is that he planned from the beginning to hurt me, but he started to like me. My brother, in the meantime, had been dating this girl who was way older and everyone knew it. What I didn't know was that Matt and Jason got into a big fight at school, right at the end of the semester. Matt got suspended for three days, missed some finals, and had to take summer school, so he was pissed and wanted to get even with Jason." Audrey's voice cracked and Erin handed her a bottle of water.

"Audrey, you're doing great. Do you want to keep going?"

Audrey nodded. "So, Matt planned an end-of-the-school-year party." She paused, looking down at her hands. "And he told all his friends that I was going to give them all head, kind of an end-of-the-school-year present. He gave me a weird drug, so I was out of it, and that night all of his friends... one after another ..."

"Is this the first time you've told anyone the story?" Erin asked, holding Audrey's hand.

Audrey nodded, tears flowing.

Erin wrapped her arms around Audrey. "You did amazing. Thank you for trusting us. I know that's hard to do after something like this happens."

"It's not fair!" Audrey sobbed. "Why me? What did I do to them?"

Audrey crumpled into Erin's lap. Wiping away tears of her own, Erin spoke words of comfort to Audrey and the other group members. The fourteen-year-old's pain was too much for them to handle, and most were crying along with her, reliving their own nightmares once again.

"Let the pain out. In time you'll realize you did nothing to deserve this. Matt is a weak, cruel person. But for now you need to know that what you're feeling is absolutely normal." Erin helped Audrey sit up. "Audrey, look at us. We're all crying with you, because we feel what you do. We have been exactly where you are. And together we will get you to a place where you can be okay with what happened. You can be in a place where you live from strength, not as a victim. Does that make sense?"

Audrey nodded, wiping her tears. Just telling what had happened had lifted a great weight from her chest, as if she'd been carrying around a water balloon that had finally burst. Now there was room for her to breathe.

CHAPTER 57

Lauren stood in the waiting room, admiring the view of Lake Michigan. She was early for her appointment with Erin. With a week left in their vacation, Lauren contemplated the events of the summer. She doubted if she had succeeded in achieving her goal or made any progress toward bringing her family closer together. It seemed as if her plans had backfired, and the vacation had driven them further apart. Certainly there was a wedge between David and her. If she were honest with herself, that wedge had a name on it. Did she regret meeting Rick? Lost in thought, she didn't hear Erin approaching.

"Mrs. Breckenridge?" Lauren practically jumped through the window. "Oh, I'm sorry. I didn't mean to startle you."

"It's okay. I was admiring the view and became lost in thought."

"The view is amazing. I get lost in it all the time," Erin said. "Do you want to come to my office or stay here in the lounge?"

"The office is fine, really. I was just thinking about the changes we've been through with the kids this spring and summer." Lauren followed Erin down the hall.

"Your family has been through a lot."

"I suppose Audrey talks about it." Lauren was suddenly hit with the realization that this young woman knew all of her family's dirty little secrets. At least most of them.

"We encourage our members to share what is troubling them," Erin said. "And, truthfully, this is what I want to talk to you about. I have grave concerns about what is going to happen with Audrey when you go back to New York. You're leaving in a week, correct?"

Lauren nodded. "I've been thinking about the same thing. Audrey doesn't talk to me in any great detail about what happens in your group. It's obvious she considers it a positive experience, but that's all I can tell, to be honest."

"Yes, well, the participants share some intensely personal experiences, and we have an agreement not to discuss what happens in group outside of the room."

"Right. I'm not asking about the other participants, but Audrey?"

"That's up to Audrey. She may or may not share her feelings with you. It depends on how the process goes." Erin leaned forward. "Mrs. Breckenridge, I'm afraid of what might happen when she goes home without a support mechanism in place. And worse than that, what happens when she is back in the same environment with her abusers. Without breaking her trust, it's a bad idea. It's setting her up for certain failure."

"What do you mean?" Lauren asked, fear gripping her chest, making it hard to breathe.

"Well, her trust in people is absolutely destroyed, and she is only now starting to open up in group. Without an outlet, I'm afraid she'll shut down forever."

"That sounds ominous," Lauren said.

"She's... fragile." Erin tried to be gentle. "She puts on a fierce act, but deep down she's much more delicate and, frankly, needs to be treated that way."

"What do you recommend?"

"Well, there are a couple options—boarding school, for one. It would get her away from the kids who attacked her. Apparently, quite a few of the boys in her class were involved. Unfortunately, from a legal point of view, there is nothing we can do about prosecuting them."

Guilt overwhelmed Lauren. Would things have been different if she'd been paying attention that morning last spring? As if she were reading Lauren's mind, Erin jumped in. "You need to understand, with the nature of the attack, even if we had been there the next day, prosecution would have been almost impossible, and we probably would not have prevailed in court. It's really unfair, but there was little evidence, and the fact is, the so-called witnesses would more than likely have stuck together." Erin crossed the room to the mini fridge, grabbed two bottles of water, and handed one to Lauren. "In all likelihood a prosecutor wouldn't have filed a case."

Lauren wasn't sure if this information made her feel better or worse. "So what are you doing with your patients? What will you do for Audrey?" Lauren felt as if she'd been run over by a freight train. Her mind was racing, directionless. The situation seemed hopeless.

"We work with the girls and try our hardest to undo the damage done. Our success rate is pretty good." Erin said. "I'm going to be honest with you; we have an idea for Audrey. It's pretty unique, and we hope you're open to listening to it."

"Of course I'll listen. I'm at a loss. I want what's best for Audrey and our family."

"You're familiar with Claire Hawkins. As you know, she recommended our program initially." Erin watched Lauren carefully but didn't wait for a response.

"She approached me about Audrey's situation as well. Obviously, I wasn't able to break confidence with her either, but she expressed concern about Audrey's environment. Apparently, Audrey shared a little of what happened with Claire." Lauren tried hard not to let the shock show on her face.

"Claire offered an alternative to boarding school. Audrey could participate in a work/study program created specifically for her under Claire's guidance. She would attend the local high school and enroll in a medical magnate program. She would work after school in Claire's practice, and her class schedule would be worked around attending group for the same three weekly sessions." Erin paused, letting the idea sink in.

Lauren was speechless but not for long. "Stay here? Wait, where would she live?"

"With Claire and her daughter."

"I didn't know she had a daughter."

"Yes, she's been downstate for the summer at an internship. As a matter of fact, Audrey took over her job in the practice. She'll be a junior in high school this year. We both felt having an older girl around as a mentor of sorts might make a difference in Audrey's recovery and development. It would give her someone to bond with in order to rebuild trust."

"This is quite a lot to think about. Does Audrey know about this?"

"Actually, the idea was Audrey's. She expressed a strong desire to avoid returning to her previous school, for obvious reasons. And she mentioned not wanting to leave the group or her job at Claire's. It started the discussion, and we found a practical and clinical way to make it work."

"So the two of you are taking direction from a fourteen-year-old girl?" Lauren could no longer keep her defensive nature in check.

"Not at all. We were afraid it would seem that way if we brought Audrey in on the planning stages. She expressed a wish; that's all she knows. We didn't want to build up her hopes and then leave her hugely disappointed. It's feasible, so now we're bringing the idea to you for discussion. In fact, unless you're amenable to the idea, Audrey will never know we tried to make it happen."

"Well, her father would need to be part of this decision," Lauren said as she began to consider the prospect. "And we would have to meet with Claire."

Erin took a deep breath. The look of relief on her face was palpable. "I'm so glad you're willing to consider the idea. I honestly believe this is the best thing for her. Sending her back to school with the boys who attacked her... . Well, I can't predict the outcome, but it seems pretty clear the results would be horrific for her."

CHAPTER 58

"I'm sorry Mr. Jason, she said she's not going to come down to talk to you."

"Manuela, please. I need to talk to her. Our family is leaving in less than a week." Jason stood on Morgan's doorstep, pleading with their housekeeper. He'd heard Morgan had returned from the tennis tournament the day before, but she hadn't come to the beach as usual.

Manuela had been with Morgan's family since she was a little girl, and her heart ached for her. In her opinion, Jason seemed like a decent boy, and he did seem to care for Morgan. She could tell Morgan had fallen for him.

"Now, Mr. Jason, Miss Morgan is not coming out of her room, and I can't fix that. But when I turn my back, if I don't see you run up the stairs then I can't stop you, can I?"

"Manuela, you're the best!" Jason said as he kissed her on the cheek.

"Now get out of here, and don't get into trouble."

Jason took the stairs two at a time. In a flash he was knocking on Morgan's door. "I'm not going away until you let me in," he demanded.

Morgan yanked the door open. "What are you doing in my house?" she demanded. "I don't want to talk to you!"

"Fine." Jason pushed his way into the room and walked over to the window seat. "But what about me? Don't I get a say in any of this?"

"Jason, there is nothing you can say to fix this."

"You need to hear my side of things. You heard a snippet of a conversation from my mother and made a lot of assumptions. Now you're killing our relationship because of something you think happened last spring? How fair is that?"

"And I suppose the fact that you had sex with Kylie on the dock right after I left doesn't matter?"

"Wait, how do you know about that?"

"At least you're not denying it."

"No, I'm not, but it's not like I'm in love with her. She completely came on to me at the beach when I was drunk."

"So a simple *no* wasn't in your vocabulary then?"

"Jesus, Morgan. You dumped me and she was all over me. I didn't think it was a big deal."

"Except now she's bragging all over that she slept with you. It didn't exactly make me feel better about our situation, you know."

"Well, I suppose the good news is you're still thinking about 'our situation'."

"Of course I'm thinking about it. I can't think about anything else. It upset me." Morgan became quiet.

"Morgan, I'm sorry. I didn't want to hurt you. The whole thing with Karen last spring was a mistake; it wasn't my fault. My mom says she should be in jail for what she did to me. And, besides that, she wasn't pregnant. She was lying because she's completely crazy and obsessed with me. The whole thing is out of control. But it's over; Dad took care of everything." Jason walked over and stood in front of Morgan, looking down on her. "Besides, it happened way before I met you. You're amazing."

"And yet the first thing you do is have sex with another girl as soon as I leave."

"Kylie? Oh my God, Morgan, she really threw herself at me. I shouldn't have done anything. I was miserable, sitting on the dock drinking. I thought I'd lost you. I regretted it as soon as it happened, and it's not like I started dating her. She was on a mission. She and the other girls have spent the summer trying to get into my pants and she won. I didn't know it was some sort of bet."

"Well, it hurts."

"Because you still like me?" Jason put his arms around Morgan. "Come on, give me another chance."

Morgan wriggled a little, trying to get away. But she didn't try hard. Being this close to him felt good, and what she really wanted was to kiss him. Jason pulled her tight against him and lowered his lips to hers. What started as a soft, tender kiss grew heated as he hungered for her. Morgan responded, wrapping her arms around him as his lips found her neck.

Jason picked Morgan up with ease, peppering her with kisses as she wrapped her legs around his waist. He lowered her gently to the bed and hovered above her, continuing to kiss her as he slowly let the full weight of his body come to rest on hers. He was determined to pace himself. This time, he was not going to rush her or let her go. But Jason need not have worried. Morgan had already made up her mind. She was not going to college a virgin.

CHAPTER 59

"David, I think we need to consider this option," Lauren implored as the two drove to Dr. Hawkins' practice.

"I agreed to the meeting because it's Audrey's counselor, but this plan seems ridiculous. I can't believe you, of all people, are considering it."

"I'm so glad you have an open mind," Lauren countered.

"I don't have an open mind, and I'm not pretending that I do."

David had been dismissive of the idea from the moment Lauren brought it up, insisting that his daughter needed to be home with her family. David refused to acknowledge the seriousness of the situation. It took a great deal of cajoling for Lauren to convince him to meet with Claire and Erin. Lauren wasn't completely sold on the idea either, but David's overwhelming negativity pushed her into siding with the two women. Lauren wondered why she and David were not naturally on the same side. Why were they arguing about what was in the best interest of their daughter?

"Oh look! The Vespa is here; Audrey must be working today. I wasn't expecting that," Lauren said as David parked.

The two were greeted by Claire who led them to a parlor room on the far side of the building away from the practice. Erin was already seated. "I thought we would have more privacy in my residence," Claire said after introductions were made. "I told Audrey you were coming in today."

Lauren spoke first, looking at David. "We have differing opinions on the necessity of a step like this, so we thought it best to have this meeting without getting Audrey's hopes up."

The subtext was clear. Erin and Claire exchanged a glance, but Lauren was certain David missed the nonverbal communication.

"Let's all sit down and discuss the issues," Claire said with calm authority. Lauren was impressed with how easily she took command of the strong personalities in the room. "David, I want to thank you for listening to us today. I know this is probably not something you are particularly interested in." David acknowledged

Claire's direct approach with a nod. "I feel it's best for Erin, who holds an advanced degree in psychotrauma from Duke with a fellowship in developmental psychology at Yale, to lead the discussion."

"You have an impressive resume, young lady. I'm just not sure what this has to do with my daughter." David backpedaled from his entirely negative and arrogant position.

"Mr. Breckenridge, I'm sure you know your daughter was in a situation where she was sexually abused last spring." Erin picked her words with caution. "I've worked with her for five sessions. When I combine this information with the notes from her hospital visit and Dr. Hawkins' observations, it is my clinical opinion that Audrey should not return to the environment where the abuse took place."

"Your clinical opinion is to teach my girl she can run away from her problems?" David asked, his face flushed. "And that living with strangers is better for her than being with a family who loves her? I'm not sure I follow your logic."

Lauren expected the discussion to end right there. David typically got whatever he wanted when it came to debate or negotiations. Perhaps these women would know of programs close to their home where she could take Audrey as soon as they got back.

"David, in some cases I would completely agree with you," Erin said, "but treatment plans need to be developed based on the individual, not lumped together based on a clinical diagnosis."

"My daughter is not weak. She's a strong girl and doesn't run away from her problems."

"You're right; she is exceptionally strong, which is how we've managed to get this far. She tried to take care of the situation herself rather than getting immediate help. Let me reassure you; a girl of fourteen, no matter how strong, would never be emotionally equipped to handle something like this."

"Then I'll help her. Now that we know, I'll go with her, have her confront this boy and make him apologize. We'll hold him accountable."

"I wish it were that simple." Erin nodded to Claire who quietly slipped out of the room. "The damage is far more traumatic. It's not something a single apology or, for that matter, even multiple apologies will fix. Audrey has given me permission to give you some details you need to know. She was raped by a number of boys who sequentially forced themselves on her, orally, while she was under the influence of a drug that rendered her unable to control her responses. We believe the number of boys to be as many as fifteen or twenty. All of them attend the high school where she would be starting in the fall." Erin paused to let her words sink in.

David sat there, speechless, his face ghostly white. A minute passed before he was able to say anything. "Oh my God!" he whispered.

"Daddy?" Audrey tiptoed into the room, tears in her eyes.

"Pumpkin?" David looked up, his voice barely audible. Audrey hurried across the room and crawled into David's lap. "I didn't know. What can I do?" David sobbed, his face buried in his daughter's hair.

"I'll be okay, Daddy. Really. Erin is showing me how, I promise." Audrey sounded so young. Lauren's heart ached for both of them. She knew, without question, Audrey needed to stay in the care of Claire and Erin. It was the right thing to do.

"Do you really want to stay here, Audrey?" David whispered.

"I do, Daddy. I feel comfortable and safe in Erin's group, and I love working at Claire's. I can't go back to that high school; I just can't."

"Okay, honey. If it's what you want, we'll make it work. But you need to know how much I'm going to miss my little girl. It's going to break my heart not having you around."

"Dad, we can text each other all the time, and I'll come home for holidays and stuff. And you still have to buy me an ugly sweater for Christmas... which I'll never wear, of course."

David laughed as he wiped away the tears spilling down his cheeks. He held Audrey as tight as he could. In that moment he knew this decision was the right one.

CHAPTER 60

David put the Vespa into the back of the Escalade, and the three of them drove back to the cottage in silence. The emotions of the afternoon and subsequent logistical planning had left them exhausted. During the wait for the ferry, Audrey fell asleep. David reached out and held Lauren's hand.

Lauren's heart ached for her husband. She could only imagine what was going through his head. He was the type of man who protected his family at all costs. She wondered if this would break his spirit.

Jason was just getting home as they pulled into the driveway.

"How about you give your old man a hand with this scooter and then have a drink with me out back after we put it away?" David called to Jason.

"Sure thing, Dad." Jason wasn't in the mood for another lecture about his relationship with Karen but couldn't think of a way to avoid it.

David and Jason carried their sodas to the back porch. David took a good look at his boy, realizing he had become a young man before his eyes. He thought about the weight of responsibility becoming a father at seventeen would hold, and his first instinct was to protect his son from such a life-altering event. He wanted Jason to enjoy the pleasures of youth, college, and the first steps into adulthood.

Thrusting him into the responsibilities of a family too soon would completely eliminate all of his fun. Yet, in the back of his mind, David realized he needed to teach Jason some sort of responsibility. There needed to be consequence to his action. David was confounded; there were no good options. But one thing was crystal clear: he had to keep the secret about the baby and his support of Karen. Any further relationship between his son and Karen was out of the question.

"I'm glad to see you've been enjoying your summer," David said.

"It's been great."

"And you've been dating Morgan?"

"I guess so."

"Jason, this is awkward for me. I guess I need to just come out and ask if you and Morgan have been using protection."

"Dad, it's not like that."

"Don't go there, and don't try to hide from the conversation. We need to talk about the fact that you impregnated a woman. I honestly thought you knew better."

"I did! I do. It's just that—"

"There is no 'it's just that', son. You dodged a life-altering bullet, and you have no idea how close you actually came." Jason grunted and squirmed in his chair. "I can't protect you your entire life. You're sixteen and, for the most part, I can step in and fix a mistake. But you'll be a senior this year, and you're going to be making some huge decisions soon, ones which will affect your future. The following year you'll be off on your own without parental supervision. What then?"

"Dad, I'm really sorry about what happened. I was being careful. I think that girl was kinda crazy and made the whole thing up."

"Jason, I can guarantee you she was not making anything up," David said, anger seeping into his voice as he fought back the urge to protect Karen. "You need to take responsibility for your part of this, son. It is only out of sheer luck that you're not becoming a father in a few months. Do you understand the magnitude of what that would have meant?"

"I guess I didn't really think about it all that much, Dad."

"No, you really didn't. Not only would a baby have changed your life forever, but it would have changed the life of the young woman you were sleeping with. Have you given her any consideration at all? She is a person with feelings, and you were using her. For what purpose? Sexual gratification?" David forged ahead without waiting for a response. "I remember what it's like to be young, when the desire is irresistible, all-consuming. But you have to think with your head! You can't go ruining your life before it starts. Do you hear me, son?"

"I don't understand why you're getting so worked up. I thought you said Karen isn't pregnant."

David paused, trying to get his passion in check. He wondered for a minute if he'd gone too far, given something away. "You're missing the point. What if she were still pregnant, Jason? What then?"

"I don't know, but if it were up to Mom, Karen would go to jail."

"Yes, but you and I both know you have quite a bit to do with this. Your mom looks at you as her little boy, not as a young man who was in control of what he was doing. You can't convince me you didn't enjoy every second of your time with Karen. Do you honestly think it would be right to send her to jail?"

Jason looked at his feet. "No, that doesn't seem fair. I knew what I was doing."

"That's right. Now, legally, she is responsible and what she did was wrong. And she should have known better. But you lied and manipulated her for one goal. And you did it intentionally. You tell me which one of you is more at fault—the one who knew what he was doing was wrong or the one who didn't know but inadvertently broke the law because of your actions."

"I guess I got lucky."

"I guess you did."

"Dad, I feel kind of bad for Karen. I really pushed it."

"Now you're getting to some understanding, the real truth. You need to learn from it. You need to respect women. One day you're going to meet a woman who you love so deeply that you want to spend the rest of your life with her. It will hit you like a ton of bricks."

"Is that how you felt about Mom?"

"Very much so. When it happens, you can't be encumbered with a family, having to explain why you already have a kid or a long history. The woman you fall for will want you to be free to start your life with her. The two of you will want to build a history together."

"Do you still love Mom that way?" Jason asked.

"Jase, the thing about relationships is that they grow and change over the years. Passion changes over time; it's a natural part of marriage. Then when you have kids, you get so wrapped up in the day-to-day matters of life that it's easy to forget what is really important. But, in all honesty, when I step back and take a look at the life your mother and I have together, I realize I'm still completely in love with her. Sometimes I focus on other things and forget to show her. That's my mistake, one I need to fix. You need to learn from the beginning. Complacency is a hard thing to avoid."

"I guess we both kinda screwed up, Dad."

"Yes, but nothing that can't be fixed."

Jason gulped down the rest of his Coke, still avoiding his dad's eyes. He thought about Kylie and Morgan. He'd had unprotected sex with both girls without considering the potential consequences.

"Dad, the next time you head into town can I catch a lift? I need to go to the drugstore."

"I think that's a good idea."

Jason was relieved when his dad didn't question him.

Chapter 61

As Rick and Lauren walked along the rocky shore of Hemmingway Point, Lauren caught him up on the details of David's New York trip and the recommendations for Audrey. Rick was surprised she was considering it.

"Honestly, we don't have a choice," Lauren said as she bent over to pick up a Petoskey stone. "The abuse she's been dealing with is almost inconceivable. It's a wonder she's held it together this long."

"What about you?" Rick asked.

"What do you mean?"

"Well, I'm not a mother, but I can't imagine it's easy learning your daughter went through all this. It must be taking a toll on you."

Lauren looked at Rick. She had been focused on Audrey and what she needed. She didn't want to think about her own feelings. "It's kind of you to ask, but I'm fine," she said, trying her best to brush off Rick's question.

"I'm not letting you off so easily," Rick said. "Talk to me. Honestly, I'm here and I want to help you handle this. It's got to be overwhelming."

Tears welled up in Lauren's eyes as Rick put his arm around her shoulder. "I don't know what to say," she said, wiping a stray tear away.

"Well, you can tell me anything. I'm your friend."

Lauren couldn't hold her feelings in any longer. She let loose without thinking about how her words might make him feel. "Honestly, I feel like a failure. This spring when everything started falling apart, I had this stupid idea that if we went away together on a family vacation we would become close again." Lauren glanced at Rick, holding his gaze for a moment, a great sadness in her eyes. "Sorry."

"It's okay. Please go on."

"Apparently I underestimated how bad everything really was—or how much worse it was going to get. I certainly didn't expect any of the problems with Audrey, not to mention Jason's issues. And my marriage seems... well, I have no idea who I'm married to, if you want to know the truth. It felt empty when we came up here." Lauren felt relief having said it all out loud.

"You're allowed to have feelings."

Lauren laughed. "Not in my world. I take care of everyone else and make sure we run efficiently, but my feelings are not... encouraged, shall we say."

"Well, that isn't fair," Rick said. "It's disrespectful. They take advantage of you."

"I don't really think of it that way," Lauren said, a bit defensive.

"Of course you don't, because you're in the middle of it." Rick reached for her hand. "Lauren, your daughter got gang-raped. That's horrific! You're expected to feel something, for Christ's sake! You should be talking to a professional about those feelings, not trying to pretend they don't even exist."

"I'm scared, Rick. I'm scared for her. What if she can't get beyond this? What if it haunts her for the rest of her life? I don't know if I can handle the thought. It breaks my heart." Lauren broke down and cried in his arms. It was the first time she let herself really feel the effects of what had happened to Audrey, and she was overwhelmed with grief.

"Of course you're scared for her. What mother wouldn't be? Honestly, Lauren, you seem like a caring mother who has been through a lot. I don't know many women who could handle this much pressure."

"I don't feel like I've handled it very well," Lauren said, wiping the tears from her eyes.

"Really? What exactly is 'handling it well' then?"

"I don't know. I just wish I'd recognized Audrey's issue sooner. It took a couple months, which was way too long."

"This is going to sound harsh, but she tried her hardest to hide it from you. Audrey used her brother's turmoil as camouflage. Who knows, if the timing had been different, you may have picked up on it immediately."

"That makes me feel a little better."

"And as soon as you got the full picture, you got Audrey the help she needed. If you ask me, you're sacrificing your own desires to give her what she needs, right? Please tell me how you could handle this any better." Rick led Lauren to sit with him on a the trunk of a fallen tree "Can I be honest with you?"

"Of course."

"I think the only problem you have, which really isn't being addressed, is your unsupportive husband. I know I really should keep my mouth shut about him. I'm the worst person to talk about your relationship with your husband."

"Why do you say that?"

"It's not obvious?" Rick couldn't hide his surprise. This was his opening. He took a deep breath. "Lauren, I'm in love with you."

Lauren looked at Rick in disbelief, not sure if she'd heard him correctly.

"It's true. I've been trying to deny it for a while. I keep reminding myself you're married, but it's not working. So, I decided the other day to go for it. What have I got to lose? My pride?"

"I'm not sure if I'm following you."

"Lauren, I've never been in love. I've had lovers and a handful of relationships that lasted a little longer. But I've always held something back. I never let a woman see the real me… that is, until I met you." Rick looked out at the lake and focused on a distant sailboat. "Liza saw it right away. She's been all over me about you. I kept denying it, until the day you and I got really drunk. I thought she was going to kill me. Liza accused me of ruining her renter-family. She thought we were having a summer fling. Little did she know I wanted more."

"More?"

"Lauren, I want to be with you for the rest of my life. I want you to leave your husband and marry me."

"I don't know what to say."

"Don't say anything; just listen. I'm comfortable with you. I can let my guard down and just be myself. I've never had that with a woman… or at least not like this. I've always known it was possible because of my friendship with Liza. I've been looking for that level of intimacy with a romantic partner my whole life. I knew it was you when we went sailing."

"Honestly, it sounds like you're in love with Liza," Lauren said, trying hard to deflect Rick's advances.

"You would think so, and I do love her, endlessly. She's like my sister, and that is never going to change. Who knows, maybe because of my relationship with Liza I didn't let my guard down with other women. I was looking for something unattainable. Or so I thought. And here you are. The spark… it's not there with Liza, but with you it's undeniable. I know you felt it."

"Rick, I'm so confused right now; I don't know what I feel."

"I know my timing is terrible; it's why I've been so hesitant to say anything. But I know you're going back to New York soon. I can't just let you walk out of my life."

Lauren looked at Rick. The pull on her heart practically made her knees weak. It was hard to breathe. "I would be sad if you weren't part of my life," Lauren said.

Rick took a step closer and put his arm around her waist. Pulling her to him he murmured, "I need to kiss you." Lauren willingly lifted her head to meet him halfway.

Chapter 62

David sat on the back porch waiting for his wife to come home from her walk. He'd been thinking about the conversation he'd had with Jason and the questions his son asked about his relationship with Lauren. He knew he'd made mistakes. In the rush of life he'd forgotten to pay attention to the one person who meant more to him than anyone else. Lauren was his rock. She made everything work in the family. She took care of all of them, and he'd taken her for granted.

David was acutely aware of the divide between them. He wondered how much damage he'd done. When he heard her footsteps in the hallway, he made a promise to himself to do whatever it took to fix the situation. David was determined to repair their relationship.

"I'm out here," he called to his wife.

"What are you doing?"

"I've been thinking. Come sit with me. I'd like to talk to you."

Lauren obeyed out of habit more than any real interest in what David had to say. She expected he wanted to talk about Audrey and her schooling for the next year. She was tired and uninterested in debating the topic again. In her mind, the conversation was over. The decision was made.

"Hon, I'm sorry."

Lauren looked at David. "What for?"

"I've screwed up."

Lauren's heart skipped a beat as she wondered what he'd done. "What are you talking about?" She could barely breathe and didn't think she could handle any more bombshells.

"It's us. I really messed us up, and I feel bad about it." David held out his hand, gesturing for her to come sit with him. "I need you to listen to me, really listen."

"Have you been drinking, David?"

"Not a drop, but it's scary that your mind goes there. It just shows how distant we've become." Lauren sat down in one of the chairs near her husband and looked at him.

"I had a long talk with Jason about responsibility. We talked about his part in this mess with Karen." David tried to ignore Lauren's wince upon hearing her name. "And I think he understands he needs to deal with the consequences of his own actions. But more importantly, we ended up talking about how crucial it is to have a clean slate when he finally meets the right woman, the woman he wants to spend his life with."

"Great. This is all important stuff, but why are you telling me this now?" Lauren was becoming uncomfortable.

"Because he asked if I still loved you like I did when we met in college. He asked how our relationship had changed over the years, and we got on the topic of the difference between new love and mature love. It really hit me how far off track we've gotten, and I feel responsible."

David looked at his wife for some sort of clue as to how she felt. Lauren appeared impassive. She had little emotional response toward him. He wondered how long she had been this way.

"Lauren, I need you to know I've never stopped loving you. I just stopped showing it. And, if it's not too late, I want to make up for it."

Lauren was stunned. Impassioned professions of undying love from two men in the space of an hour? It was hard to fathom.

"David, what are you going to do that will be so different from how you've been for years?" Lauren asked, not exactly confirming his beliefs but not telling him otherwise either. "I've been trying to get your attention for a long time, and now all of a sudden you want to do something different. Honestly, it's a little hard to believe."

"I know. And it's going to be up to me to show you. I need to prove to you our relationship can be the way it was. I need to do it for us. I need to do it for the kids. I mean, so long as you let me."

"David, I don't know what you're asking. I've always been right here. Do you need my permission?"

"No, I guess I don't. I guess I'm just trying to tell you I'm aware of my mistakes and I'm sorry."

"Look, I'm tired. The past couple days have been exhausting. I'm going to bed. I don't know what you want me to say." Lauren stood and headed into the house. When she got to the door she turned to look at him. "While you're sitting there thinking, try to remember last spring and why I brought us up here in the first place. I think I was trying to send a message to you then."

CHAPTER 63

"Hey, Morgan! Can we walk down to the beach or something?" The two were standing on her doorstep, Jason glancing around to see if her father was nearby. "Dad's packing up the car. We're going to be leaving in a couple hours."

"You're leaving? So soon? Okay, let me grab a sweatshirt."

Jason took Morgan's hand as they walked down the path to the beach. "I had a long talk with my dad. He's pretty smart about relationships and stuff."

"Really? Did you talk about us?"

"Not exactly, just in general. But I learned some things."

"Like what?"

"Well, for one thing, I made you go too fast... you know, sexually. I wanted to be with you so bad, and I let it get in the way. I didn't think about how things could have turned out. I should have respected you more. I'm sorry about that, Morgan."

"I didn't do anything I didn't want to do."

"I know, but in the beginning I was pushy. If I could do it over again, I would be a lot different."

The two reached the end of the dock and sat down, their feet dangling in the warm water. The lake was dotted with sailboats and jet skis. They could hear laughter in the distance, but somehow Jason and Morgan were alone, isolated from the world.

"How would you be different?" Morgan asked.

"I would be more patient, for one thing. It would have been okay to wait longer. I really like you—a lot. And I still want to see you."

"That's impossible, Jason. I'm going to college in California, and you live in New York. You don't even come to the club every summer. How are we going to see each other again?"

"Well, I was thinking, I'm applying to colleges in the fall. What if I applied to ones near you in California?"

"You would do that?" Morgan said, astonished.

"Sure, why not? And in the meantime, we could text and FaceTime once in a while, if you want to."

"I won't sit in my dorm room doing nothing, waiting for you." Morgan was skeptical.

"Of course not. I don't even know if I can get into any colleges out there. But we could keep in touch, as friends, and then see what happens later on."

"I think that sounds really nice. I would like that." Morgan smiled at Jason. "After all, you're my first boyfriend. I'm sad you're leaving. I'm going to miss you so much."

Jason leaned over and kissed Morgan gently. "You feel like my first real girlfriend, too. It's so hard to say good-bye to you."

"Do you think your parents would mind if I walked you back to the car?" Morgan asked.

"I was hoping you would say that. I want to spend every second with you."

The two walked back to the cottage holding hands without saying a word, neither wanting to let go. Both secretly feared, despite their plans, they may never see each other again.

Chapter 64

Lauren looked around the clubhouse, her stomach churning. Rick said he would meet her here, but he was late, and now she was beginning to lose her nerve. Finally, she heard the screen door open and his footsteps approach. Her heart raced.

"Good morning, beautiful," Rick whispered, kissing her on the cheek. "Tell me something that will fill my heart with joy."

"Rick, there is so much I need to tell you, and I don't have a lot of time."

"Okay, I'll be serious. Please, go ahead."

"I haven't stopped thinking about what you proposed. Honestly, it makes me happy just thinking about it," Lauren said.

"That's a good thing. You should be happy."

"Thank you. But there are things I still need to do. My son needs me at home while he applies to college. It's his senior year of high school. And Audrey... even if I'm not physically in the same location with her, she needs me to be available for her mentally. I need to put my kids first."

Lauren could see a shadow of unhappiness pass over Rick's face. Watching his pain hurt her. She put her hand on his arm. "Rick, I don't want you to underestimate how important you are to me. I feel so much for you, and I know how cliché this sounds, but I'm begging you to still be my friend."

"Seriously? You're handing me the 'let's be friends' thing? That's my line, Lauren."

"It's not a line, Rick. I mean it. I couldn't leave David now, even if I wanted to. The kids are in precarious positions and you know it. You saw what happened this summer. They need stability. It would be completely irresponsible of me to run away right now. That's not who I am, and I don't think you would respect me if I did."

Rick stepped back a moment and looked at Lauren. He was trying to think logically and not act like a petulant child. "You're probably right. I'm thinking about my desires rather than the big picture. You wouldn't be who you are if you abandoned your kids when they needed you most. I'm sorry for being so selfish."

"We've known each other for such a short time. I was hoping we could spend more time getting to know each other, as friends. You once said you come to Manhattan on a regular basis. I can meet you there..."

"It's not perfect, but what choice do I have? If time is what it takes for me to win you over, then okay; I'm willing to wait. I'm not going anywhere."

Lauren breathed an obvious sigh of relief. "Thank you. I couldn't breathe just thinking about what you were going to say." Lauren paused. "I need to go now. David was almost finishing packing the car. I told him I was returning a library book. I don't know when I'll see you again." Distress rose to her throat, threatening to choke her.

"I'll come to the city next month. How does that sound?"

Lauren smiled. "Perfect."

Rick wrapped his arms around Lauren, not wanting to let her go. "I promise this is not an ending; it's just the beginning," he said, tilting her face to his for one last kiss. "I'll see you soon, okay?"

Lauren nodded and rushed out the door. She didn't look back. She couldn't risk it.

Chapter 65

"Are you sure this is what you want to do?" David asked Audrey one last time. "You can still change your mind, you know." Claire and Lauren were talking in the kitchen, going over last minute details while David and Jason helped Audrey move her stuff into what would be her room.

"Dad, I'm sure," Audrey said over her shoulder. "Dr. Hawkins got me into the medical magnet program and everything. The math is going to be hard, but she found a senior to be my tutor. The rest of the classes will be about the same. Plus, I get credit for working in the animal hospital, and I get to help out in the surgery center in Petoskey. It's all worked out, Dad."

David's heart was heavy. The changes happening this fall were dramatic, and he wasn't sure if he and Lauren were ready for them. He would be helping his son look at colleges, and his daughter was basically gone. He thought they had years left before they became empty nesters.

"Dad, I'll come home for vacations. Plus, we can text and email. It'll be like I'm still home. You'll see. And if you really, really miss me, you can always come for a visit."

"You don't have to sound so grown up, you know. You're still my little girl." David set a suitcase near the dresser.

When the three of them had everything safely stashed in Audrey's room, they went to join Lauren in the kitchen. Erin showed up to finalize the details about who would ultimately be responsible for the individual parts of Audrey's care.

Good-byes were said and Lauren gave David a knowing glance; they could delay the inevitable no longer.

Claire reached out and hugged Lauren. "I know how hard this is for you. Thank you for putting your trust in me. I promise I won't let you down. I'll care for Audrey as if she were my own."

Lauren knew this was the truth. "Thank you for everything, Claire." Lauren had grown to trust and respect Claire over the past couple weeks. There was no doubt Claire cared a great deal for Audrey and would have her best interests at heart.

As Lauren, David, and Jason walked to the car, Lauren heard Audrey call out to her. "Mom, wait!" She turned to see her daughter running toward her in the parking lot, tears streaming down her face. She wrapped her arms around her mother. "Thanks, Mom. I love you so much. I'm going to miss you."

Lauren broke down in tears. "Oh honey, I'm going to miss you, too. I love you more than you can ever imagine. I'd do anything for you." The two stood wrapped in each other's arms for a minute before Audrey broke away.

"I know, Mom. Thank you... for everything."

Lauren looked in her mirror as they drove away. She saw Claire put her arm around Audrey while Erin stood by her side. Leaving Audrey was the hardest thing she'd ever done.

While Lauren knew her daughter was in a safe place and she would be getting the help she needed, her heart longed to stay in Michigan to look after Audrey. No matter how hard she tried to convince herself otherwise, part of her felt as if she were abandoning her only daughter. Lauren glanced at Jason in the backseat. He was already deep into his electronic world, disconnected by the earbud barrier. Did he need her, really? David was satisfied so long as the family and house ran smoothly. No, she couldn't kick the feeling that her place was with her daughter.

Lauren took a deep breath and tried to put her thoughts into perspective. Erin and Claire had bent over backwards putting the plan into action. If they felt she was needed, they would have said so. Wouldn't they?

CHAPTER 66

Alice squealed with excitement when she saw Lauren. It was as if the two women had become teenage girls again.

"I missed you so much! This summer was excruciating," Alice said, about to bubble over. "I had nobody to talk to. Tell me everything."

Lauren was happy to be home again, to be with her friend. Most of the events of the summer still seemed unreal. Over coffee, Lauren slowly unraveled the story, lingering over every single detail.

"How old was this man who kissed you?"

Lauren giggled. "I don't know... maybe ten years younger than me."

"Are you serious about him?"

"That's the real question. I don't know the answer, Alice."

"When are you going to see him again? Wait, *are* you going to see him again?" Alice peppered Lauren with questions about Rick, about what was happening with Audrey and, finally, Karen. Those were the hardest questions for Lauren to answer. She still had a difficult time accepting that her son had been involved with an older woman.

"Ha! You're doing the same thing Jason did." Alice quipped when they got into the details of Jason and Karen's relationship.

"Excuse me? I don't see how you can say that!"

"What do you mean? Aren't you ten years older than the man you're interested in? How is that any different?"

Lauren was flabbergasted. "Well, for one thing, we're both consenting adults. And I didn't sleep with Rick; I didn't cheat on David."

"Oh honey, calm down! Of course I see the difference, but you've got to admit there's a definite similarity. You need to get over the anger you feel about this Karen issue. It's consuming you."

"He's my son."

"And he's growing up. You need to take a good look at him, Lauren. He's a boy in a man's body, and he's going to want things every red-blooded man wants—and

I'm including Rick in that list. He wants the same damn thing, you know."

"The world doesn't revolve around sex, Alice. There are other things to think about."

"Maybe," Alice said knowingly, kissing Lauren on the temple. "Sweetie, I'm so glad you're home. Now things can get back to normal. After all, David is a pretty good guy. Anyway, let's do our run in the morning. It'll be good for both of us."

Alice trotted out the door, leaving Lauren alone to ruminate on their conversation. It was hard for her to accept any similarity between her relationship with Rick and what had happened to her son. Leave it to Alice to come up with some unusual way of looking at a situation. But somehow, her friendship with Rick suddenly felt awkward.

She tried to put Rick out of her mind. In truth, Lauren doubted she would hear from him again.

CHAPTER 67

David picked Karen up for her prenatal appointment. When she scheduled the ultrasound appointment, she had not anticipated he would be involved in any way. This was the appointment where she would most likely find out the sex of the baby. When David got home from Michigan, he phoned her and insisted on coming along.

Karen was still unsure of his intentions. She was not used to the idea of him wanting to be part of the baby's life, although the money helped significantly. She was trying to relax about the whole thing and enjoy the process. This baby was coming, and crying about it was only going to make it worse.

David seemed positively giddy as they drove to the appointment. They talked about baby names, and Karen found herself laughing for the first time in months.

"I have a good view. Would the proud parents like to know the sex of the baby?" the ultrasound tech asked. Karen looked over at David in a panic.

"Absolutely!" David said as he winked at Karen, grinning ear to ear.

"I'm pretty sure it's a girl."

David took Karen's elbow as they walked to the car. He helped her inside before climbing into the driver's seat.

"I think she's got your nose," David said as they took another look at the ultrasound photos. Karen couldn't help herself. She started laughing and joined in on the merriment.

"What do you say we go shopping and get some stuff for the baby's room?" David said, not quite ready for the excitement to end.

"David, you've already done so much."

"Nonsense. This is my granddaughter; she deserves everything I can give her." David brushed off Karen's concerns as he tucked the ultrasound pictures into a folder the tech had given them. He insisted they head to Babies 'R Us.

Two hours later, they were back at Karen's apartment. David insisted she rest while he carried the packages inside. He made himself at home and started putting the crib together in Karen's spare bedroom.

In the excitement of the day, neither of them had eaten. Karen made sandwiches which they ate while sitting on the floor of a room which was well on its way to becoming a nursery. David was so focused on the prospect of a new baby that he lost all perspective on the time. Looking out of the window, he suddenly realized it was dark.

"Shit, I'm so sorry, I've got to finish this room up next time." David grabbed his jacket and kissed Karen on top of her head. "I'm really late."

"I'm grateful for what you've done."

"Not to worry, I'll be back next week." David dashed out the door in a rush. He didn't give a second thought to his double life or its ramifications. He was caught up in the excitement of his grandchild.

CHAPTER 68

David sat in the driveway trying to collect his thoughts. He could see Lauren through the kitchen window. He was feeling satisfied with himself; everything was falling into place. The only challenge that remained was to make Lauren feel his love for her. He watched her for a minute longer. She was so beautiful.

David grabbed the flowers he'd picked up at the grocery store on the way home and went inside. Coming up behind her, he wrapped his arms around her and kissed her neck. "Flowers for my amazing wife."

"Thank you, David. You're later than I expected. Things go okay at work?" Lauren tried her best to sound enthusiastic.

"Everything's fine. I got distracted and didn't notice the time. Sorry about that."

"Don't worry. I spent quite a bit of time catching up with Alice."

"I can only imagine. How did she manage without you this summer?" David said, tried to keep things light. "Dinner smells great. Do I have time to change?"

"Plenty. Take your time. Jason will be home in half an hour."

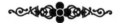

Lauren was surprised at how quickly they fell back into their routine. The house felt empty without Audrey, but the three of them soon fell into a predictable rhythm. Jason's birthday came and went, and he passed his driver's license test. He no longer relied on Lauren to take him to his preseason water polo practice or college application prep classes. His senior year would start in another week. David bought him a used car to ensure his complete independence. Lauren rarely saw him unless he was hungry.

Although David spent a lot of time at work, he was highly attentive and animated when he was home. He seemed to listen when Lauren talked about whatever she'd done during the day. When she expressed an interest in taking a class at the local community college, he was supportive. Audrey texted her almost every day, and she received regular emails from both Claire and Erin, so she never

felt out of touch. Lauren reached a level of complacency; her life was acceptable. She didn't expect to feel true happiness.

In early September, she checked her emails after her run with Alice. There was a note from Rick. Lauren was caught completely off guard; she'd heard nothing from him since leaving Charlevoix weeks before. He'd become less real with each passing day. She read the note four times before responding.

Hope you haven't forgotten about me. I'll be in New York on Thursday. Meet me. You promised. Rick.

Lauren was bewildered. She had not forgotten about him, but after almost a month she'd assumed he'd moved on. She hadn't expected to hear from him again. Her fingers flew across the keyboard.

You're not easily forgotten. I'll take the train in. How do you feel about the Metropolitan Museum of Art? Lauren.

The reply was almost instantaneous.

Take the 9:04 train. I'll meet you on the steps of the Met at 11:30. Rick

Lauren's face flushed. How did he know the train schedule? Was he checking up on her? Her stomach fluttered in anticipation. And, feeling like a teenager, she started thinking about what to wear.

Chapter 69

The Metro-North train into the city seemed to take forever. Normally Lauren would read a book during the ride, but today she was too nervous to focus on anything, including the magazine left in the seat pocket. When the train reached its destination, she took a cab instead of enjoying the walk from Grand Central Station up 5th Avenue, along Central Park to 68th Street. She arrived at the Met twenty minutes early. To her surprise, Rick was waiting for her.

Rick trotted down the steps as she paid the cab. "It's so good to see you, Lauren. I've..." He stopped short, not sure just how much he should say.

Lauren beamed. "I'm happy to see you, too." They stood together on the steps for a few awkward moments, together for the first time outside the sheltered environment where they'd met.

"Are you hungry? Do you want to get lunch somewhere, or do you want to go inside?" Rick asked.

Lauren laughed, amused by his obvious nervousness. She was used to him being in charge and leading her to all of his chosen places. For once they seemed on equal footing.

"I have a guilty secret," she said, almost embarrassed.

"Oh, I need to hear this. I'm in, whatever it is."

"When I come to The Met, I always get lunch from that hot dog vendor." Lauren pointed to a stand on the corner, its blue-and-gold umbrella visible above the throng of passersby. "I crave one with onions and mustard."

"You're kidding." Rick chuckled. "Far be it from me to deny a woman her favorite lunch spot in all of Manhattan."

"I didn't exactly say it was my favorite place," Lauren said with a laugh. "There's a really good pretzel cart in front of the New York Public Library."

The two relaxed and fell into a comfortable pace together. After the hot dogs, they went into the museum. Their conversation flowed easily, from playful banter to thoughtful discussion about their impressions of the European paintings, sculpture, and decorative arts exhibits. The time flew by, and soon it was late afternoon.

Lauren had told David not to expect her until the evening, but she really needed to catch a train by six p.m. Rick suggested they walk together to Grand Central. Lauren agreed, eager to spend every possible moment enjoying Rick's company. He accompanied her all the way to the track, until they were standing next to her train.

"I feel like I'm in an old black-and-white movie. I should be wearing a pencil skirt and a hat," Lauren said, trying to make light of the sudden awkwardness between them.

"You'd look amazing in that getup. I'd play Bogie to your Bacall any day."

"Thanks." Lauren smiled and looked away.

"Lauren, today was... perfect. Oh hell, I promised myself I wouldn't put pressure on you. I've missed you. Not a day went by that I didn't wonder what you were doing. I've been dying to come see you. I didn't know how long to wait."

"That means a lot to me. I've thought about you, too. Every day."

Just then, the conductor called "All Aboard."

"Can I come back in a couple weeks?"

"That would be great."

As Lauren stepped away from him, Rick reached out to her.

"Wait," Rick said as he pulled her close. He brushed his lips against hers and trailed one finger down her cheek. "Until next time."

Lauren blushed and boarded the train, waving to Rick from her seat by the window as the train pulled out of the station.

CHAPTER 70

Lauren woke early on Sunday morning. David and Jason were still asleep, and she didn't want to disturb either of them. Lauren took a cup of coffee to her computer and opened the last email from Erin, written on Friday. All was well and Audrey was making good progress, adjusting nicely. She suggested Lauren come visit soon so Audrey would feel her family's love. The plan was working better than they'd anticipated.

As good as the news was, her heart ached for her daughter. She missed having her around the house. Jason's life was on a fast track. He gave her updates at dinnertime, but it seemed like he had grown up into a young man overnight. Lauren felt loved and appreciated at home, but she wasn't really needed. It seemed to her that the only place where she was actually needed was in Michigan—with Audrey. After all, Erin *had* suggested Audrey could use a visit from her mother...

Lauren pushed away from the computer. "I need to do something productive," she muttered as she paced the kitchen. She decided to do a bagel run for the boys. She knew David would appreciate the Sunday paper. As she headed out the door, she noticed David's car blocking hers in the driveway. Now that Jason had a car, they were constantly juggling parking places. Lauren fished David's keys out of the bowl by the door and took his car instead of hers.

Driving David's car was an adjustment. She was used to driving the Escalade, and switching to a smaller, sporty car always made her feel uncomfortable. On the drive home, Lauren misjudged her speed in a curve and had to slam on the brakes, skidding off the road into a grassy area. Her heart pounded as the bagels and newspaper flew off the passenger seat. Fortunately, the only thing damaged was her ego.

Lauren reached over to gather the scattered newspaper from the floorboard. As she shuffled the sections back into order, she found a folder crammed between them. As she pulled it out, annoyed at David for leaving paperwork tossed haphazardly in the car, a photograph fell onto the seat.

Lauren picked it up, her hand trembling. She could not believe her eyes. How was this remotely possible? An ultrasound picture with Karen's name on it, dated a week ago.

Lauren picked up the unmarked folder. In it she found receipts from a medical clinic, bank deposit records, and a receipt from the baby store. The evidence was overwhelming. Karen was obviously still pregnant and David knew about it.

Her hands were shaking so hard she could barely get the papers back into the folder. She tried to start the car, but the engine wouldn't start. After three tries, Lauren broke down in tears.

Sobbing, Lauren called Alice. She was only a mile or so from home, so Alice told her to hang on; she would jog down to the car and drive her home.

Alice arrived in no time and slid into the car next to her distraught friend.

"Okay, this looks really bad, Lauren," Alice said as she thumbed through the folder. But you need to calm down before you confront David about it."

"Why?" Lauren shrieked. "He's been lying the whole time. Why should I give that bastard anything?"

"I know. I really feel bad for you, honey. I'd be upset, too. But I'm hoping there's some explanation, that it isn't as bad as it looks here. Because this looks horrible."

"I don't see how there can be any explanation other than she's still pregnant, and he knows about it. He's supporting her. There are fucking bank deposits, Alice! He's been lying about all of it."

"Yeah, I don't know what I would do, to be honest. Come on, let's get you home. I'll drive."

"Thanks. I don't know what I'd do without you." Lauren reached out and held Alice's hand as her friend pulled the car back onto the road.

Chapter 71

Jason's car was gone when Alice pulled into the driveway. Lauren was relieved. She didn't want her son to hear any part of the argument she knew was about to happen. She was still in denial, trying to believe there was some way to protect him from the fact that at seventeen years old, her boy was going to become a father. It was too much for her to accept.

Lauren walked into the kitchen to find David standing near the coffee pot.

"You son of a bitch!" she yelled as she hurled the bag of bagels at him.

"What the hell?" David ducked, spilling coffee on the counter. "Have you lost your mind?" Lauren saw the look of panic on his face as he spotted the folder in her hand.

"That's right, David. I know. I fucking know." Lauren broke down into sobs as she slumped into one of the kitchen chairs.

"Lauren, honey, it's not what it looks like."

"Really David? You mean that woman isn't pregnant, and you haven't been giving her money and lying about it all this time?" Lauren seethed, her anger burning through her tears.

"Oh God, help me," David whispered. "Lauren, what was I supposed to do? She's carrying our granddaughter. Like it or not, she's real and not going away. I wanted to protect you and Jason. I thought if I could just keep it separate, everything would be okay."

"So you lied to me?"

"Lauren, you wouldn't have accepted the truth. You wanted our granddaughter to be born in prison."

"Stop saying that! Stop calling that thing our granddaughter."

"See? Right there—that's the whole truth, Lauren. You are unwilling to face the fact that Karen is a person; she has feelings. Yes, she made a bad mistake, and now she's pregnant with our son's baby. I'm trying to minimize the damage. How am I the bad guy here?"

"And I suppose laws don't mean anything to you, do they, David? I suppose they're just suggestions. What if it was the other way around, and, God forbid, it had been Audrey who had gotten pregnant? Would you have been so forgiving? I don't think so. This is some manly, my-son-got-laid kind of thing, and you don't see the damage it did to our boy."

"Damage? What damage? He's fine."

"Really, David? I caught him being sexual with that Morgan girl this summer."

"So what? That's normal teenage boy behavior."

"Is it, David? So every boy should have multiple sex partners before he graduates from high school? And how many children should he have? Because I'm not so sure he was practicing safe sex on the living room floor in the cottage."

"You can't keep him from growing up, Lauren."

"You know something, David? Growing up, as you put it, is not about sticking your dick into everything that walks. And I sure as hell hope you've done your job teaching him about love, responsibility, and loyalty."

"Of course I have. How can you say that?"

"Well, you haven't demonstrated it, because you didn't show loyalty to me when you lied about the pregnancy." Lauren was hurt and angry. "Tell me something. What else have you lied about over the years? How do I trust you, David?"

David moved to the table and looked at Lauren with tears in his eyes. "Lauren, I love you, and if I made the wrong decision, I'm sorry. I wanted to protect you and Jason. There was nothing I could do to change what happened. I can't change the facts. I just wanted to shield you and our son, keep you both from being hurt." Tears rolled down David's face.

"Well, your plan didn't work." Lauren reached for a napkin to wipe away her tears. "And now, not only do we have the utter disasters of our kids' lives; we don't have much of a marriage left either. I honestly don't know what hurts worse, feeling like you left the marriage years ago, because you paid attention to everything else *but* our marriage, or the realization that I can't trust you."

"Lauren—"

"What do you want me to say? It's the truth and you know it. The only question now is what do we do about it?"

CHAPTER 72

David balanced two cups of coffee as he knocked on the door of their bedroom. He waited for Lauren to answer before entering. The previous night he stayed on the couch in the living room, although he didn't actually sleep.

"Thanks." Lauren sat up in the bed and accepted the cup. She hadn't slept much either.

They looked at each other, and both began to speak.

"You go first," David said, settling across from her at the foot of the bed.

"I think I should go back to Michigan to be with Audrey for the rest of the school year." Lauren's tone was flat. "Last night I thought about everything. About what has happened and how it tore through this family. I've been wondering where I need to be right now. I think it's best for me to be with Audrey. Jason doesn't need me while he's applying to colleges; you can certainly handle that. He and I can text each other. It's practically all we do now anyway. And I think it would be best for us to be apart from each other for the time being."

"You're talking about a separation."

"Not a legal one but, yes, I'm basically saying we need to be separated. Until June, when Audrey is done with her school year. We'll come back for Jason's graduation and see what happens then."

"Lauren, I'm not giving up on our marriage. I love you too much. I've made some bad decisions for what I thought were the right reasons."

"I understand, David. Maybe I'm not thinking clearly about this baby. I can't bring myself to accept it the way you have. And I certainly can't accept that woman. But I think I understand why you did it. You've always been protective of your family. I guess I can't fault you for that. It's who you are."

"How do we get back to where we used to be when we were kids, Lauren? Do you remember how great we were together?"

"I remember being dazzled by you, David. It's like you took me over and swallowed me whole, and I loved every second of being with you. But I was never your equal. I've always felt more like your supporting cast. I don't think it's your fault. I stopped developing as a person and rode your coattails, content to be your wife and a mother to your kids. I didn't develop my own interests along the way. I think that makes me a weak person."

"That's not how I see you."

"Of course not. Why would you? You see me as your wife. I'm a possession."

"But you *are* my wife. I need you, Lauren. I'm sorry about how I handled the pregnancy. I should have been more upfront with you. It seems obvious now. It would have been more respectful if I'd told you the truth. We should have faced the problem together."

Lauren nodded. "Yes, that would have been the better plan. But I didn't make it easy for you either. We both made mistakes."

"Will you forgive me, please? Will you give me a chance to make it up to you, to us? For our family?"

"I honestly don't know. Right now, I'm going to Michigan. For Audrey, for me. I need some time for figure out what I want. But, one thing I know for certain is Audrey needs me. That is the true priority in this situation, everything else can wait, including you."

EPILOGUE

Lauren's flight sat on the tarmac at JFK, seventh in line for takeoff. She marveled at how complicated it was to fly to Northern Michigan. A train to New York City, the first flight to Chicago, a commuter to Traverse City, and an hour drive to Charlevoix made for a long day. When she'd sent Liza an email asking questions about the winter in Charlevoix, she'd received an immediate response. Lauren could stay in her cottage until mid-November. The caretakers would show her how to heat the rooms so it would be comfortable. She would have plenty of time to find a place to stay for the duration of the winter. Liza said she would have the hard top put on the Jeep for her. Lauren was touched by her generosity. She marveled how the two had truly become good friends in such a short amount of time, despite how vastly different their worlds were.

Jason had almost seemed relieved she was going up to Michigan. He'd admitted that Audrey and he had been texting on occasion. He thought she'd sounded a little lonely but hadn't said anything to Lauren because he didn't want to worry her. Lauren had made him promise to communicate with her about his senior year and the college application process. She'd also begged him to consider schools outside Northern California. She hoped he would listen to her words of advice—to find a school which fit his interests rather than simply following a girl. Lauren had stayed clear of the topic of Karen. David had convinced her he was better served not knowing about the baby for the time being. It would not be possible for him to actually take responsibility for the baby; he was far too young to be a father. David had told Lauren he would set up a trust fund for the baby, but he was still unwilling to go to the police. It was clear they would never agree on this issue, so they'd dropped the subject rather than rehash it for the thousandth time.

Lauren wanted to be a part of Audrey's recovery. She knew Erin was working with her on how to develop healthy relationships. In their sessions they worked on when and how to trust people and the importance of following her instincts. According to Erin, Audrey was doing fine and was making friends in high school. Dylan was understanding and, despite the incident over the summer, still wanted to be friends. Audrey invited him to group a few times, and the two seemed to be able to open up to each other. When Lauren called to tell Audrey she was coming to Michigan for the year, her relief was palpable. As much as Audrey enjoyed living with Claire, she admitted she really missed Lauren and wanted to be home at the same time. This gave her the opportunity to have both.

David and Lauren both realized this was the right thing to do for their family. In some odd way, Lauren's decision to move to Michigan brought David and Lauren a little bit closer. In the days before she left, they talked in a way they hadn't done in years, open and honest about their situation.

Lauren wondered if their marriage finally had a real chance of surviving the chaos they'd been through. She wondered if any marriage could survive this level of turmoil. Her family was torn to shreds by events so utterly disruptive they changed the entire course of everyone's lives.

Eventually, Lauren's thoughts turned to Rick. Certainly he was a good friend when she needed one. And when she was with him, she felt a much-needed peace. But was that love? He seemed to respect her opinions and treated her much more like an equal than David ever did. But she made a commitment to David when she married him. She had a family with David, and he was not wavering on his commitment to making their marriage work. Lauren thought about what she owed to David and the kids.

As her plane lifted into the air she knew one thing for certain: she wasn't going to rush into anything. There was no reason to tell Rick she'd left her husband—at least not right away. It was time to build a connection with her daughter and maybe reconnect with the person she once was a long time ago.

Kayaking on

A Guide to

Advanced

Technique

for Experienced

Paddlers

By Ben Solomon

Menasha Ridge Press
Birmingham, Alabama

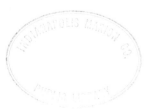

Excerpt from *Into the Wilds* by John Krakauer reprinted
with permission of Bantam/Doubleday books; Quote
from Coran Addison and Gordon Grant reprinted with
permission from *Canoe & Kayak Magazine*/Whitewater
Paddling (800) MY CANOE.

Manufactured in the United States
Published by Menasha Ridge Press
First edition, first printing

Library of Congress
Cataloging-in-Publication Data:
Kayaking on the edge: a guide to advanced
technique for experienced paddlers /
by Ben Solomon
p.   cm.
ISBN 0-89732-309-2
1. Kayaking. I. Title
GV783.S573 1999
797.1'224—dc21
99-37815
CIP

Cover and text design by Grant Tatum
Cover photgraphy by Ben Solomon
Unless otherwise noted, all photographs are by Ben
    Solomon, © 1999.

Menasha Ridge Press
700 South 28th Street, Suite 206
Birmingham, Alabama 35233-3417
800.247.9437
www.menasharidge.com

Table of Contents

Dedication

For Mom, Dad, Ali, Echo, & Molly

Acknowledgments

I'd like to express thanks to the following people for all their help: Derek Cummings, Cathy Clark, Bryan Jennings, Darryl Knudsen, Chuck DeRosa, Cathy Clark, Bill Hester, Tom & Ellen DeCuir, Mike Jones, Bud Zehmer, Craig Parks, Shane Williams, John Miller, Barbara Beran, Jay Maroney, Chris Ennis, Laura Hayes, Jon Wilkinson, the Blatts, Aaron Napoleon, and everyone at NOC.

I would also like to thank the following companies who have sponsored me during the whitewater rodeo season: Dagger, Wyoming Wear, Smith, Croakies, and Crazy Creek.

Finally, special thanks go to Land Heflin, who showed enormous patience in teaching this fee-bleminded writer to do rock spins, and to Brian Totten, who spins in places that make me feel ill to even think about.

Introduction

Every once in a while, I spend a few weeks out
of my boat. It's usually a great time: I'm able to
visit my family and see friends who have moved
far away. My shoulders get a much-needed rest,
and the bruises and cuts all over my body finally
start to heal. I'm even able to deal with the truly
exciting parts of life, like figuring out how to pay
off my credit card bills and whether or not I can
afford health insurance.

As nice as it is to be able to do all these things,
I'm always antsy within a few days. I miss the
rush of throwing myself off a huge vertical drop,
the sensation of actually being airborne for a second, falling toward the froth. I miss slicing the

bow of my boat into a pourover, feeling the boat rotating around me as it cartwheels end-over-end. I miss the camaraderie, arguing with my friends about the best line in a scary rapid, telling awful carnage stories, and sharing tips about how to do certain hot new moves. I miss paddling through an incredible gorge, looking up at the thick forest, and feeling I'm in a holy place that few people have been lucky enough to see. I even miss stopping at some backwoods gas station with boats on my truck and having the locals laugh at the moron who plans on getting in a barely accessible creek in the middle of winter.

There are easily a million more things I miss. In short, kayaking is just about the most wonderful, unbelievably fun thing I've ever done. Over the years, I've learned more and more (at least, I hope so). I remember finally figuring out how to do a roll, learning to surf on a teeny little wave, popping my first ender (wow!!), and running my first Class V rapid (I was totally, absolutely, 100 percent sure I would die). As I slowly figured out each new move, each different skill, I realized the first rule of kayaking:

Rule 1: The better you are, the more fun you'll have.

This book is based on Rule 1. In this book you'll find a semi-organized compendium of tips, suggestions, and advice aimed at giving you some new ideas and maximizing the fun you have on the river. Hopefully, these ideas will help you perform old moves better, learn new tricks, and therefore have so much fun it'll be almost nauseating.

Most of the instructional books I've come across are really excellent. However, these books tend to be aimed toward beginning paddlers or folks who have heard a little bit about kayaking and want to learn more. These books (see list of suggested reading at the end for more information) give very detailed information about the

RULE 1

The better you are, the more fun you'll have.

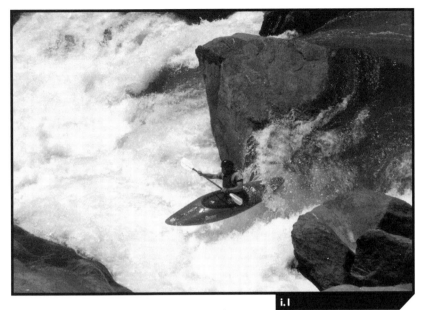

basics: specifically, how to do each stroke, how to pick a first boat, and so on. Instead, this book targets those kayakers who have slightly more experience, people who are already starting to get a grip on the sport and who wish to push things farther. Therefore, I assume my readers have a good grasp on fundamental kayak techniques such as peel-outs, rolls, eddy-turns, and a bit of basic playing. I've spent more time on the skills which come next, like getting better at reading water, running harder rapids, and figuring out some of the latest freestyle moves so you can show off for your pals.

Before we start, I want to make a point that the methods I discuss aren't the only ones out there. A different instructor might use an entirely different way of explaining a certain aspect of paddling. Or some readers might disagree with my suggestions about how to pull off a certain move. If you feel that you have a better method for teaching anything mentioned here, or that some of my ideas are just plain wrong, you may very well be correct—I sincerely wish

i.1 Better than a real job. Boater: Ben Solomon

that you would write and tell me so that I don't keep making the same dumb mistakes.

I hope this book helps your paddling so much that the next time you see me on the river you'll laugh in disgust at my pathetic attempts to boat (don't feel bad—I'm used to it by now). To further help you toward this goal, I've included a list of resources at the end of the book. Good luck!

Some Paddling Basics

OK, so maybe I lied a little bit when I said we'd jump right into all the hottest moves out there. Patience, patience—we'll get to that soon. For now, I want to briefly touch on some fundamental elements that all kayakers should keep in mind, whether it's your first day on whitewater or your thousandth.

Boring? Well, maybe. But I just want to make sure we're all together before we work on our eighty-point cartwheels or figure out the optimal entry angle when running hundred-foot waterfalls. The best paddlers all have one thing in common (besides their offensive odor): excellent basic technique. Having solid fundamentals will be an enormous help when you're ready to try harder moves.

POSTURE

First, sit back and relax in your boat—really get that slouch going. Ahhhh. Nice, huh? Imagine that you're kicking back on your couch after a long day at work, a beer (your fourth of the night) in one hand, the remote in the other. You've got "The Best of NASCAR" on the tube and life is good. We'll call this the classic "Bubba Position." Now, while in Bubba Position, try to move around a little bit: try to rock your boat back and forth with your knees; try to rotate your body from side to side; try to bend forward and kiss the deck. Hmmm. Not too mobile, huh?

OK, enough of that silliness. Sit up nice and tall now. Imagine there's a string attached to your belly button, and that someone's pulling that

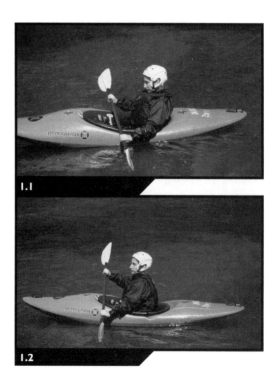

1.1 *Like this boater, bad posture is an embarrasment to us all.*

1.2 *Sitting up tall will help all aspects of your kayaking. Boater: Alice Solomon*

string straight forward until you're sitting upright. Your weight should now be on the front part of your butt, instead of the back. You should feel a slight arch in your lower back, and your chest should be puffed out like you're proud of what you're doing: "Look, Ma! I'm kayaking!" Now go through those ranges of motion again. You'll feel a great increase in flexibility. That is, you now have a much wider range of motion: you can move your body and the boat a lot more. You can try this exercise without a boat: just sit on the floor and imagine you're in a kayak while you go through the motions—first in the Bubba Position, then while sitting up nice and tall.

When we're out on the river, we tend to get lazy and slide toward Bubba Position. Not a big deal if you're hanging out in an eddy telling some beautiful person that you'd love to spend the weekend helping him or her install new roof-racks. But if you're becoming Bubba as you go for that must-make eddy above a rapid called White-Hot-Screaming-Death, things might not go so nicely. In order to kayak well, you need to be able to move your body well. It all boils down to having good posture.

Posture does a lot more than increase range of motion, though. With good posture comes good balance. Sitting up tall will also help you see the rapids better. And good posture translates to confident body language: your body will feel happier about throwing itself off that big waterfall, so it will perform better. Plus, of course, you look far cooler if you're sitting up tall than if you're hunched over like you're trying to hide from the big, scary river.

At first, sitting up nice and tall probably won't feel too great. Most of us have had pretty sloppy posture for years. Our cushy office chairs, car seats, and sofas have conditioned us to be slouching losers. To be blunt, our lower back muscles are pathetic. So paddling with good posture is

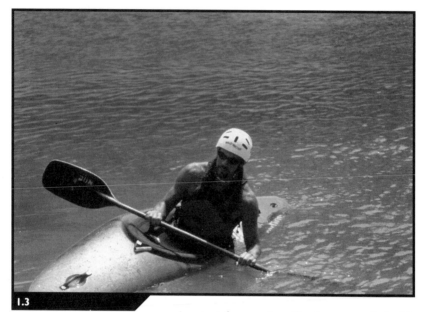

1.3

1.3 *The Terrible-Lean-of-Humiliating-Agony. Boater: Jimmy Leithauser*

going to take practice. Don't worry—it builds character, as well as stronger back muscles.

BODY MOVEMENT: EDGES

Now that we look good in our boats, we want to consider how we move our kayak around. The paddle is a great tool; good paddling technique can really help our boating. However, our body motion is just as important; how we use our bodies affects how we control our kayaks.

One important example of body motion at work is how we lean our boats. A number of outdoor sports these days involve moving your chosen vehicle—whether it's a surfboard, a snowboard, or a kayak—while on edge. Each of these sports involve a similar technique of edging through a turn; one way to spot experts is by the way they use their edges.

When people initially try to edge their kayak, they usually accomplish an edge by simply throwing their upper-body weight toward one side. For example, if I want to edge my boat to

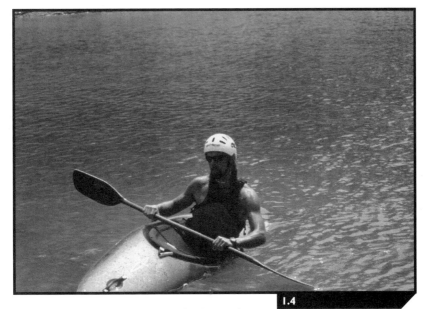

1.4

the right, I simply lean my upper-body weight to
the right. This will do the trick—the boat will be
on edge—but the edge won't be too steady, and
I won't feel in control. Let's call this the Body-
Lean, or the Terrible-Lean-of-Humiliating-
Agony.

1.4 The J-Lean. Boater:
Jimmy Leithauser

In order to show our expertise, we actually
want to keep our upper body over our boats.
Instead of just chucking our upper-body weight
around, we'll use what's inside our boats in order
to edge. To edge, simply sink your weight into
one butt cheek. Relax your torso and gently
allow your head to drop toward the other butt
cheek (the one you're not sinking into). So, if
you're edging to the right, sink your weight into
your right butt cheek and let your head relax and
drop toward the left shoulder.

This edge, called the "J-Lean" because of the
shape of your body, should feel much steadier
than the Body-Lean. You can hold the J-Lean
almost indefinitely. If you want more of an edge,
simply increase upward pressure with the knee
opposite the butt cheek on which you're putting

weight. If you want to enhance an edge to the right, pick up your left knee. By applying different amounts of pressure with your knee, you can vary the degree of edge, from a barely perceptible lean to being right on the brink of going over. The key is that the upper body isn't doing much; you're establishing an edge with your butt, hips, and knees.

When you're edging, it's not essential to get the most radical lean possible; you don't want to be constantly on the verge of tipping over. Rather, what matters is that you can hold a slight but steady edge for at least ten seconds or so. To test how healthy your edge is, try this: on flatwater, see if you can steadily hold a slight edge (you shouldn't be applying much pressure with your knee) on each side for at least ten seconds. When this is so easy you're about to pass out from boredom, try to hold this edge while you paddle forward and backward. Not so simple now, tough guy!

You want to be able to hold an edge, because you edge while you turn. For example, when you're peeling out of an eddy, you'll edge downstream throughout the turn. To stay upright, you'll want to hold that edge during the entire turn, until your boat is pointing downstream. Most of us have experienced what

Advanced Tip

Dealing with edges brings up a very important point in boating. Use what's inside the boat! When we kayak, we're holding a large, impressive-looking paddle. Since we have this cool (and expensive) tool, we feel that we need to use it and ignore everything else. No, no. When you're kayaking, you're actually doing a lot of work with your knees, hips, and feet. Edging is a great example.

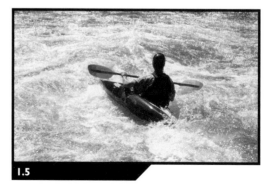

1.5 *Edging while leaving an eddy. Boater: Matt Jennings*

1.5

happens when we don't hold the edge long enough: we end up performing a quick biological survey on the local fish populations.

STROKES

Again, I promise I won't dwell on the basics too much. I won't go over individual strokes, but I will discuss some fundamentals common to all strokes. Whether you're performing a stern draw to angle your boat away from a rock, executing a duffek as you swing into an eddy, or planting your blade in order to initiate a cartwheel, each kayaking stroke is built on the same ideas.

First, plant your blade in the water so it will be effective. Don't just splash your paddle into the river. If you decide to use a stroke, use it well!

Here's a common scenario:

Rupert drifts into the top of a rapid; he's a little nervous, but feeling OK. He's starting left and knows he has to move right. In order to angle his boat to the right, he uses a stern draw on the left. But, to our utter dismay, he just splashes the stroke down. Aahg! It's ineffective! Finally, after three more tries, Rupert manages to turn his boat to the right. But by now, he's been pushed too far downstream, so it's time to crank out some good hard forward strokes. Rupert starts to paddle as quickly as possible, but his strokes are, for lack of a better description, spastic and irregular. Bad leads to worse, and Rupert ends up in a terrible place at the bottom of the rapid: he drifts into the big rodeo hole, collides with the beautiful girl who was working on her ten-point cartwheels, flips over, and swims, while she laughs hysterically.

Poor Rupert. When we get scared, or nervous, or are generally unsure of ourselves, we tend not to concentrate on how we place our

A Fancy Explanation

Splash occurs because of a phenomenon known as cavitation. When you put the paddle in the water, a tiny air pocket forms around the blade. If you take a stroke before letting that air pocket fill in with water, you'll generate splash. So if you see splash, you know that your stroke is, for an instant, pulling air, not water—and that's way less powerful. The solution? After you place your stroke, let it settle for a split second before you move the blade.

strokes. This can be bad, since these are usually the times when we really need good strokes. The moral is that we should plant our strokes deliberately. A good thing to look for is splash. If your strokes generate lots of splash, chances are that you aren't paddling very smoothly. Make sure that you place the entire blade in the water, and that you place the blade intentionally, not just slapping it down. Paddle smoooothly.

In other words, think about paddling with quality, not just quantity. One well-placed, effective stroke will do much more than a bunch of quick, sloppy ones. Take the time to commit to a good stroke.

Second, remember this magic word: rotate. The driving power behind your strokes should not come from your puny little arms. Instead, use larger muscle groups like your back muscles and abdominals. This will do three good things:

1. Larger muscle groups give you stronger, more efficient strokes.

2. Larger muscle groups can take more stress than smaller, more vulnerable areas. Moving the work load to these more powerful groups will help you avoid injury.

3. That person at the bottom might still laugh hysterically, but they will comment on your "great rotation!" as they help tow you into a nearby eddy.

So how do we access these larger muscle groups? How do we rotate? There are two basic ways in which we can rotate. The first way involves turning strokes, like sweeps and stern draws. To start, hold the paddle in front of you with elbows relatively straight. Hold the paddle horizontal, low to the water. An obvious square should be formed, bounded by your chest, arms, and the paddle shaft. When trying to turn the boat with a sweep or stern draw, focus on maintaining this square, often called the "paddler's box." When learning, you can ensure rotation by watching the working blade—your shoulders and arms should rotate with the paddle.

Later, on the river, you'll find that you might not want to look so intently at your paddle, no matter how much you paid for it. That rock approaching your bow at the speed of sound is suddenly a little more interesting. That's fine— watching your paddle in practice is just a way to train your body to rotate with the turning stroke. As long as your chest and shoulders turn with the stroke, you don't need the head, too. Fancier turning strokes, like the duffek, work the same way, though the shaft position changes; just think about rotating your torso with the stroke.

The second way in which we rotate involves the forward stroke. This is a slightly trickier motion, one which can take a long time to pick up. But the same ideas apply. With the forward stroke, the arms should be fairly straight and relaxed. To access good rotation, follow this nifty recipe:

1. Sit up straight; use that beautiful posture to your advantage. Remember, you can't move well unless you have good posture.

2. Reach your hand forward as if reaching into the plant position of the forward stroke. The paddle shaft should be fairly vertical. Ideally, the blade should reach past your feet, but it probably doesn't yet.

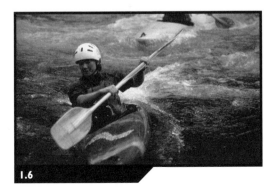

1.6 *Rotating in order to plant a forward sweep. Notice that the paddler keeps her chest parallel to the paddle shaft in order to maintain the paddler's box. Boater: Juliet Kastorff*

3. Rrrrrrrrrotate! Pivot the working shoulder (the shoulder on the side on which you're planning to paddle) forward, and drop the other shoulder back. You should have gained almost a foot of reach; the paddle should now reach, magically, past your feet. Astound your pals.

4. Simply unwind from this position. Draw the paddle back until you're in the neutral position, with both shoulders facing forward. Don't overdo it; unwind just enough so that you end up taking a short stroke. You want the paddle to exit the water just past the knee. If you take the paddle out any farther back, you're just lifting water—wasting energy.

5. Now you're ready for the other side. Repeat steps two through four, paddling on the opposite side.

Don't worry if forward stroke rotation doesn't feel natural at first; like anything new, it will take time before this rotation feels normal. Here's a tip that really helped me: loosen up your arms as much as possible and consciously think of them as limp sticks holding the paddle, while your abs and back do the work. If you keep your arms loose and relatively straight, you'll be forced to use larger, more effective muscle groups in order to move the paddle.

Third, think about your pivot point, your center of gravity. Without going into too many details, think about a pivot point in terms of a seesaw. The pivot point is the fulcrum, right in the middle. Where do you want to apply pressure to have a lot of effect on the seesaw? Obviously, as far from the pivot point as possible. The farther from the pivot point you apply pressure, the easier it is to move the seesaw. Force applied farther from the pivot point simply means more leverage.

So, let's apply this to turning our boat. When we're not moving in any one direction, our pivot point lies right under our butt. So, we want our powerful turning strokes to reach out far from us. To do this, we simply keep the paddle low, especially the nonworking hand. When we move forward, our pivot point moves farther forward, up past our feet. So, the easiest way to turn the boat will be toward the back, and far from the boat.

Conversely, there are times when we just want to go in a straight line, when we don't want our strokes to turn the boat at all. No problem: we just paddle close to that pivot point, keeping the paddle far forward and near the center line of the boat. We keep the paddle close to the center line by keeping the paddle shaft fairly vertical. If we keep the nonworking hand high (about eye level), the shaft will automatically be fairly vertical; we'll be applying force close to the pivot point, so the boat won't turn.

So now you're an expert with the mechanics of forward strokes versus turning strokes. I just

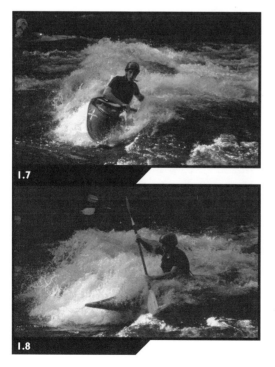

1.7 *A low stroke is used to turn the boat. Boater: Scott Collins*

1.8 *A vertical stroke is used to power the boat forward, back onto the wave. Boater: Scott Collins*

want to mention one other important facet of kayaking strokes.

There are a number of clues that help us discern a really good paddler from one with less experience. One clue is the use of negative strokes—the little back sweeps used to turn the boat. A good boater minimizes the use of negative strokes; she only uses a back stroke when she consciously wants to slow herself down or move backwards while she turns.

Small back sweeps can be really effective when you're trying to change your angle. The problem is that these back sweeps kill all your momentum—they drive you backwards, away from your target. This is fine if you're too close to a rock, but its not so great if you're ferrying or trying to set your angle in order to punch into an eddy. In general, minimize the use of negative strokes. If you want to turn to the right, use a forward sweep or a stern draw on the left—these are positive strokes. Don't give in to temptation and stick in that little back sweep. It ain't worth it.

ROLLING

To a nonkayaker, the roll seems like absolute magic, an inexplicable phenomenon somewhere along the lines of sword swallowing or walking on water. In fact, the roll still feels this way to some kayakers. The kayak roll can be tough to learn because you've got to force yourself to do a lot of unnatural things. For example, when rolling, your head should come out of the water last, but keeping your head down is completely counterintuitive: you want air now!

Without going into too much detail, let me outline a few points that are central to having a good roll.

Advanced Tip

A great way to become a better boater is to watch other people's styles. Analyze exactly what they are doing well, and what they could improve. Being conscious of these fine points will help make you more aware of your own technique. A word of warning: it's not considered tactful to voice aloud your opinions about others' paddling. "Hey, you. Yeah, you. Your forward stroke looks OK, but those turning strokes really stink." Not a good way to make new friends.

Relax your upper body. A lot of us are more comfortable answering any physical challenge by using our upper body. But rolling is not accomplished with your bulging biceps. Instead, try to think of your upper body as a jellyfish, a wet noodle. Your hips and knees will do the work; your upper body will merely follow the motion that you create with your lower body.

Relax your noggin. Let it flop like a rag doll's head. When you decide it's time to stop all the upside-down foolishness, simply let your head flop toward the "working shoulder." If you're rolling on the right, allow your head to gently fall to your right shoulder. This will allow your body to do what it needs to do to get upright.

Relax! If you're tense, worried, and scared, that's normal. But try not to let these feelings affect your roll. Take a deep breath (before you've flipped over, please), let it out, and imagine yourself as no more than a blob of jelly. Think "loose and easy."

PLANNING

So far, we've talked about what to do when you're already in the water. But let's turn back the clock just a bit. Before we even get into that hairy drop, it's necessary to make a plan. In the next chapter, I spend a little more time on how exactly one goes about making that plan. But for now, let's contrast two styles of boating.

Exhibit A: Here, ladies and gentlemen, we once again encounter the hapless Rupert. Rupert tends to do fairly well when he goes boating. He doesn't usually come back with a serious injury, and he's very good at coagulating. Rupert's problem is that he simply drifts wherever

A Commercial Break

Time for a short break. Whether you want it or not, I've been dying to share my collection of really bad kayaking jokes. If you're ever feeling really unhappy, think back to when you first read these jokes. You'll feel better immediately because you'll remember a time when you felt even more miserable.

Q: How many kayakers does it take to change a light bulb?

A: Four. One to unscrew the bulb, and three to stand around and talk about how gnarly the hole is.

Q: What's the difference between a kayak instructor and a U.S. Savings Bond?

A: A savings bond matures after twenty-five years.

Q: What's the difference between a kayaker and a catfish?

A: One has whiskers and smells bad; the other one's a fish.

the water wants to take him. Once he's in the meat of the rapid, he just hangs on and tries to survive. Let's call Rupert's style reactive—he simply tries to deal with what the river hands to him.

Exhibit B: On the other hand, Molly carefully decides what to do before she does it. In some cases, she gets out to look at a rapid if she's unsure. Sometimes, she'll scout on the fly; by looking way ahead, she can figure out where she wants to go and can use certain strokes to get her to that place. Molly's style is proactive. (Isn't that great? Simply by using that word, I feel like a powerful executive instead of a dirty, smelly, kayaking bum.) Molly chooses her destiny—she doesn't simply let the river decide.

The lesson is that we need to plan way ahead. When we don't have too much experience boating, we tend to get fixated on our bow grab loop. I admit, those grab loops are lovely. But you'd probably boat much better if you looked way downstream. The same rule applies whenever you're moving. If you're skiing, driving, or even walking, you don't look just a foot in front of you. You look way downslope, or road, or whatever, so that you'll be ready for what's ahead. In kayaking, likewise, the earlier you can plan and start to execute a move, the better your runs will be.

In the next chapter, we'll talk a lot more about specific river features. So wake up! Wipe that drool away! The excitement has barely begun.

Advanced Tip

Here's a tip that a good friend of mine, a great instructor, told me. A good way to understand whitewater (which will allow you to make a plan) is to concentrate when you're on rapids that aren't really hard for you. When you're on these oh-so-easy sections, really try to figure out exactly how each feature (each eddy line, each wave, each small hole, for example) is going to affect your boat. Don't just bob down these easy rapids; use them to learn how the river works.

2

Where Do I Go?
Reading the River

You can be the most naturally adept kayaker to ever hit the river. You can wear the fanciest gear, paddle the hottest boat on the market, and even have enough gas money for for the drive home. But no matter how smooth your strokes are, or how many points you can link in some gigantic hole, things will get tough if you don't know where you should put your boat in the first place. Life won't be too good unless you can read the water (look at a certain area of the river and figure out how it will affect a kayak) and know what you need to do in order to end up safe and sound.

Unfortunately, reading water is like any other

skill—some bad news comes into play here. This bad news is the second rule of kayaking:

Rule 2: The more time you spend in your boat, the better you become.

In just about any sport, it's hard to come up with a substitute for countless hours of practice. Kayaking is no exception. The more time you spend in your kayak, the better you'll be. No matter how much natural talent you have, it will be just about impossible to run a hard rapid well without a basic foundation. An important part of this foundation is a good understanding of how water works and how it affects your boat.

The good news is that there are, of course, shortcuts. There's no trick to the shortcuts: simply learn from others. Hang out with more experienced people. Watch where they go and how they boat. Ask them lots and lots of questions. Usually, they'll be more than happy to help you out; it gives them a chance to show off how incredibly cool they are.

Before you do head for the river, there's one more very, very important rule to think about. It's mostly important because I get a chance to use italics again. Here we go:

Rule 3: Be afraid of commitment: don't leap before you look.

In other words, don't commit yourself to running a rapid until you feel pretty certain that

RULE 2

The more time you spend in your boat, the better you become.

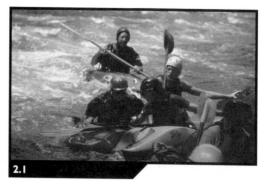

2.1 *Discussing life, love, and the art of the cartwheel. Boaters talking: Maria Noakes and Kim Jordan*

2.1

you'll be a happy camper at the bottom. Make sure that you can stop in time to make a fairly informed decision about where you want to go. Mike Hipsher, former Wildwater World Champion, used to say, "You only have one chance to run a rapid blind." While this is true, and it is often fun to just figure things out on the move, there are often times when it's a good idea to be a little more careful (especially if you don't happen to be a former Wildwater World Champion). For example, little-known creeks, rivers after big rains (which can wash logs into new places), and runs which seem like they'll really push a person's limits deserve some extra consideration.

So stop before you're halfway down a 20-foot vertical drop that lands on a rock. And stop in a place where you can get out of your boat, look at the rapid, and walk around it if necessary.

RULE 3

Be afraid of commitment: don't leap before you look.

SCOUTING

Now that you're not heading blindly over a Class VI rapid, you can start working on making a plan. There are obviously two ways to read water: from the seat of your boat, or from out of your kayak (perhaps from shore, or from a rock in the middle of the river). First, we'll discuss scouting from out of the boat. Then we'll talk about scouting "on the fly"—scouting without leaving your kayak.

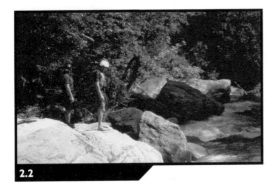

2.2

2.2 *Taking time to look. Scouter: Chuck DeRosa*

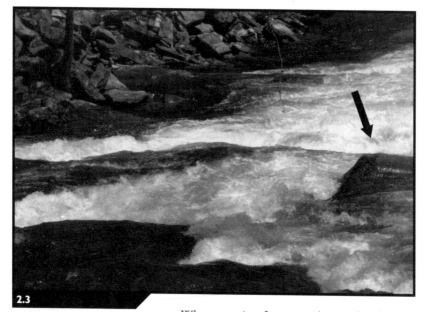

2.3

2.3 A rapid as seen from a scouting position above.

When scouting from outside your kayak, realize that you're going to have to figure out how things will look from your boat. A rapid looks very different when you're standing above it compared to seeing it from your kayak. In the following pictures, notice how the rapid's appearance changes from different vantage points.

In general, you can't see nearly as much when you're in your boat: you're too close to the water to see past any significant horizon line. Therefore, look for features that are obvious enough to key off of when you're in a kayak. Rocks, tree branches, waves, eddy lines, and so on, all work well as reference points. A feature that occurs after any kind of vertical drop, even a small one, will be hard to see from a boat.

While this lack of height can make things more difficult, there's an easy way to reduce this problem. As I've mentioned before, there are tons of reasons to sit up straight in your boat. In addition to increasing your range of motion and your muscle powers, sitting up will make you taller and will give you a better view of the rapid.

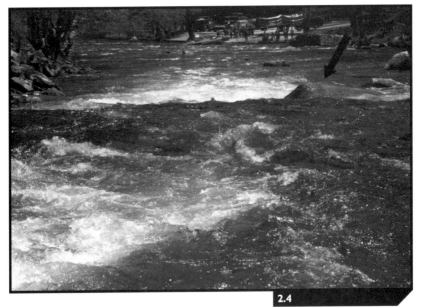

2.4

You'll be able to see what's over the edge of that monstrous-looking horizon line a little better. Also, your kayaking will be much improved, and that's always a plus.

So how do you decide where to go? How do you choose a line? There are tons of ways to break down a rapid. Here's one: the basic idea is to plan your run backwards.

One: Decide where you'll end up. Hopefully, the answer to this won't be "gasping on shore, trying to figure out where my teeth went." If you honestly feel that things could easily end up this way, think about walking. I know, I know. You want to go for it. Especially since that know-it-all you're with said he didn't think you could handle it. But remember, you'll have plenty of other chances to hurt yourself. And a stop at Taco Bell on the way home is no fun without your incisors. So figure out a good place to finish the rapid, some place where you can stop and either celebrate or regroup.

Two: How are you going to get to that safe place at the end? Here's the hard part. Pick a line,

2.4 *The same rapid seen from a boater about to run the drop.*

and pick it specifically. Don't plan vaguely: "Oh, I guess I'll kind of go by that strainer, try to avoid the sieve, and then sort of slide past the hole." Choose exactly where you want to be in relation to specific reference points, like rocks or waves. Decide which strokes you're going to use and where you'll use them. If possible, see if you can break up the rapid into stages. If the structure of the river allows, eddy-hop down the rapid instead of running it in one fell swoop. This will give you a chance to relax and keep things from getting out of control.

Next, pick a line where the water will help you. In other words, let the river be your friend. Try to get on a piece of water that is moving toward your goal. This may take a little work initially, but an early effort is better than later trying to escape from the current flowing right into the man-eating hole.

Three: Decide where you'll start. As mentioned above, start at a point that will make it as easy as possible to get where you're going. Put your kayak on some water that's flowing toward a good place. And, just as importantly, start with your boat angled in such a way that it will help get you where you want to be.

Backwards planning will work whether you're checking out a rapid from shore or from your boat. You just won't have quite as good a view of the rapid from inside your boat. The main idea, though, is to take your time and to

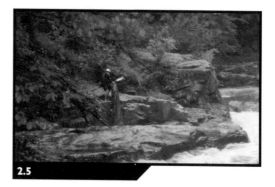

2.5 *Not today. Sometimes the best run is the dry one.*

2.5

consider how to run the rapid, whether that means running the big boof in the middle or walking your boat down the left-hand shore.

But how do we know if we can handle a certain rapid? There's no sure way to know; you have to evaluate the rapid and your skills and make the choice. Still, we can try to make the decision process a little more scientific. In *Canoe and Kayak Magazine*, Gordon Grant does a great job describing one way to decide whether or not to run that frightening drop. Grant writes that we have to consider four questions:

1. *What moves are required of me?*

2. *Can I do these moves?*

3. *What are the consequences if I fail to do those moves?*

4. *Am I willing to accept those consequences?*

According to Grant, we shouldn't run any rapid unless we feel confident about the responses to each of these questions (and he doesn't mean that you should feel confident that you are really going to hurt yourself). Don't let other people pressure you into running. It's probably more fun to keep your vertebral column intact than your pride.

READING WHITEWATER

OK, so we have a better idea about how to decide if we want to head down a certain rapid. But what do we do if we are going to run? We still don't have a very good understanding of how the water's going to affect our boats. In order to understand the interaction between the river and our kayaks, let's get into some more specifics.

First, look at where the water in a rapid is flowing. This seems obvious, but we often forget when confronted with the chaos of whitewater. At first glance, a rapid can seem like a mess of out-of-control currents. On closer inspection, you can usually see which way the water "pushes." That is, you can tell where most of the water goes. Sometimes throwing a stick in the rapid and seeing where it ends up can help determine the direction the current is moving. This is probably (though not always) where you'll go if you drift through the rapid without paddling. Think of this as the "Tuber's Line."

Second, look at where the water in a rapid isn't flowing downstream. In other words, where are the eddies? Eddies can be big, catchable pieces of still water behind a rock, or just a patch of slower-moving water behind a small hole or wave. You can use eddies to stop or to move your boat to where it needs to be.

Third, think about those edges. As you improve, you won't have to concentrate on edging your boat, but there are some moves in which it will help to plan ahead of time exactly how to edge your boat. In general, you always want to keep water flowing under your boat: edge away from the flow. If the kayak is edged toward the flow, the water can catch the edge of the boat and—whammo—roll practice. Edging away from the flow can mean leaning downstream when coming out of an eddy, leaning upstream when entering an eddy, or leaning into a hole when hitting it with a bit of angle.

Does this mean that we must always edge our boats? If we're floating sideways in uniform current (it can be pretty strong current), should we edge our boats downstream the entire time? Naah—too much work. And it would be hard to feel stable if you were constantly on edge.

In the kayaking days of yore, a popular adage was kicked around: "Always lean downstream." This saying isn't entirely wrong, but it gets misinterpreted. Actually, as long as you're moving with the speed of the current, you can lean any way you want, and, barring any cosmic weirdness, you'll be A-OK. We only need to edge our boats when we move from a current of one speed to a current moving at a different speed, such as from an eddy into the main current, or from the main flow into a hole or a wave.

No more dwelling on this edge stuff. But to reiterate, think about your edges and how you'll use them to keep yourself upright when running a certain rapid. Runs are usually more successful if you do them right-side-up.

Finally, look carefully for hazards. Is that wall undercut? How far underwater do those strainers extend? Are you going to punch that hole, or are you going to do an unintentional Marc Lyle imitation? In looking at possible hazards, we want to consider two things:

Plan A: Decide how you plan to avoid those unfriendly looking features.

Plan B: Decide what you'll do if you end up getting a little too intimate with those hazards.

Don't dwell on Plan B; just realize that things don't always go right. You need to know what to do in case of a mistake. Sometimes, this means setting up safety—for example, telling your kayaking buddies to hang out below with a rope.

Advanced Tip

In general, edging only makes a big difference when you move from one speed of current to another.

SCOUTING "ON THE FLY"

By now, you've figured out a general strategy for scouting rapids and deciding where to go. Sometimes, though, we do just head down without too much overt scouting; we stay in our boats and figure out the rapids as they come. Watching a highly experienced boater can make this look like the easiest thing in the world. Watching folks with a little less time in the kayak shows how scouting on the fly can be incredibly frustrating.

I remember my first trip down the Nolichucky River, a beautiful run right on the North Carolina–Tennessee border. I was with a group of people who were much better kayakers than I was (and pretty much anyone fit the bill at that point). The water was pretty low (thankfully—otherwise, I would have been pummeled), and I felt like I got stuck on every rock in the river. I couldn't figure out how everyone else seemed to glide effortlessly by the rocks. Of course, I blamed it on my lousy gear, despite the fact that we were all using pretty much the same stuff. Which leads us to a very important lesson: always blame mistakes on something else.

Can you sympathize with my day as a rock magnet? Here are some things to look for while you're in your boat. These tips might not be too applicable when you're trying to figure out where to go on the flooded Class XX section of the Upper North Branch of South Death Creek. But if you want to make life a little better on the smaller stuff, check out these tips.

- You're above a rapid with no earthly idea where to go. Don't fret. First, look where the water's going. If you can see a line of continuous flow of water from the top of the rapid to the bottom (or at least to the next eddy), chances are that you've found a good line. This unbroken chain of water has a steady loss of gradient—there will be fewer sudden drops. More importantly, you won't be going unawares into a big hole or onto a poorly padded rock. You'll know what you're getting yourself into, and, just as importantly, you'll be

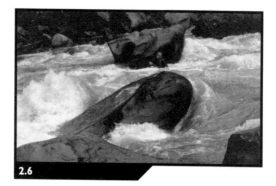

2.6 *A paddler follows a steady line of water. Photo: Craig Parks*

2.6

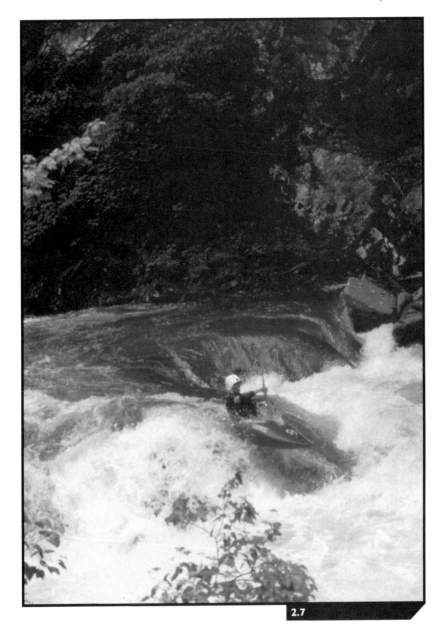

2.7

2.7 *Heading down a tongue.*
Photo: Ryan Boudrand.
Boater: Craig Parks

going where the water is going—with less chance of getting stuck.

- Second, that unbroken chain of water will often contain what's called a "tongue," or a "downstream-**V**." A tongue is simply a relatively deep, unobstructed channel of water. Tongues are wide at the top and narrow as they move downstream, hence the name "**V**." **V**s are formed by two places where there is a differential in current; the **V** is simply the smooth water between two eddy lines. You'll often find a series of waves at the end of a tongue, where the two eddy lines converge. Known as a wave train, these waves are usually deep and fun, just a roller-coaster ride.

- Another feature to look at is the surface of the water. Unless you managed to pick up X-ray vision from your parents back on Krypton, it can be hard to figure out where the best, least obstructed route is. Look for dark, smooth water. Water that looks like this tends to be deep. Go there.

- Also, look for water with small, irregular ripples on top. These ripples usually indicate rocks just below the surface. Don't go there. Random patterns of white froth indicate a bad place to practice that roll.

- It's also important to keep your eyes out for smooth, rounded-looking mounds of water.

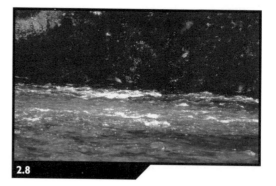

2.8 The white froth shows where those sneaky rocks are hiding.

These formations usually indicate a rock with a little water flowing over it. Waves will generally have more of a crest. But a slightly covered rock, though hard to see, could cause some problems.

- Finally, look for small eddies. These are just big versions of the ripples. If you see a small eddy, you can bet there's something just upstream creating it, something that is dying to get you stuck. These mini-eddies are probably fine to go through—just avoid whatever's upstream creating them. Another name for these mini-eddies is "upstream **V**s." From upstream, these mini-eddies have a **V**-shape, with the point of the **V** closest to you, and the rest extending downstream away from you.

One more river feature deserves a little extra coverage: the hole. Holes can be great play spots. Holes can also be potentially deadly monsters. It's

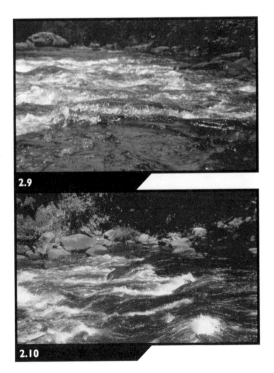

2.9 *The small, rounded humps indicate rocks.*

2.10 *The same hidden rocks are easily apparent from a side view.*

up to you to tell the difference. There are a number of ways to decide. If in doubt, the best thing to do is to ask someone you trust. But the main clue in looking at a hole is how long the tail, or backwash, is. The backwash is the water downstream of a hole that's flowing back into the hole. If the backwash is ten feet long, it'd be tough to break through that hole. But if the hole's tail is only a foot or so, you can probably make it through.

In judging a hole, there are a number of other factors to keep in mind. A ragged, uneven-looking hole will probably contain some weak spots, unlike a smoother, "cleaner" hole. Also, a hole with edges downstream of its center will tend to hold a boat better than a hole with edges upstream of its center. Don't dwell on trying to develop a fail-safe hole-rating system. There are hundreds of factors involved. Just remember that discretion is the better part of valor.

I trust that these hints will help you pick more pleasant lines than I found that day on the Nolichucky. Hopefully, this chapter has helped you get better at one of the fundamental skills in boating: making a plan. Again, a great deal of your ability to scout will simply come as a result of experience. The first time a person looks at whitewater, the rapid can look like a crazy, out-of-control mess. It's the same as if a semi-educated dolt like myself were to look at a complicated math equation. But if I were a trained mathematician, I could make sense out of that convoluted formula. The same holds true of whitewater. Once you've been trained, you'll understand how the river works. And this will allow you a much better opportunity to put your boat in a good place. (No. "Good place" does not mean "in the back of your garage, gathering dust.")

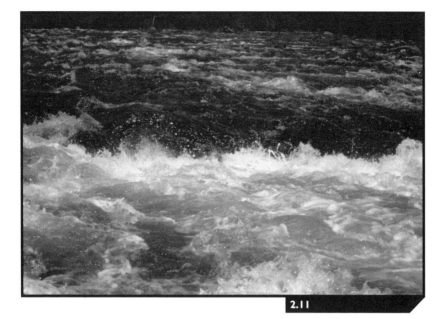

2.11 *The appropriately named "Lost Guide" hole on the Pidgeon River.*

3

Pushing the Limits: Running the Tough Stuff

Sorry. This section won't tell you how to ensure beautiful runs down any Class VI rapid you happen to encounter. There's no way to do that. The exciting thing about rapids that really push your personal envelope is that you are not completely safe. Kayaking involves genuine risk. There's no stop button to push when things are no longer going your way. If you're going to run difficult rapids, you've got to feel that you can handle what the river will deal you.

This chapter discusses some tips aimed at helping you run hard rapids succesfully. By hard, I mean any rapid that challenges you. Whether you're starting to check out technical Class III

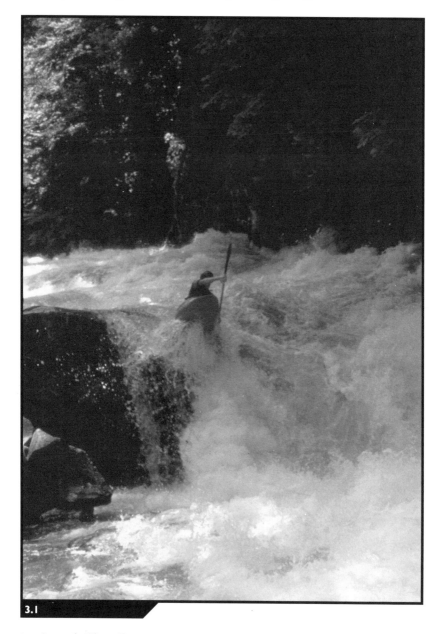

3.1

3.1 *Aw, yeah. Photo: Ryan Boudrand. Boater: Doug Geiger* rapids or are throwing yourself off marginally runnable waterfalls, I've tried to bring together some ideas to make sure you have a grand ol' time.

But first of all, why do we run the scary stuff? Difficult water has a strong draw, an almost frightening magnetism. This will seem very pretentious coming from me, a person who has trouble not sticking himself in the eye with his silverware, but I think that in "Kubla Khan," Samuel Taylor Coleridge describes perfectly the beauty and majesty we feel when we encounter the power of the river:

> But oh! that deep romantic chasm which slanted
> Down the green hill athwart a cedarn cover!
> A savage place! As holy and enchanted
> As e'er beneath a waning moon was haunted
> By woman wailing for her demon lover!
> And from this chasm, with ceaseless turmoil seething,
> As if this earth in fast thick pants were breathing,
> A mighty fountain momently was forced:
> Amid whose swift half-intermitted burst
> Huge fragments vaulted like rebounding hail,
> Or chaffy grain beneath the thresher's flail:
> And 'mid these dancing rocks at once and ever
> It flung up momently the sacred river. (lines 12-24)

If you were to ask what nonboaters thought about going down insane-looking drops, their reactions could usually be grouped into one of two categories:

The Mom Reaction: "Oh, dear. Are you sure it's safe? It doesn't look safe. Can't you do easier things? That nice boy next door doesn't kayak. He has a good job. And he doesn't smell. It's not that we don't approve, honey, we're just concerned. Are you careful?" And so on.

The Drunk-Local Reaction: "Sheee-it. Me and my cousin Bo went down that in tubes when we was ten!"

Out of curiosity, I asked a number of "expert kayakers" (whatever that means) how they feel about running rapids that push their limits. Here are some responses:

Why do I run hard rapids? They're a lot more fun because they usually involve adrenaline, falling, acceleration, tight places, or a lot of water hitting your body . . . it sucks that they can be really not-fun when you mess up.
—Brian Totten, Team Prijon

I run hard stuff because it's difficult to walk around . . . Some days "hard stuff" doesn't seem so hard, and other days it seems impossible.
—Sarah Foreman, NOC Kayak Instructor

I run difficult rapids for the focus they give me. Since they demand total concentration, I find running them almost meditative. Then, of course, there's the adrenaline rush at the bottom.
—Bruce Lessels, President, Zoar Outdoor

RULE 4

Don't do it if it's not fun.

Remember that kayaking is not a Mountain Dew commercial. The idea is not to see how much you can scare and amaze your viewers. Here, we come to another wonderful rule of kayaking:

Rule 4: Don't do it if it's not fun.

There's no need to earn a nickname like "Kamikaze Karl" or "Hospital Heather." If a rapid is so scary that you won't enjoy anything until you're safe at the bottom, don't run it! What a novel idea.

THE HEAD GAME: MENTAL PREPARATIONS

Sometimes, though, you'll decide to go for it. It's time to run that drop you've been considering for years. When this time comes, first make sure that your trusty pals are hanging out below the rapid in case your run doesn't work out as well as planned.

Second, you need to be mentally ready. When paddling something that frightens you, get in the right frame of mind. Concentrate! Look at the drop, pick your line carefully, and style your way down the rapid.

Chris Ennis, a member of Team Dagger and the U.S. National Team, has been a slalom racer ever since he was a wee lad. During a run down a local creek, he mentioned something he still uses from his racing background (besides his rotting PFD): whenever Chris is about to run a tough rapid, he envisions himself having a perfect run from top to bottom. If he has trouble picturing this run, he'll carry around the drop.

Imagine yourself running the rapid perfectly, then run it. Don't spend hours staring at the drop. It's easy to look at a rapid way too long and get what kayak guru Tommy DeCuir calls "Paralysis through Analysis."

Once you start down the rapid, your worries and fears will disappear—you'll be perfectly absorbed in the instant. This is one of the most beautiful moments in kayaking. Thoughts drop away. There is no more "What if I miss the eddy?" No more worries about that funny knocking noise your car's starting to make or if the new McDonald's burger really measures up to the Whopper. It's only you and the majesty of a river falling off a mountain. No matter how incredibly petrified I am above a rapid, I'm calm the second I start paddling. It's not until the bottom that I'm aware how fast my heart is racing.

This same feeling, the sensation of awareness

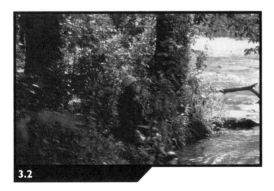

3.2 *Alice Solomon becomes one with the river.*

of only the moment, is a common theme in meditation traditions. I don't want to dwell on this too much, but I'll briefly quote a passage from *The Experience of Insight*, written by Joseph Goldstein, a teacher of Vipassana meditation. While you read Goldstein's words, I think you'll be struck by the way in which they so accurately describe certain kayaking moments:

> *Our minds are mostly dwelling in the past, thinking about things that have already happened, or planning for the future, imagining what is about to happen, often with anxiety or worry. Reminiscing about the past, fantasizing about the future; it is generally very difficult to stay grounded in the present moment.*
>
> *Bare attention is that quality of awareness which keeps us alive and awake in the here and now. Settling back into the moment, experiencing fully what it is that's happening.*

Jon Krakauer in *Into the Wild*, describes a similar feeling in relation to his sport of choice, climbing:

> *Hours slide by like minutes. The accumulated clutter of day-to-day existence—the lapses of conscience, the unpaid bills, the bungled opportunities, the dust under the couch, the inescapable prison of your genes—all of it is temporarily forgotten, crowded from your thoughts by an overpowering clarity of purpose and by the seriousness of the task at hand.*

Despite the fact that we can tap into this feeling of "bare attention," there are definitely times when it's hard to concentrate. If there's too much pressure, we can become too worried or distracted to focus on the

My Personal Ritual

This is going to be a little embarrassing, but I'm nothing if not embarrassing, so here goes. Every time before I run a rapid that scares me silly, I go through a short ritual: I sing a song for luck. I learned this song from a woman in the first kayak clinic I ever taught. I'm somewhat superstitious, but not too bad—the song simply gives me a little time to relax and loosen up. I've sung it enough times that it works as a trigger. As soon as I sing it, my body knows that it's time to shake off the jitters, get the job done, and have some fun in the meantime. Here are the words to the song, though it's not the same without the melody:

> The river, She is flowing,
> Flowing and growing,
> The river, She is flowing,
> Down to the sea.
> Mother, carry me,
> Your child I will always be,
> Mother, carry me,
> Down to the sea.

Doing the same ritual every time you are about to run something that requires focus will send your mind and body a message: "OK, settle down, time to get ready." NBA fans may have noticed that the players often go through a short routine when taking free throws. We can overcome our nerves by settling into a routine. But don't take my word for it—try it out. I guarantee you won't be nervous when you're hopping around naked, chanting in ancient Tibetan, and sprinkling snake blood all over your paddle.

moment at hand. To help yourself get mentally prepared, go through a quick, pre-scary-rapid ritual.

TOUGH-WATER TECHNIQUES

By now, we've all achieved a state of kayaking nirvana. Let's get in our boats and focus on some specifics.

First, when you're running that rapid, your vision is very important. Too often we tend to fixate on where we don't want to go. We keep our eyes glued to the boat-eating undercut on the left or on the strainer below. Don't do that, silly paddler! When you scouted, you picked out a point where you wanted to finish. So during your actual run, look at that place. Chances for a good run are much better if you look toward a positive goal. Time for another rule:

RULE 5

Look where you want to go: "Eyes on the Prize."

Rule 5: Look where you want to go: "Eyes on the Prize."

Along these lines, be specific about where you look. If you want to catch a certain eddy, don't just look at the eddy in general. Find an exact spot in that eddy where you want to put your boat. On one of the harder rapids that folks from my neck of the woods run, the most difficult part of the drop is making a small, turbulent eddy just above the main drop. There's a certain leaf hanging down the rock wall at the back of that eddy.

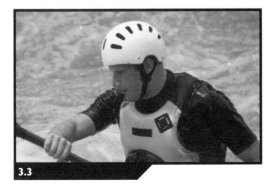
3.3

3.3 *Keep those "Eyes on the Prize." This kayaker looks toward his goal.*

Every time I run that drop, I first find that leaf. Before I even start my run, I'm looking at that leaf. I don't stop looking until I'm in the eddy, ready to run the rest of the rapid. Looking at the leaf makes it tough to run shuttle, but it's worth it (ha, ha, ha . . .).

Second, remember to get the job done. Often, when we become nervous or frightened, we just freeze up and let the river take us where it will. Sometimes, you can get away with this "deer in headlights" reaction. But not always. The first time I ran an infamous big drop in North Carolina, I was scared to pieces. I drifted through the entrance, barely paddling, just bracing to stay upright. Things went fine, except that I flipped, rolled up just in time to go over the main drop backwards, snapped my paddle in two on the way down, and got ripped out of my boat at the bottom. How embarassing.

We have a saying in kayaking that's especially applicable when you're nervous: when in doubt, crank it out. As Corran Addison says in *Canoe and Kayak's Whitewater Paddling* issue, "You can only have so much technique. After that, you just have to pull harder." If you're scared, get moving. You'll relax because you'll be too busy concentrating on what you're doing. You won't think to worry about how they'll get your boat out from under that rock. Since you're actively working toward where you want to be, instead of just floating, chances are that you'll have a better run. And, if you have some speed going, the water won't have as much of a chance to mess with you.

Third, there are some specific "tricks" that often come into play when running challenging rapids. Here are some of those tricks.

True Story Time

Once upon a time, Carol was just learning to kayak. Her boyfriend, Tom, was teaching her. One day, they were on the river, a section which was pretty challenging for Carol. At the bottom of one rapid, Tom turned to Carol and suggested, "You need to relax!" Carol glared at him and shot back, "I am f---ing relaxed!"

The Moral? You can't force yourself to be relaxed and loose. Feeling at ease comes from not trying to push yourself too hard. Know your limits. Don't run Niagara until you are genuinely good and ready.

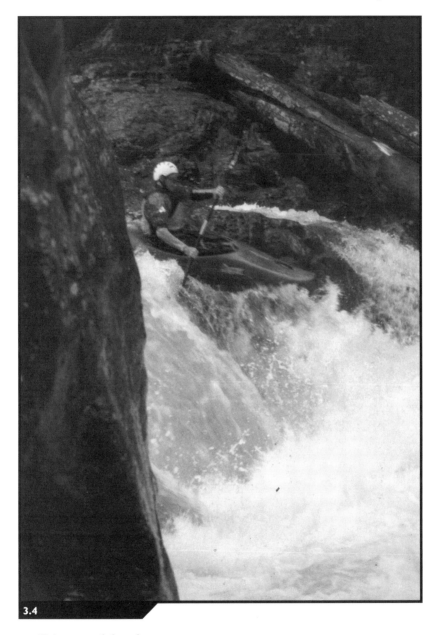

3.4

3.4 *Going over a ledge takes guts, commitment, and sometimes a good boof. Boater: Land Heflin*

DA BOOF

Ledges

To quote the Fresh Prince, "OK, here's the situation": we have a solid Class IV rapid in front of us. Most of the water pushes to the left, where there are some ugly undercuts, strainers, and a few man-eating sharks. The only real line is on the right—a small vertical drop, about five feet high, a slot between two huge rocks. No problem, except that the drop lands on a big flat rock only a few feet below the surface. Alas! What shall we do?

Simple. We boof the slot. Our boats sail through the air like vomit at a frat party, landing flat well beyond that pesky underwater rock. Life is good. And when you buy this fancy new tool, you get even more! Boofing can be useful in any number of situations, whether you're avoiding a shallow rock below a drop, avoiding a particularly sticky hole, or simply choosing the only safe line (which is over a rock).

The boof isn't very hard, but it can take a little time to figure out. It's worth it, though. Boofing can be really useful, especially as you start to run steeper and more technical rivers. For starters, let's learn how to boof off a vertical ledge. To practice, you don't need to head to your local three-thousand-foot waterfall. A small pour-over will do the trick.

An Enthralling Tidbit of Kayaking Etymology

We call this move a "boof" because that's the sound our boat makes as it lands. If your boat doesn't make this exact sound, you're obviously doing something terribly, horrendously wrong, and are endangering yourself and your paddling partners.

1. To begin, get some momentum going as you approach the lip of the drop. Why the need for speed? Simple—we want to finish the drop and keep moving away from the nasty stuff at the bottom. It's hard to give high-fives to your pals while you're surfing in the hole at the bottom of the ledge.

2. Now here's the crux move. As you near the lip, lean forward aggressively to hook the paddle over the ledge. This stroke should be vertical and as close to the front of your boat as possible. As you pull back on the stroke, you should feel like you're launching yourself over the lip. In order to help keep the bow from sinking as you go over the drop, shift your weight back with the stroke and think about pulling your knees up to your chest. As

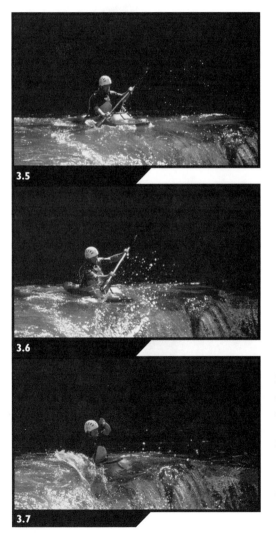

3.5 *The boater builds up speed as he approaches a small ledge.*

3.6 *He then reaches forward to plant the boof stroke . . .*

3.7 *. . . brings the stroke back while lifting his knees . . .*

you finish the stroke, you should be leaning back.

3. Perfect. A+ for boofing. But lifting the bow is just one note in the huge symphony you're creating. Don't make that note stand alone. In order to put the icing on the cake, hit the ground running. In other words, don't just land flat, only to let yourself wash into the strainer downstream. You want to land paddling and with your weight forward so that your momentum keeps going away from that terrifying rapid you just ran.

Think of the boof as a two-stroke combo with three body-weight positions (sounds fancy, huh?). First, you reach for the boof stroke with weight forward. Second, as you bring the stroke back, you lean back. Third, you land with weight forward and plant a stroke on the other side.

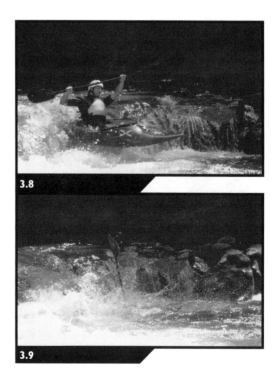

3.8 . . . *and keeps the bow up.*

3.9 *The boater lands with his weight forward, taking a powerful forward stroke as he lands. Boater: Chuck DeRosa*

Boofing Rocks

While we can boof off vertical ledges, it's also useful to be able to land flat by using handy obstructions, like rocks. Here's the story. Imagine you have
a vertical slot bordered by small rocks (small
enough to drive your boat onto). You could just
run the slot straight, but you would risk diving
straight to the river bottom. In order to keep your
bow from dropping, you can drive the front of

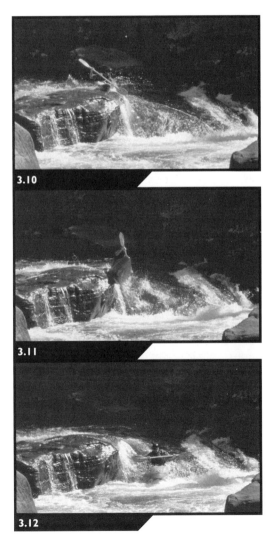

3.10 *To boof a rock, our fear-
less boater first drives his boat
up onto a rock.*

3.11 *He takes a big boof
stroke on the side opposite the
rock . . .*

3.12 *. . . and lands flat to
crazy applause and hundreds
of desperate, scantily clad
groupies. Boater unknown.*

your boat partly onto one of the rocks that border the slot. The friction between the boat and the rock slows the bow down, letting the the stern, which is still in the fast-moving water, catch up. The bow and stern go over together, which allows you to come off the drop flat. Nifty. This will work with many types of obstructions—anything from rocks to trees to your pal's head.

As you boof the rock, you'll use that same boof stroke that you used with a ledge. Simply reach forward with your paddle (usually with the blade on the opposite side of the rock) and yank your bow up. Try to plant your stroke even with the downstream edge of the rock. Proceed as before: pull the stroke back, lift your knees, and smile like you just won the lottery.

Boofing Holes

Sometimes we have to deal with one more problem: the hole. Very scary. But no big deal at all. We can take what we already know about the boof and apply this technique to punching holes. Just before the edge of a hole, reach forward and pull your bow up with a boof-type stroke. As you land in the hole, shift your weight forward and plant a strong stroke on the other side to keep pulling you through the hole.

In general, keep a few ideas in mind: keep paddling, keep your weight forward rather than back, and try to hit the hole relatively straight. It may also help to edge your boat in order to slice through the hole more easily, though be careful that you don't make yourself unsteady.

Big Ol' Drops

When we think of the boof, the classic picture that comes to mind is some drugged teenager in sparkly gear and a helmet roughly the size of a yarmulke, soaring off a waterfall the size of the Empire State Building. So, for those kids, let's talk about waterfalls.

If Hamlet were a loser kayaking bum like the rest of us, his defining existential question might be reduced to "To boof or not to boof?" There are definitely times when it's not a great idea to land flat; vertebral fusion sounds a lot cooler than it feels. There's no set rule about when you should land flat, or vertical, or somewhere in between. Every boater has an opinion. I try not to land totally flat if the drop is more than about fifteen feet high. Landing flat on even a ten-foot drop can feel not-so-good to your back. So be careful—it's hard to find a new spine.

On the other hand, it's usually not great to drop in completely vertically. If you land vertical, you'll go deep, which means you could hit things lurking on the bottom. Also, you won't be able to paddle away from the drop; you might spend some time freestyling in a hole at the bottom of a fall. Finally, it'll take you a little longer to recover, which might not be good if there's another demanding move right away.

So with fairly decent-sized verticals, use your judgement. Again, there's no perfect way to decide. Just realize that there are potential dangers with either extreme—landing flat or penciling.

There it is, folks. Some advice on how to run tough rapids. I want to point out that when I say tough rapids, I don't mean the hardest rapids available. People are definitely running rapids out there that I don't want to have any part of. A tough rapid is whatever type of water pushes your abilities, whether it's Class II or Class VI. Don't adopt another person's limits as your own. Run only what you feel is right for you.

So how do you know what's right for you? There's a fine line between pushing yourself enough to make things exciting, and running stuff that's just plain dangerous for your skill level. When in doubt, be conservative. It's OK not to be the craziest person out there.

In terms of general decisions, a good way to know that you're ready for more difficult water is when you feel totally at ease on slightly easier rapids. For example, if you're able to catch tough eddies, play, and make the hardest moves you can find on Class II water, try some Class III. Remember: you can make just about any run as difficult as you want. Go for that tiny eddy. See if you can attain all the way back up a rapid. And so on. A rapid doesn't have to be dangerous to be challenging. Don't just survive the river— finesse it.

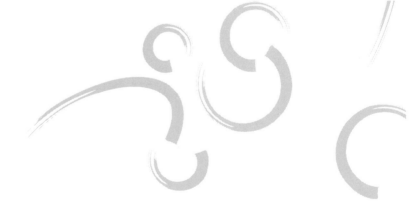

4

Getting Fancy: Basic Playing Techniques

Even if we totally ignore technique, it's easy to tell a really good kayaker from someone who's not quite as experienced. Just compare what they do within a rapid. Typically, Rupert, the less-experienced boater, will start at the top of a rapid, point downstream, and go as fast as possible to the pool at the bottom, eyes big as dinner plates, hands holding the paddle so tightly that if it were coal, it'd be ready for a ring by the end of the run. Rupert will make it down the rapid, but he won't exactly have a good time.

Molly, a better boater, will do much more with the rapid. She'll catch tons of eddies. She'll surf a few waves and stern-squirt on an eddy line.

She might even throw a few quick points in a good-looking pourover. And she'll have a huge smile on her face the whole time. Remember Rule 1? Of course you don't. Here it is again:

Rule 1: The better you are, the more fun you'll have.

An experienced kayaker like Molly can turn an easy rapid into an incredible playground. Molly doesn't just survive the river—she styles it.

With that in mind, this chapter focuses on the fancy moves and little tricks that will have other boaters looking at you in awe, jealousy, and abject slobbering worship. Guaranteed.

For many people, playing is a huge part of the appeal of kayaking. Whether you're carving up a big glassy wave or cartwheeling in a huge hole, there's a sense of exhilaration, excitement, and challenge. Play-boating is incredibly addictive. It's easy to become what people call a "hole troll" or a "destination boater," a person who heads to one prime spot and stays there for hours and hours.

Playing is good for another reason, too. Not only is it intrinsically fun, playing forces you to become a much better boater. Playing demands a great deal of boat control. In general, the more you play, the more you learn about the way your boat reacts to the water, and the more your all-around kayaking improves. Also, you'll find that you'll be able to use certain play moves when running rapids. For example, if you need to head over to the other side of the river, you'll find a wave or a hole and surf it on over. If you feel yourself get back-endered, your experience with stern-squirting could help you twist around in order to stay upright.

If there's one move that's basic to almost all of freestyle paddling, it's surfing. Surfing is the key ingredient to a number of more complicated skills. If you have good control while you front- or side-surf, you'll have a much easier time when you start getting fancy. Long ago in the days of

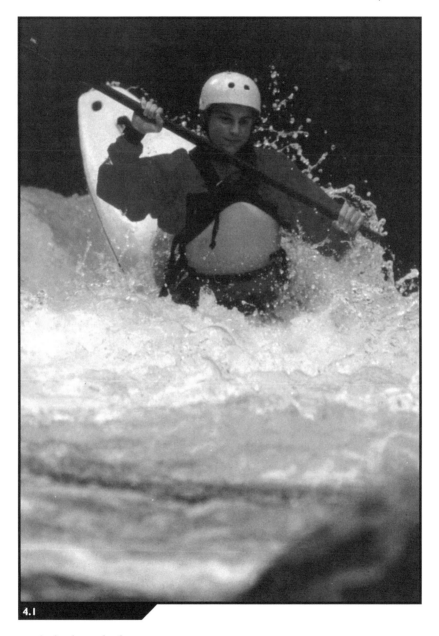

4.1

4.1 *A play-boater hard at work. Photo: Benjamin Miller. Boater: Mike Blatt* yore, you'd head out in your forty-foot boat to side-surf holes and front- or back-surf waves. No longer are we so limited! Now, you can surf either feature just about any way you want.

FRONT-SURFING

Often, the hardest part about front-surfing is getting on the wave or hole. There are three basic ways to start your ride.

Method one: Slide onto the target wave or hole from directly upstream. Select a lovely feature (let's imagine it's a wave for now) and turn around so that you are facing upstream. As the current starts to carry you closer to the target wave, paddle forward to slow yourself down. If you slow down enough, the wave will hold you as you drop into it. However, there's a drawback to this method: as your boat picks up momentum from the water in front of the wave you're trying to surf, you could miss the wave entirely, especially if you're in the middle of a big wave train—it's tough to overcome a powerful current by simply paddling upstream.

Method two: Ferry onto the target wave from an adjacent eddy. From the eddy, enter the current and begin your ferry. While you're ferrying, make sure to keep your eyes on the wave, so that you're aware of where you are relative to it. As soon as you're on the wave, use a little corrective stroke (usually on the side you were coming from) to adjust your angle—otherwise the wave will simply ferry you all the way across to the other side.

Method three: Combine aspects of methods one and two. As in method one, face upstream and paddle forward to kill your speed as you approach the wave. As in method two, you'll start slightly to the side of the wave so that paddling upstream will effectively ferry you toward the wave. Since you're ferrying to the wave, you'll be approaching the wave from the side—not from directly above it. Cut behind the wave in front of your target wave so that it won't mess up your speed or angle. This method takes a little practice, but it tends to work really well. You'll find it easy to catch waves even if there aren't any good eddies nearby.

So you've caught that perfect wave. Uh-oh— immediately, you encounter another problem. That wave just won't cooperate. Maybe your bow immediately gets sucked underwater. Or maybe you go flying off one edge of the wave at roughly the speed of sound. So what do you do in order to stay on the wave? And no, shrieking and screaming at the wave won't help. Believe me.

Surfing Tips

1. Relax.

2. Find the wave's "balance point," the place where you can sit still and make small adjustments without having to paddle frantically. There might not be much of a balance point on steeper, faster, or more irregular waves. But on the more user-friendly waves that you'll probably begin on, it shouldn't be too tough to find. As you improve, you'll have an easier time locking in on the balance point. This will make surfing much easier; you won't be working so hard to stay on the wave.

3. As soon as you start moving in one direction, use a correcting stroke (such as a stern draw or a pry) to bring your boat back the other way. If your strokes feel ineffective—if they don't bring you back like you want and you ferry off the wave—the problem probably isn't the stroke itself. Rather, the problem is that you've waited too long before making the correction. If you wait too long, too much turning momentum will build up. Once the boat starts moving in one direction, it's

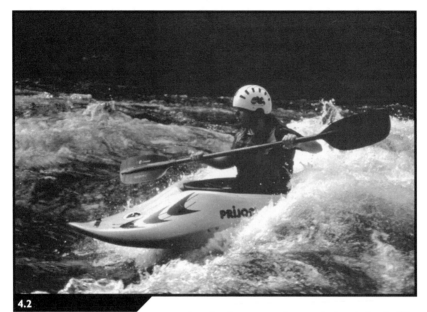

4.2

4.2 *After work on "The Wave." This kayaker keeps her weight forward to keep herself on the wave. Boater: Barbara Beran*

already almost too late to bring it back. The corrective stroke must be put in place immediately, or it's too late. In brief, you need to anticipate.

4. Remember your body. Keep your weight over the middle of your boat. If you're moving your upper body from side to side a lot, you'll have a tough time controlling the boat.

You don't want to just toss your weight around to either side, but there are times when shifting your weight *forward* or *back* can help. You can lean way back to keep your bow from dropping underwater. You'll still slide into the trough, but your bow will stay up. Or, you can lean way forward to keep the boat on the wave if it seems like the wave doesn't want to keep you.

5. Paddle less when you're on the wave. Instead of using lots of fast strokes, see how long you can keep one stroke in the water. By leaving the paddle in the water, you can keep adjusting your position without using lots of energy.

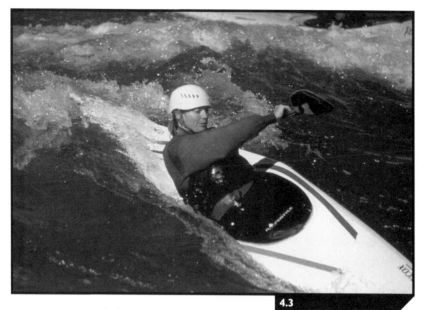

4.3

6. As you start to feel in control, close your eyes. This'll be weird at first, but bear with it. You'll get a much better feel for the interaction between your boat and the water.

7. Hand-surf. This will force you to do less with that pesky paddle.

You can also use your boat's edges. On steep waves, the boat sometimes "pearls"—it slides too far forward down the face of the wave, the bow catches, and you get endered off the wave. Alas. Carving can help fix this. If you angle the boat slightly to one side, and edge downstream, the boat won't pearl so easily; you'll simply carve from one side of the wave to the other. As soon as you stop carving in one direction, carve the other way; use a stroke (usually a back rudder on the side you want to go toward) to turn the boat, then edge the other way.

Have you ever skied down a mountain way too fast and felt out-of-control? (To be honest, I don't think I've ever skied and not felt like this.) To control your downhill speed, you can carve

4.3 This kayaker carves back and forth to keep from pearling. As she carves to her right, she keeps her left blade in the water in order to start carving back to the left. Photo: Philip Hart. Boater: Eileen Ash

from side to side, edging and turning in order to keep things in check. Surfing a wave works the same way—we edge and carve so that we don't fly down the face of the wave too quickly.

Carving up a big wave can be incredibly fun, especially in today's flat-bottomed, hard-chined boats. Like a slalom water-skier, you can actually send up big waves of spray. Everyone waiting in line to get on that great wave you're hogging will think this is the neatest thing since sliced bread, though they'll still want you to get off the wave so badly they'd physically hurt you if they thought they could get away with it.

A Fascinating Bit of Kayaking Etymology

"Pearling" refers to the practice of diving for pearls and other treasure. When a kayak is on a particularly steep wave, the end of the boat can pearl, or dive into the current.

BACK-SURFING

You'll be happy to know that back-surfing works the exact same way as front-surfing. You'll be sad to know it's a lot harder to do. With front-surfing, you're used to seeing what's going on while controlling your boat. No such luck in back-surfing. If you want to get better at back-surfing, it will help to simply do more moves backwards when you're just messing around in a rapid. Practice catching eddies backwards, do back-ferries, and so on. The more you get used to controlling your boat backwards, the easier it will be to back surf.

There's another hurdle to leap when you're trying to back-surf. A lot of boats today have a low-volume stern that just aches to sink underwater. The low stern can make things tough when back-surfing; it tends to catch and send you into a nice-looking but unintentional back-ender. The main thing you can do to prevent this is to keep your weight way forward--think about putting you chest to you skirt. you can also carve. Backwards. Use little forward strokes to keep from dropping too far into the trough. To change

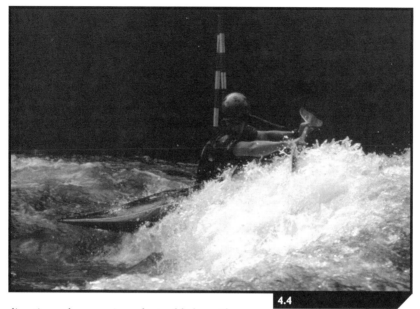

4.4

direction when carving, plant a blade as if starting a forward sweep (you'll want to plant the
blade on the side toward which you want to
move), then pull the stroke a few inches out,
away from the boat. This will turn the back of
the boat (we're back-surfing, remember?) in the
direction in which you wish to carve.

When back-surfing with a boat that doesn't
have a low-volume stern, the same rules apply. You
won't have to be so careful about pearling, but
everything works the same way—you'll just get an
extra chance to laugh at your pals who have been
stern-squirting on every single little insignificant
eddy line while you sat in the eddy glaring.

4.4 *The back-surfer keeps his
eyes on his stern as he surfs.
Photo: Steve Blatt. Boater:
Larry Norman*

SIDE-SURFING

Side-surfing can be a fun, bouncy, exciting ride
in which the boater controls one of the river's
scarier features—the hole. (Although we can
side-surf waves in many of the new boats out
there, I'm going to discuss side-surfing in holes,
just for the sake of that whole learning thing.)

Side-surfing can also be a frightening, unintentional thrashing in which a kayaker feels like a tiny piece of flotsam being slowly digested by a monster that makes the Sarlakian Pit (a dorky allusion to *Return of the Jedi*) look comical. Wherein lies the difference?

First of all, the kayaker (just for kicks, we'll call her Molly) chooses a user-friendly hole. The hole isn't too wide, probably isn't huge and violent-looking, and most importantly, does not have an extremely long backwash area. That is, the water that's recirculating back into the hole doesn't extend ten feet downstream of the hole.

Second, Molly is relaxed. Her hips are loose, her arms are held low, and, most importantly, she's smiling.

Third, Molly isn't trying to do all the work with her paddle. She's edging downstream just enough so that her upstream side doesn't get caught by the water coming into the hole from above. She's not edging downstream as far as possible, nor is she putting lots of pressure on a huge brace. Since she's balancing so wonderfully without her paddle, she's able to use her paddle to move around in the hole. She can take backstrokes if she wants to move backwards, or forward strokes if she wants to move ahead. In other words, Molly's weight is over her boat, not resting on her blades.

Remember: When you side-surf, you don't want to depend on your paddle for balance. If you lean on your paddle, you will be stuck! You won't be able to use your paddle to move in the hole. You'll be a great side-surfer because you won't be able to stop. Ever. Your friends will have to come back to the hole every few days to bring you sandwiches.

The trick to balanced side-surfing goes back to the edging technique described in the first chapter. To edge her boat, Molly uses her lower body. When side-surfing, Molly sinks into her downstream butt cheek, but lets her head tilt

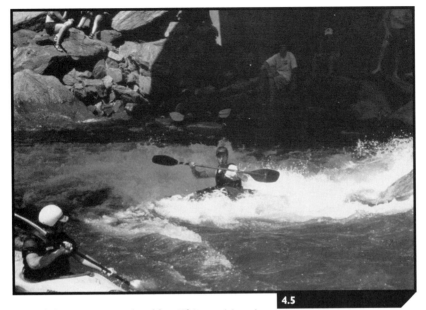

4.5

toward her upstream shoulder. This position is called the J-Lean because her body is in the shape of a **J**.

Learning to apply a steady J-Lean can be a wee bit hard, so here are some incredibly fun and fulfilling drills to help convince you that you can side-surf with the best of them without using your paddle for balance:

As in Chapter One, practice holding an edge on flatwater. See if you can hold an edge for fifteen seconds without using your paddle for support.

Once you've mastered this, try to move forward and back while holding your edge. Paddle forward for fifteen seconds then back for fifteen seconds while holding a steady edge. Only use the blade on the side you're edging toward.

Side-surf without that silly paddle. Hand-surfing will eliminate embarassing paddle dependence. If the idea of being in a hole without a paddle terrifies you, keep the paddle, but don't let it touch the water. Just hold the paddle low and loose.

4.5 *You don't need to use no stinkin' paddle when you side-surf! Boater: Aaron Napoleon*

Back to Molly and her incredible display of side-surfing excellence. There's one final thing at which Molly excels: she knows how to get out of that hole when she decides to allow someone else to have a turn. There are lots of ways to get out of a hole, some more embarassing than others. Often, the hole will let you go if you don't do anything to keep yourself in there. Sometimes flipping over will cause the water going under the hole to push against your body, sending you out of the hole. You might simply pull yourself forward or back until one end of your boat enters the current going around the hole; that end of your boat (the one in the current) will swing downstream, and you'll be able to paddle out. Or, if you're feeling especially cool, you can turn this into a 360-surf.

360-SURFING MADNESS

So let us commence. The trick to 360-surfing, like the trick to a lot of kayaking, is realizing that it's easy. If you can front-surf, side-surf, and do a little back-surfing, you're all set. You just have to combine these skills. First find a hole that will hold you, but one that is not so sticky that you can't move around in it. Ledge holes usually won't cut it. Look for a deep, fluffy hole with a decent amount of backwash (water flowing back into the hole). Once you've found that nice hole, here are some tips to make your quest for 360-surfing godliness all that much easier.

- For the most part, let the water do the work. When 360-surfing, all that you're doing is putting your boat in a good spot and staying upright. The only work necessary is an occasional stroke to keep yourself in the hole. This occasional stroke is usually necessary when going from a side-surf to a front- or back-surf. This is simply because a boat that is turned sideways doesn't move downstream as quickly as a boat pointing forward or backward. So, as you start back-surfing, you may need to take a few back-strokes to keep from washing out of the hole. And as you begin to front-surf, some strong forward strokes will help keep you in the hole.

- So where exactly is that "good spot"? This took me a long, painful time to learn, and it should for you, too. Ha, ha, ha, ha. No, no. Just a silly joke. In order to 360-surf, pick a spot where water kicks out of the hole, usually on one edge of the hole. If the hole is angled at all, use the upstream corner of the hole, which tends to be a little stickier.

- When you side-surf, make sure that you're moving slowly across the hole. If you let yourself gather too much speed, you'll simply end up rocketing out into the current. To slow your side-surf, simply take back-strokes on your downstream side.

- Keep looking at the water flowing into the middle of the hole. This will help orient you.

- Sit up tall and think about keeping your weight centered—no weight allowed on those blades, y'all.

- In general, use only your downstream blade. Taking an upstream stroke in the water flowing into the hole might teach you a really cool move: the window-shade, in which you do an upstream barrel roll at the speed of light.

Now that we've gone over some basic tips, it's time to get going.

Side-surf to back-surf. So, you're in the hole, side-surfing like you're sponsored. Start by facing the edge of the hole where you want to start your 360. Let the boat move slowly toward the hole's edge. If you're in a sticky hole, you'll have to paddle forward on your downstream side, but remember, don't let your boat move too quickly. The current going around the hole will grab the bow of your boat and swing you into a back-surf. Pretty nifty. Notice that you are not doing any stroke to turn yourself—the current going around the hole is making things happen. As the bow starts to swing downstream, take a big back-stroke on your downstream side to keep you from shooting out of the hole. Begin to lean forward and keep looking at the hole.

Back-surf to side-surf. In an ideal spot, you might have already set yourself up for a perfect 360. But if the hole (or your technique) is less than perfect, you might need to take a few strokes to make sure you don't wash out of the hole. Now you should have established yourself in a back-surf. Remember to keep looking at the hole, and keep your weight way forward (put

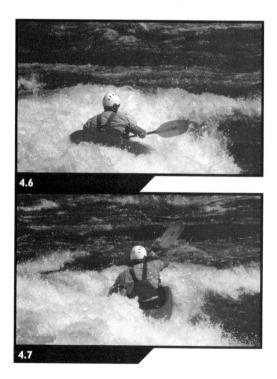

4.6 *The boater starts working his way toward the side of the hole. At first, he is on his left edge.*

4.7 *As his bow starts to swing downstream, he pushes back with his left paddle to keep himself in the hole.*

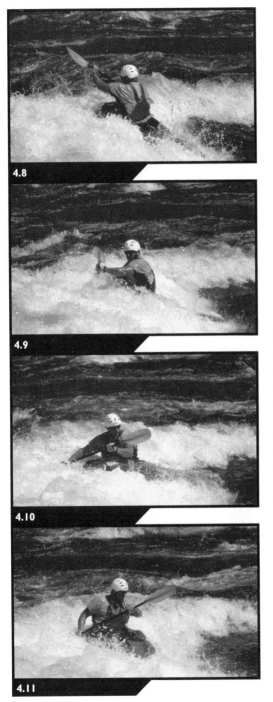

4.8 *As he starts to back-surf, he plants his right blade to keep the spin going. At the same time, he switches from his left to his right edge.*

4.9 *The boater keeps looking at the hole as he starts side-surfing on the right.*

4.10 *Using a sweep stroke on the right, he keeps himself in the hole as he swings back toward a front-surf.*

4.11 *When the boat comes back into the front-surf, the kayaker flattens the boat out. If he wants to spin again, he'll simply keep swinging the bow to his left and start edging left. Boater: Marc Lyle* your chest on your sprayskirt) so your stern doesn't go deep.

In order to complete the first half of the 360, take a strong forward sweep on the downstream. Make sure this is a sweep (keep the paddle low), not a simple forward stroke (which will tend to pull you out of the hole). Taa-daa! You're now side-surfing on the other side. In order to stay upright, you will need to have switched edges so that you're always edging downstream.

Knowing the proper timing for switching edges can be tricky. Erring in either direction can result in impromptu roll practice. Here's a good rule of thumb: as long as you can see the middle of the hole over your right shoulder, you should be edged left; as soon as you have to turn your head and look over the left shoulder in order to see the hole, you should edge to the right.

Side-surf to front-surf. Simply repeat what you did earlier, but backwards (gulp). Work the stern of your boat toward that magical place where the water kicks past the hole. To move your stern to the edge of the hole, you may have to paddle backwards. Let the current grab the stern and swing it downstream. Presto, you're front-surfing. You might need to take a few strokes in order to make sure you're still in the hole. Hopefully, you've remembered to switch edges. To go back to that original side-surf position, use a reverse sweep on the side where the hole is. You are now the proud owner of a beautiful new 360-surf.

Phew. That's a tough one to explain. If you don't feel like you caught all that, don't feel bad. Just send me lots of hate mail.

STERN-SQUIRTING

I love to stern-squirt. It's super fun, looks cool, and once you have the hang of it, is one of the easier play moves. It takes a wee bit of time to learn, though, because the stern-squirt is based on the opposite of what people learn when they start boating. Here's the general idea: as a boater crosses an eddy line, she edges her boat the "wrong" way (upstream if leaving an eddy, downstream if entering an eddy) then uses a strong back sweep to start moving the stern underwater.

In theory, you could stern-squirt in just about any boat design. In practice, however, a kayak with a sharp-edged, low-volume stern will make life much easier (and it won't have the annoying tendency to rip your shoulders out of their sockets). Any of today's play-boats will do fine.

Here's how it works:

1. Approach an eddy line. It's easier to learn by starting in an eddy and paddling toward the current, rather than the reverse. As you approach the eddy line, get some speed going. Try to hit the eddy line just a bit upstream of perpendicular. If you plan to err one way, point a bit further downstream than you think (the opposite is true when stern-squirting into an eddy). We want to cross the eddy line with a radical angle so that a lot of current hits the kayak at once, making this crazy move a bit easier. Also, exit the eddy close to the obstruction that creates it; the eddy line is usually more powerful there.

2. As you cross the eddy line, keep those eyes glued to the stern. The current will swing the bow of your boat downstream. As the stern crosses the eddy line, you will perform two moves simultaneously (if you had trouble with that whole chewing gum and walking thing, now's the time to head downstream to warm up the car for your pals). First, sink into your upstream butt cheek (that J-Lean again) so that your boat is edged upstream—the opposite of everything you know about leav-

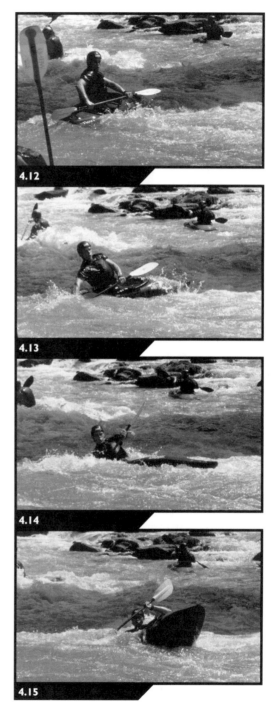

4.12 *Our stern-squirter has built up speed and is just about to cross the eddy line.*

4.13-4.15 *He pushes out with his reverse sweep in order to slice the stern underwater . . .*

ing eddies. Don't, don't, don't throw your body weight upstream. Just edge your boat by shifting your weight onto that upstream butt cheek. It's important to make sure that you hold this edge throughout the process. If you let it go too early, your stern-squirt will collapse. Second, at the same time as you edge, twist your body toward the stern on the downstream side and plant a big ol' reverse sweep. Make sure your body is really rotated toward that reverse sweep. In order to ensure rotation, keep looking at your stern. If you've really rotated into this stroke, you should be able to drop your paddle without it hitting your boat.

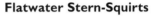

Flatwater Stern-Squirts

To reduce your already-astronomical stress levels, you can get a feel for the stern-squirt on flatwater. Get some speed going, then take a big reverse sweep while edging away from the stroke (if you reverse sweep on the right, edge toward the left). In order to make things easier, fill your boat partway up with water (don't use air bags, or the water will go to the bow).

3. By now, you should be starting to go vertical. Keep looking back at the stern, and keep your blades in the water for control.

Just as you can stern-squirt coming out of an eddy, you can squirt on the way in. The process is exactly the same, except reversed. Going into an eddy, you'll reverse sweep on the upstream side while sinking into your downstream butt cheek. It'll take some practice to get the timing down, but once you've got it, you'll be amazed by how effortless it is to get your boat vertical.

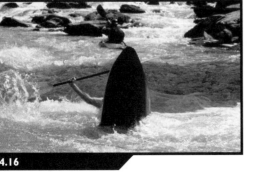

4.16 . . . *and the boat goes vertical. Boater: Rob Kelly*

How to Make That Already Insanely Cool Stern-Squirt into Pure Heaven

One of the neat things about stern-squirting is that you can combine the stern-squirt with some other moves in order to do some really great tricks. All of these tricks use the basic technique of the stern-squirt, with a few easy additions just for show. So, once you get the stern-squirt down, these moves will be so effortless you'll be bored. Here are a few tricks to try out:

Spinning on the Stern-Squirt. As you initiate the stern-squirt and begin to go vertical, your boat will start to turn. To keep the spin going, look over the shoulder in the direction that you are rotating. To prolong it, slice the paddle from the reverse sweep position to the bow-draw position. Now, simply use bow draws to keep spinning.

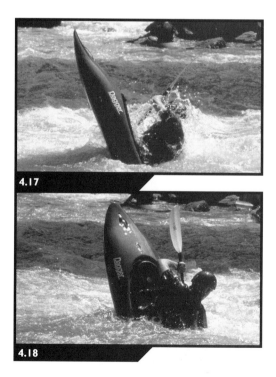

4.17 *Our loyal stern-squirter rotates while vertical by using a duffek on the side he spins toward. Note the lovely body rotation.*

4.18 *Rob keeps looking in the direction of the turn.*

The Screw-up. Easy. While you start to stern-squirt, smash your paddle as hard as you can across the bridge of your nose. Within a few seconds, you should be bleeding and semiconscious—very hip. No, no—please don't do this. I'll feel terrible. Actually the screw-up is not too tough, though it may look hard. With a normal stern-squirt, you can easily fall all the way over backwards as you spin on your axis. No big deal, but you can do a screw-up to get upright more quickly. As you feel yourself begin to flop over, start a roll. If timed correctly, you'll roll upright just as you fall over. Make sure that you're rolling on the side that will allow you to keep the momentum of your rotation going. That is, don't try to roll going the opposite way from the way your boat is spinning.

Splatting. Again, not hard. Approach a benign-looking rock (one that you won't get pinned on or under) with some current pushing into it. There are a number of ways to splat, but here's the easiest. Paddle toward the rock at about a 45-degree angle. Just before you would hit the rock, sink into your upstream butt cheek (remember, don't lean your upper body weight upstream) and use a big forward sweep on your upstream side. As your bow rides up on the rock, stop edging so that your kayak lands on the rock flat. Presto! You're splatted against the rock like a bug on a windshield. Again, make sure you pick a

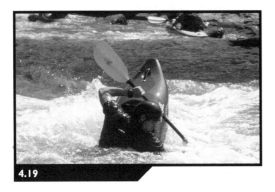

4.19

4.19 *He draws his right blade to the boat in order to make his boat spin. Boater: Rob Kelly*

4.20 – 4.23 *As the boater nears the rock, he edges slightly upstream and sweeps to sink his stern.*

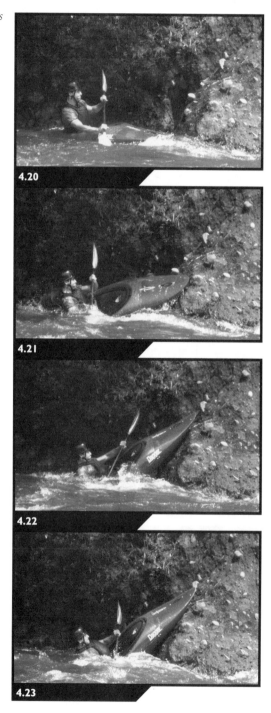

4.20

4.21

4.22

4.23

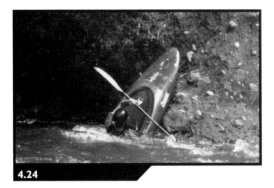

4.24 *Once vertical, he uses his paddle blades to maintain control. Boater: Ben Solomon.*

good rock; if in doubt about a certain place, don't try it! Trying to splat is not worth getting sucked under an undercut or getting pinned above a hard rapid.

Blasting holes. This is the same move as the splat—you're just performing the move on the face of a ledge-hole, not a rock. The idea here is to get vertical in a hole so that you're facing upstream. Approach the hole from one side. You'll want to initiate the move as close to the hole as you can get without actually being right in the hole. To get vertical, use a big forward sweep on your downstream side, and edge toward that stroke. This will get you vertical. Now, to stay there, keep your weight back and use your paddle to keep you from falling toward one side.

Rocket Moves. Head downstream on a wave train. When you get to the crest of a wave, it naturally lifts the boat upwards. To get some verticality, just as you reach the crest, throw in a big ol' forward sweep while you edge your boat toward that stroke. This will pull your stern down, and you'll go vertical as you pass over the wave's peak.

That's enough for now. Take a well-deserved break from trying to decipher my directions. Go hit that river.

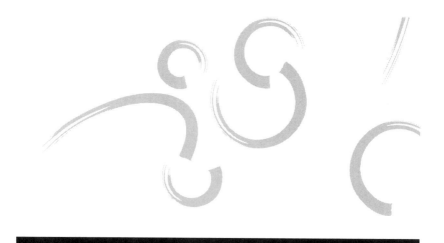

5

Still More Playing Techniques: "All's Well that *Ends* Well"

Today's funky little rodeo boats are mind-boggling. With a lot of today's designs, the craziness can go on just about anywhere in the river. These boats are begging to do all sorts of insane tricks and would love to take you along for the ride. But for the sake of learning (this is supposed to be educational, remember?), let's begin with a river feature that will make life a little easier: the hole. But before you go screaming into that hole, make sure of a few things:

- The hole's deep enough to get your bow down. Hitting rocks is no fun; you'll bang up that pretty boat, and your ankles won't feel too great either.

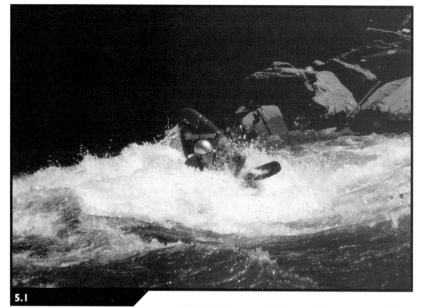

5.1

5.1 *A honed, freestyle athelete gets the point at Hell Hole. Boater: Bill Edmonds.*

- The hole's powerful enough to get your bow down. It's got to have some kick. In general, if the water pouring into the hole from upstream is relatively steep, you're good to go.

- You can get out of the hole when you want. It's no fun to be stuck doing an indefinite side-surf ten minutes after you tried to go in for a few quick cartwheels.

- An added bonus (though this isn't absolutely necessary) is easy access to the hole, such as big eddies on one or both sides. There's nothing more frustrating than being just downstream of the perfect hole, with no way to get back in. The horror. The horror.

All right. You're ready to rip that hole apart. Let's start with the easiest stuff first.

ENDER

The first step is to work on that setup. Start in the eddy and get your boat right on the edge of the hole, but not in it. You should be able to sit just outside the hole so that you only have to move your body weight forward to initiate. A common error is screaming into an ender spot at Mach Five Billion. For every action there is an equal and opposite reaction. So if you fly into the hole with tons of force, the hole will fly right back at you; you'll find it tough to control your boat.

On the other hand, be aggressive about getting into that hole. Again, that doesn't mean you have to paddle as hard as you can into the hole. Rather, stay in control of your boat; keep your paddle in the water so that the swirly water behind the hole doesn't push you off-line. A common problem that people have when going for enders is being wishy-washy. That hole seems pretty violent up close, and the eddy downstream looks awfully nice. So people don't really go for it, and the river shows them who's really in charge. You'll have to find the mean between extremes. Don't tear into the hole like a spastic buffalo. Take your time, but when you do initiate, go for it.

Now, as you initiate, keep your kayak straight. That is, you want your boat lined up so that you are parallel to the flow of the water going into the hole. If you don't enter the hole parallel to the flow, you'll be spun sideways. Sometimes the hole will be angled, so take a quick look before you hop in. Your sinuses will thank you for being patient.

The final step is to lean forward as you enter the hole. A little scary, maybe, but you've gone too far to turn back. No chickening out now. Getting your weight forward will help sink your bow. If all goes well, your bow will drop down, you'll go vertical, and then the volume of your bow will pop it up out of the water. Huge air. The crowd goes wild.

Once you've got that ender going, you can fine-tune things as you go up. If you want to go all the way over (past vertical), keep leaning

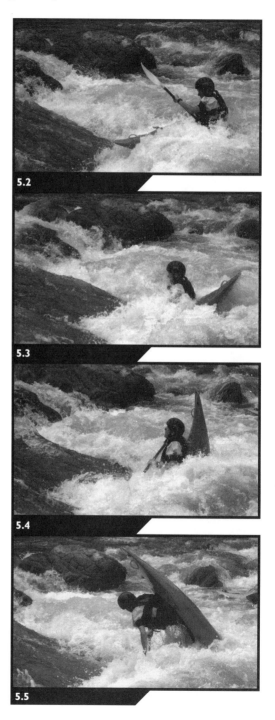

5.2 – 5.3 *To initiate an ender, the boater keeps her boat parallel with the current and leans forward, allowing the bow to sink.*

5.4 *The boater brings her weight back to slow things down . . .*

5.5 *. . . Then throws herself forward to go up and over. Photo: Ben Solomon. Boater: Laura Hayes* forward—your weight will force the boat all the way over until you flip. Or, to keep the angle of your boat less than vertical (that water's cold, right?), simply lean back once you've initiated your bow. Remember: keep your paddle in the water while you're initiating. A play-boater without a paddle is literally a ship without a rudder.

A short postscript. Obviously, a hole is not the only place to get that big ender. A steep wave will serve the purpose as well. When you front-surf on a steep wave, you've probably noticed that your boat wants to pearl, or dive, into the trough. If you want to turn this to your advantage, simply keep your boat straight, lean forward, aid the process by paddling, and get vertical. Nifty. Again, just make sure to keep the boat straight or you'll just get peeled off or end up practicing your roll.

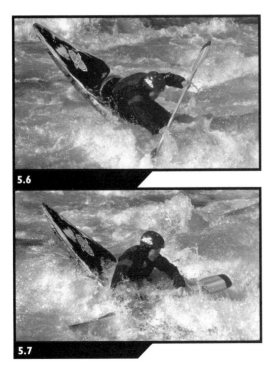

5.6 – 5.7 *For less vertical enders, this kayaker brings her weight back after she initiates. Photos: Phillip Hart. Boater: Hannah Kim*

PIROUETTE

Now we'll get a little more complicated. When we get that fancy ender, we can spin on our long axis. This move, called the pirouette, is great, but requires good control. Like a lot of kayaking, what you do with your paddle during the pirouette is important. But what you do with your body is even more important.

To start that pirouette, first you need to be able to get a solid, vertical ender on command, so you'll start things out just like you're trying to get a big ol' ender. (Hopefully, you're feeling pretty relaxed about enders. Piece of cake, right?) Here's the trick to spinning on your bow. As you begin to get vertical, simply lean back so that your back is against the deck of your boat. It will look like you're standing up, and your weight will be on your foot pegs. The reason you want to lean back against your back deck is the same reason figure skaters pull their arms in when they spin. By bringing all your weight to the center, your center of gravity isn't so spread out, and you'll be able to rotate quickly on a central point.

Now, here's the key: as you go vertical, look hard over your shoulder in the direction you want to spin. If you lead with your head, your shoulders and the rest of your body will follow; the head motion is the secret to the pirouette. When you want to spin, look as far as possible in the direction of the turn. Don't lean your body weight toward the spin—just rotate your head, like a dog trying to chase its own tail.

Which way should you try to spin? Which shoulder do you look over? Well, it depends on the way the water is pushing. If the current going into that wonderful play-hole you've found is kicking to river right (your left if you're pointing upstream), you're probably starting from river left of the hole. So the current will be naturally wanting to spin you to your left. It'd be nice of you to play along, helping the current in its quest. Look over your left shoulder. Pirouette city.

So far, we haven't even mentioned that paddle. I actually find that it's a lot easier to pirouette without a paddle; you don't have a huge stick in your way as you try to spin. But you can use your paddle to help drive that pirouette around.

There are two ways to use the paddle. We'll start with the simplest stroke, basically a reverse sweep. As your boat pops up, use a reverse sweep on the side toward which you want to spin. If you want to pirouette in a place where the water is kicking to your left, keep your left blade in the water as you initiate, and push from behind as you start to go vertical. Remember to look over your shoulder and rotate your body—that's more important than the paddle action. This stroke will help the spin a bit, but it won't do much; it's a

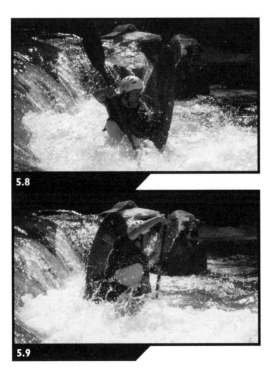

5.8 – 5.9 *To pirouette, look over your shoulder in the direction of the spin. Boater: Chuck Derosa.*

short, relatively weak movement.

We do have a more dynamic, but much more complicated, stroke at our beck and call. If you want to get really crazy, you can use a crossbow draw to get the spin going. The crossbow draw is a stroke borrowed from canoeists. The idea is to reach across your body, plant your paddle, and pull water toward the front of your boat. The stroke is basically a bow draw that uses the opposite paddle blade.

Back to the crossbow pirouette. If you're spinning to your left, you'll reach across your body and plant your right paddle blade on the left side of your boat. As you initiate, you'll pull your right blade toward the front of your boat. The trick to lovely crossbow pirouettes is anticipation: plant that crossbow stroke even before you initiate the ender. Get the crossbow in the water before you even start to get vertical.

A common crossbow ailment is leaning your body weight way over the side, toward the crossbow stroke. Letting your weight fall way over the side won't allow you to pirouette, but you will be able to do another groovy trick, the "fall-flat-on-your-face-before-you-initiate wheel." To keep in control, rotate your upper body hard with the crossbow and keep your body weight over the center of your boat.

All of this might be a little hard to visualize— and I'm sorry. In the instructional video *Retendo*, Kent Ford mentions a great way to figure the pirouette out: put yourself in less-intimidating surroundings. Head to some flatwater and fill your trusty kayak up with water. You should be able to get vertical on your bow just by leaning forward and paddling. When you're vertical, practice making yourself spin. Try to make your boat spin on end without using a paddle. Now try to pirouette using your paddle. The motion of the pirouette is the same on flatwater as in a hole—the only difference is the manner in which you got your boat vertical. Working on

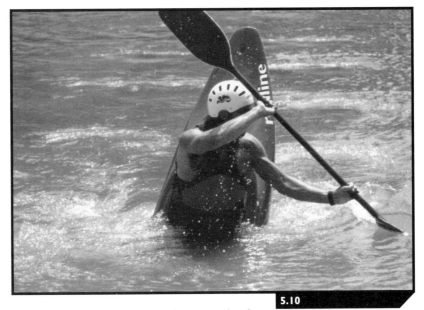

5.10

these moves in flatwater will help tremendously; without a hole trying to slap you around, you'll have the time and the nerve to learn these tricks.

5.10 *Working on vertical moves in flatwater. Boater: Jimmy Leithauser.*

ZEE CARTWHEEL

A few years back, cartwheeling became the hot new move. Instead of just trying to get big air from an ender, the idea was to get vertical on the bow, then get vertical on the stern, then on the bow, and so on, ad infinitum, ad nauseam.

Learning the cartwheel takes some time. But it's worth it—I guarantee. Once you have a good grasp on how to cartwheel, you'll be able to "throw down points" (cartwheel) in any ender spot. In fact, with today's incredible boat designs, you can cartwheel in flatwater (more about that later). In general, shorter "rodeo" boats make cartwheeling much easier, but you can do cartwheels in just about anything.

Go back to that hole where you got those great enders. A pourover-type hole will work best at first, simply because you won't be actually surfing in the hole until you initiate the cartwheel. Here's the play-by-play:

1. Initiate the ender (the bow "point") just as before.

2. As you initiate, perform the second half of a reverse sweep, starting wide at your side and pushing toward your toes. The hole will tend to push in one direction—that's the way you want to cartwheel. If the hole is pushing to your left (river right), your first stroke will also be on the left. Don't just push down. If you push down, you'll just send yourself up and out of the hole. Instead, concentrate on a wide turning-type stroke.

3. That first stroke will get you rotating in the direction of the cartwheel. As you rotate, make sure you're always looking at the hole! In our example, as you start to turn toward your left, look back over your right shoulder toward the hole. Just like 360-surfing, you want to keep those eyes on the hole. In fact, cartwheeling uses a lot of the same techniques as 360-surfing. You've just decided to elevate your boat enough to show off.

A Rodeo Boater Speaks Out:

"I'd like to say that cartwheeling stirs great emotions, but it's just plain silly fun."

—*Shane Williams, Team Perception*

4. What you've done so far will elevate the boat and turn you around so that the stern lands in the hole. As the stern starts to initiate (you will know when this happens because you will be looking at the hole!), plant the first half of a forward sweep on the other side of the reverse sweep. In our example, you're cartwheeling to the left, so you initiated with a reverse sweep on your left. Your next stroke would be the first part of a forward sweep on the right. Take this stroke early. The early bird gets the cartwheel. A common problem that people have is that as soon as they get vertical on the bow, they stop doing anything. You can

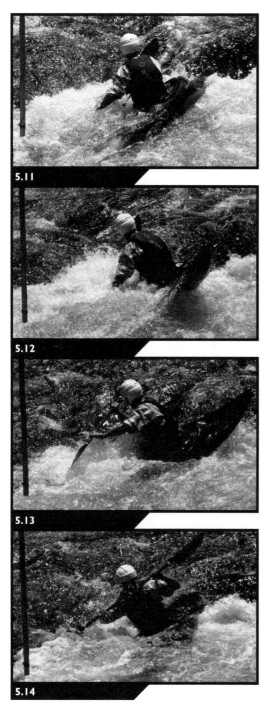

5.11 *A fast learner sets up the cartwheel. Notice the first stroke.*

5.12 – 5.13 *As he initiates, he pushes toward his toes with his left blade and keeps looking at the hole.*

5.14 *As his stern starts swinging into the hole . . .*

do one cartwheel if you initiate well and then freeze. But if you want to do more than one cartwheel, or stay in better control, you'll have to be a little more active.

5. You've entered the hallowed halls of the cartwheel. Call up your paddling buddies and gloat until they refuse to have anything to do with you. Alienating your friends is by far the best part of rodeo paddling.

6. That's one cartwheel. Multiple-point cartwheels follow the same recipe. If you executed Step 4 perfectly, your stern will swing out of the hole, and your bow will start to go back in. To keep cartwheeling, quickly shift back to the original position, placing your weight forward and planting the second half of a strong reverse sweep.

I hope that long explanation made some slight bit of sense. Here are some general ideas to keep in mind when you're throwing down points:

• Keep your eyes on the hole. I can't repeat myself enough. If you make sure you're always looking at the hole, your body naturally will be perfectly rotated to allow the boat to keep the cartwheel going. Often, cartwheeling hopefuls look downstream way too soon. If you look downstream early, you'll tend to move out of the hole, making retentive moves (like the cartwheel) tough.

• Take your time. Don't rush blindly into the hole. Be aggressive about it, but move into the hole methodically, making sure you're doing what's necessary to get a cartwheel.

• Don't get frustrated. Chances are that learning to cartwheel will take a bit of time, but it's better than sitting in a cubicle, glaring at the clock. If you're having a tough time, take a break. Rome wasn't built in a day.

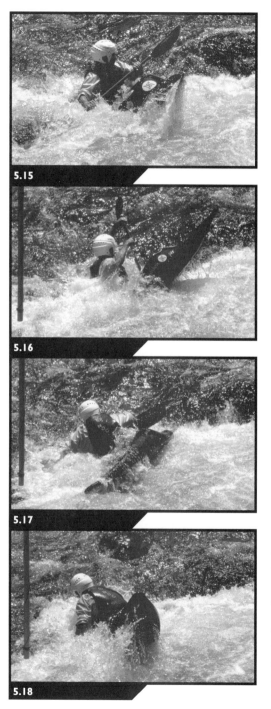

5.15 . . . *he uses the first half of a forward sweep on the right to keep the cartwheel going.*

5.16 – 5.18 *He keeps the cartwheel gong by simply coming back to Step 1. Boater: Shane Benedict*

Advancing beyond two-point cartwheels is tricky. One big stumbling block is leaning way back. Often, we try to throw our weight back to drive the stern under. This is fine for a single cartwheel, but will tend to make you back-ender all the way up and over, throwing you out of the hole. As the stern enters the hole, keep your weight way forward (as in a 360) to stay balanced.

Here's another tip to help you keep cartwheeling after two points: throw that third point *early*. As soon as you finish your second stroke (a forward sweep), go ahead and start trying to bring the bow back under: bring your weight way forward and start the back sweep. Don't wait until the bow comes all the way around to slice it under.

Let's review. So far, we've talked about a lot of things we could do in one specific place. If we found an appropriate play spot, like a deep, fluffy hole, we have a pretty big bag of tricks from which to draw. We could front-surf, side-surf, back-surf, 360-surf, ender, pirouette, and cartwheel. As they say up north, "wicked." If you've practiced a lot at any of these individual moves, you'll find that, as long as you're in a good spot, you don't have too much trouble. The problem comes when you try to stay in the hole in order to link these different moves. It takes lots of practice to be able to stay in a good play spot and combine a number of moves without getting flushed out.

I remember a fine summer day during the start of my play-boating career. I had driven over to Hell Hole in Tennessee, an absolutely terrific play spot on the Ocoee River. Hell Hole can get pretty crowded; everyone goes there to mess around, from the world's best rodeo boaters to folks who haven't quite gotten the hang of their roll. You have to time your turns between rafts going through the hole. And to top it off, since the Ocoee is a roadside run, there are usually at least a dozen spectators. Typically, the onlookers

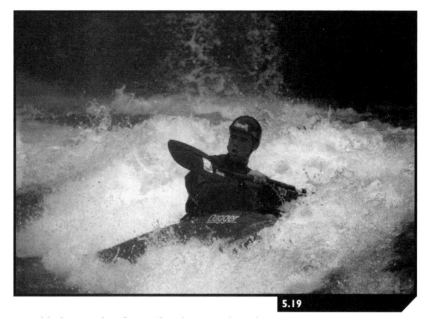

5.19

5.19 *Eyes on the hole. Boater: Rob Kelly*

are elderly couples from Florida, armed with camcorders and wearing flowered shirts, who are trying to figure out why you keep trying to go upstream. It's a zoo. On this particular day, I was doing my usual flailing, so I sidled up to one of the really amazing paddlers there and asked him for a few tips. He sneered at me from beneath his glittery helmet and said, "Stay in the hole. Here endeth the lesson."

My new pal's tip wasn't too helpful at the time, although he was absolutely right. I've thought a lot about what he said, and I've tried to come up with some more concrete tips about how exactly to stay in that hole.

- I just love to repeat myself. It takes up space, so I feel like I'm accomplishing something. Keep looking at the hole. I was having an awful time at our local rodeo spot one day, until my friend Rob Kelly, an absolutely amazing boater, pointed out that I needed to lock my eyes on the green water pouring into the hole. It's amazing what a difference just looking at the hole makes. If you don't remember this right now, don't worry. I'm sure I'll say it again several times. Except for a few moves, such as splitwheels and blunts, you should always look at the hole.

- Keep your body loose and centered above the boat. A common problem is that we let our upper-body weight rest on our blades. If you let your weight shift too far to either side, you'll tend to lose control. Don't move the boat by throwing your weight to the sides.

- Study the hole! You can further your quest for rodeo mastery by looking carefully at the hole and what others are doing in it (besides being painfully window-shaded). Figure out which side is better for cartwheels, or 360s, or whatever. Find spots that won't hold you in the hole as easily. A lot of this information is hard to deduce at first; you'll need to get in that hole for some trial-and-error work. When errors happen, use them to better understand the hole. The more you understand about the hole, the longer you'll be able to stay in and the more you'll be able to do.

- Initiate vertical moves early. In other words, initiate so that your boat doesn't go deep into the water pouring into the hole. Throw points early, while you're surfing on the top of the hole, rather than down in the trough (the bottom part of the hole). If your boat goes too deep, the water going under and out of the hole will have a better chance to push you out.

- Stay upright. If you flip, the current going underneath and out of the hole will have a good target (your body). So try not to go over. It's also harder to breathe underwater.

- If you feel that you're starting to flip, the natural instinct is to try to brace to stay upright.

In a hole, the brace might keep you upright, but you could easily get flushed out of the hole. Instead of bracing, simply go with the momentum. Do a full roll. And here we introduce a new skill: the back-deck or rodeo roll.

THE BACK-DECK ROLL

The back-deck roll is much faster than the standard C-to-C or sweep roll, but you sacrifice safety for speed: in the back-deck roll, you completely abandon your tuck so that your face and chest are exposed to nasty things lurking underwater. The bottom line is this: don't try a back-deck roll unless you're absolutely sure you're in deep water (I speak from rather miserable experience). With that in mind, let's figure out how to do this sucker.

1. Start by planting a duffek. Now lean back a bit and rotate toward the water on the side on which you've set the stroke. Cock the top wrist all the way back, like you're revving a motorcycle (otherwise, your paddle won't get any purchase from the water). As you start to flip, look back over the shoulder on the side you're flipping toward (if you're flipping to the left, look over your left shoulder). Rotate as far as possible. When you flip, your chest should hit the water first.

2. Hold this position as you roll; your body will pass under the boat.

3. You can start the actual roll even before your body comes all the way to the surface. Leaving your nonworking hand (in this case, the left) low and relaxed, pull your working blade (right) from the back to the front of your boat, and bring your body forward with the paddle. Your chest actually acts as a big planing area, another paddle blade, to torque yourself up. Make sure that you drop your head

toward the working shoulder (the right shoulder), just as you would in a boring, ordinary, everyday roll. Another way to think of the motion is that you start by twisting and leaning back. Then, as you roll, you sit up and untwist.

4. You're up! If you've done a swell job, you'll still be in the hole, about to continue shredding.

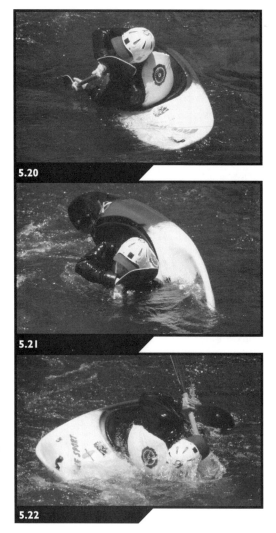

5.20 – 5.21 *As he flips, the kayaker goes into the back-deck setup.*

5.22 *The roller sweeps forward and ends up with his head to his right shoulder. Boater: Craig Parks*

The back-deck roll may seem strange at first, but it's actually just the reverse of a sweep roll. In a sweep roll, you start tucked forward, and you lean back as you bring the paddle from front to back. In a back-deck roll, you start back and sweep the paddle forward in order to come up.

I want to repeat the fact that you should only use this roll in situations where you won't hurt yourself. I know from painful experience that there are definitely times when a back-deck roll is not the best option. When I head for a creek run after I have spent too much time practicing rodeo, I tend to immediately go to a back-deck roll whenever I start to go over. While this is fine if I'm at Rock Island, I'm not quite as happy when I use that fancy back-deck roll on a shallow creek.

FLAT SPINS

Now that we've perfected our hole technique, let's move back to the wave and figure out one more move. Sometimes called wave 360s, flat spins are very similar to hole 360s. However, flat spins require more control because the wave won't hold you as well as a hole will. Flat spins are not one of the easiest play-boating moves. But they look way cool. And since the reason we paddle is to look cool, we simply must learn to flat spin.

First of all, your choice of boat can be important. It will help a lot if the boat is relatively short and wide, with a flat bottom and hard chines. Most of the new-generation rodeo boats will serve the purpose, as long as you've found a good wave.

Second, it's tough to flat spin on any wave. The wave should be pretty steep—the kind of wave that you have to be really active on in order not to get endered out. In general, the bigger the wave, the better. Naturally, the better your technique, the more waves you'll be able to 360 on.

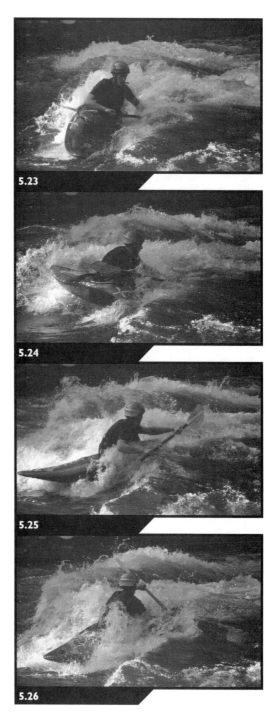

5.23 – 5.25 *Starting with a little angle toward the spin, the kayaker uses a reverse sweep to start the move.*

5.26 – 5.28 *To keep the spin going, the boater plants a forward sweep at his toes, while looking back at the wave.*

One side note: With both flat spins and 360s in holes, you may not be able to do the entire spin in one motion. Often, you'll have to spin halfway around, then pause to get your boat repositioned, and only then will you be able to do the second half of the spin. Be patient—don't force the move if you aren't in position.

The body motion when you flat spin is actually not too different from when you cartwheel. Since we are all now cartwheeling demigods, the

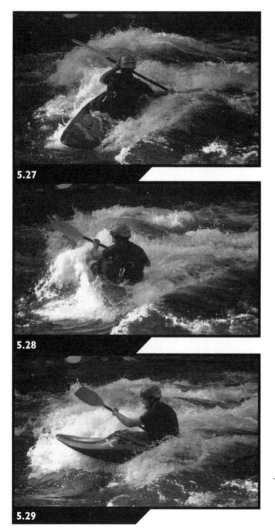

5.27

5.28

5.29

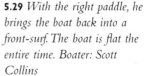

5.29 *With the right paddle, he brings the boat back into a front-surf. The boat is flat the entire time. Boater: Scott Collins*

flat spin should be no problem. Here's how to flat spin:

1. Start by front-surfing on the crest of the wave, so that when you are ready, you can slide down into the trough. In order to cheat things a bit (as my high school tennis coach used to say, "If you're not cheating, you're not trying"), have a little angle in the direction you plan to spin.

2. You want to initiate the spin as soon as you start down toward the trough. Keep your weight forward, and use a wide, powerful reverse sweep on the side to which you're spinning. This is similar to the motion that initiates a cartwheel. Keep the boat nice and flat so that it will spin easily; if you edge, your spin will be way too slow to work.

Which Way Should I Spin?

Start on the steepest part of the wave. You'll want to spin toward a part of the wave which is slightly flatter. By sticking your nose into the flatter (faster-moving) part of the wave, the water will help you spin.

3. This should get you a 180—now you're back-surfing. To keep the spin going, use a big forward sweep on the opposite side of the initial reverse sweep. Seems easy, doesn't it? The motion is no big deal; if you can keep the boat flat and do a reverse sweep on one side, then a forward sweep on the other, you've got it. The trick is timing: it's tougher to stay on the wave if you don't spin as you slide down to the trough.

4. Now you've 360ed. Congratulations. That wasn't so hard, now was it?

Typically, it's not too hard to figure out the first half of the flat spin, but the second half can be much more difficult. Here's a tip that Eric Jackson, an incredible boater, told me when I was having a tough time figuring out the flat spin: as the stern begins to come around, wait until you are almost side-surfing before making a turning stroke. The problem is that most folks are just not being patient. When you spin from the front-surf, you start with a little angle for two reasons.

First, angle allows you less distance to spin. Second, if you have angle, the turning stroke will just spin you. If you're straight, the stroke will turn you, but it will also pull you downstream, off the wave. So be patient: don't spin the boat back around until the stern has already swung pretty far in the direction of the spin.

That's all for now. Tune in next chapter for another enthralling edition of play-boating.

6

Tear the Roof Off: More Freestyle Techniques

ROCK SPINS

Rock spins, or 360-boofs, are the sick and twisted half-sister of the traditional boof. In a regular boof, the idea is to drive your boat onto an obstruction, like a rock, in order to get where you want to be. With a rock spin, the rock is where you want to be; you drive your boat onto a rock, do a full 360, and fall off. On a really great rock, you can even spin more than once. I've seen a friend get almost three full rotations on a perfectly shaped rock. Pretty impressively, compared to my meager attempts.

As usual, the first order of business is to find a

good place to ply your trade. When starting out, look for a rock with a large, flat surface area, one with a little current pushing into it (but not too much), and one that isn't too high above the water (the higher the rock is, the harder it will be to get your boat onto it in order to spin). You should feel like you can easily drive about half of your boat up onto the target rock.

Now that you've found a lovely rock, let us spin. Here's the recipe:

1. The first thing you'll want to do is get that boat up on the rock. With strong forward strokes, drive your boat onto the rock until your butt is on the rock. Your butt acts as the pivot point, the place around which you'll rotate. Getting the right amount of kayak up on the rock will take some practice. If you drive too much boat on the rock, you'll be high and dry. Too little and you won't be able to spin—you'll just fall off. In general, people

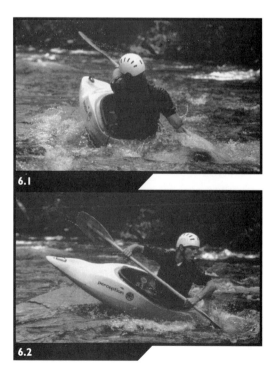

6.1 *The boater drives the boat onto the rock.*

6.2 – 6.4 *Using a powerful reverse sweep on the side toward which he will turn, the boater starts the spin. Notice his body rotation.*

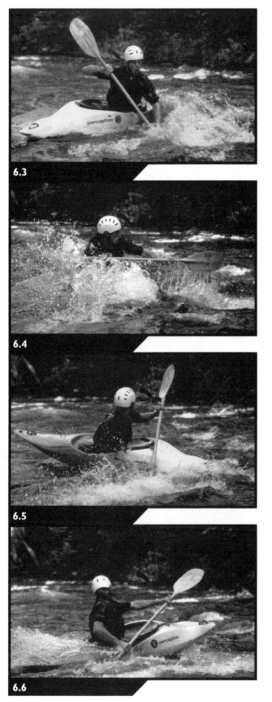

6.5 *A forward sweep keeps the boat spinning* . . .

6.6 . . . *finishing the 360.* *Boater: Bryan Jennings*

tend not to drive enough of their boat onto the rock. Be aggressive: get that kayak on that rock.

2. Cheat that spin a little bit. As you drive onto the rock, get that boat pointed hard in the direction you want to spin. If you want to spin to the right, you should have a lot of right angle as you paddle up onto the rock. To get this angle, take a forward sweep on the left as you hit the rock. This stroke will drive you further onto the rock and will give you some angle toward the spin. If you've got a lot of angle as your butt gets up on the rock, you've already performed a good bit of the spin.

3. Now you're on the rock, pointed toward the right side of the river. As soon as you get on that rock (or even an instant before), look hard in the direction of the spin so that your body is wound up, like a spring. This rotation will help the spin get going. You have a lot of energy stored up in your rotation. To unleash that energy, throw in a big reverse sweep on the upstream side. If everything has gone perfectly, you might already have the spin.

As your bow comes around so that you're facing upstream, throw your weight way forward. That way, your bow will slice underwater when it hits the current coming into the rock. If you don't lean forward, the water might hit the front of your boat and stop the spin in its tracks. As you get better, you'll be able to do fully vertical "splat-wheels," in which you cartwheel against a rock.

4. To keep that spin going, simply use a big forward sweep on the other side. Remember to keep looking in the direction of the spin.

5. Drop off the rock and head downriver, desperately scanning the horizon for more rocks to spin on.

Keep spinning until you fall off. Once you've spent a bit of time practicing this skill, you'll find that it's not too hard to get a full spin, as long as you've found a good rock. And every once in a while, you'll be able to get multiple spins.

EDDY-LINE CARTWHEEL

Once the exclusive property of squirt-boaters and folks getting trashed in Chile or Nepal, today's boats make it possible to cartwheel like a madman on eddy lines. In fact, with good technique, one can even throw points on a lake. The eddy line makes things a little easier, though: the bow will sink better in an eddy line than in flatwater.

The move is not difficult, but takes good timing and balance. You already know most of the moves required; if you can splat and cartwheel, you're all set. Here's the story:

1. Starting in an eddy, get your speed going. You'll want to leave the eddy line near the top (where it's powerful), pointed a few degrees downstream from parallel with the current. In other words, think about leaving with a conservative ferry angle.

2. Guess what? You can throw either way. If you're having trouble getting the bow down, throw toward the current (if the eddy line is on your left, throw right). If you can slam the nose down like Kobe Bryant, and you want to get tons of points, go the same direction (but not with you upper body!) as the current (if the eddy line is to your left, throw left). To throw, edge hard in one direction and take a powerful forward sweep to lift your bow up (the same motion you do when splatting a rock). Get that bow up just before you hit the eddy line. Make sure that your strokes stay up toward the front of your boat. A stroke in the back will tend to throw your timing off and cause you to bring your weight too far back.

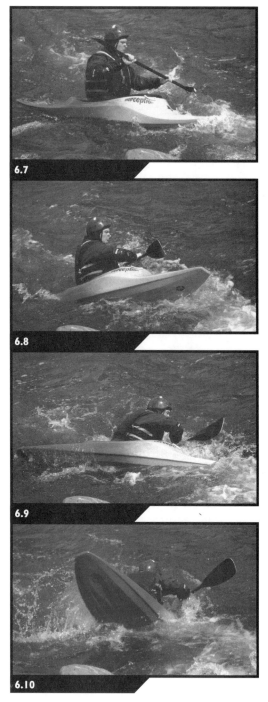

6.7 *The boater approaches the eddy-line with good speed and appropriate angle.*

6.8 *Boater lifts bow up just before eddy line . . .*

6.9 – 6.10 *. . . and slams it down with a reverse sweep. Notice the edge!*

3. Just as you cross the eddy line, slam the bow down by pushing your paddle from wide at your side in toward your toes (the first stroke in a cartwheel). As you take the stroke, throw your body weight as far forward as possible. Keep the boat edged hard, but don't lean your body weight out to the side. Thou shalt only use your lower body to lean the boat! Otherwise, you're practicing your roll.

   This should get your bow down (within about a trillion attempts, at least). One hint: don't look downstream. Instead, look at your opposite foot. So, if you're eddy-wheeling to the left, look at your right foot. This will keep your weight centered and forward.

4. As your bow drops and then starts to resurface, use a strong sweep stroke on the other side while edging toward that stroke. This is the exact same move as the second stroke in a cartwheel. And just as in a cartwheel, you'll pull the stern under with the second stroke.

5. If you're in the mood, repeat steps three and four for as many points as your heart desires. Once you know how to eddy-wheel, you can do all sorts of weird things, like free-wheels (cartwheels as you go over a waterfall) and wave-wheels (see below).

WAVE-WHEELS

The wave-wheel, one of the hot new moves on the market, is ready for your consumer enjoyment. When I first saw the wave-wheel, I was baffled. Somehow, the boat cartwheels end-over-end while cruising down a wave train. Weird. I asked my pal Jay Maroney how to wave-wheel. He answered with the classic kayaking response: "Oh, it's actually really easy. Just do this . . ." Approximately one million attempts later, I'm happy to say that Jay's lessons have paid off.

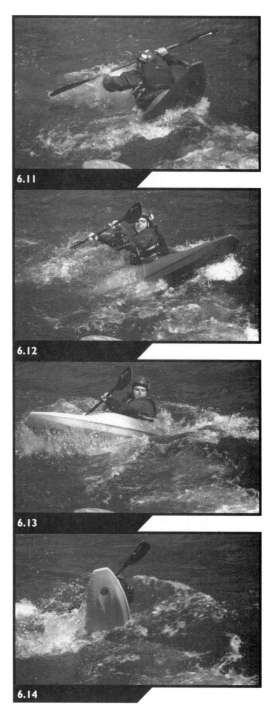

6.11 *The bow goes down . . .*

6.12 *. . . while the boater gets ready to perform a forward sweep.*

6.13 – 6.14 *As the boater does a forward sweep, the second point slices into the water. Boater: Shane Williams*

In reality, there's not much new about the wave-wheel; simply throw an eddy-line cartwheel as you head down a bunch of waves (OK, I admit, it's not that easy). A wave-wheel starts by getting the bow up—a controlled rocket move. The next point comes by throwing the bow down on the downstream side of a steep wave. You can finish things out by throwing the stern underwater again.

The location: you'll need to find a fairly sizeable wave. It's possible to wave-wheel on smaller waves, but at first, stick to bigguns. In performing the move, you'll use the front and back of one wave—the front to get the bow up, and the back to put that bow down. Ideally, the wave needs to be steep enough to do a really good rocket move, but not so steep that the wave crashes down on top of you.

The Move

1. Start by heading down the middle of that big wave train. Just as with an eddy-line cartwheel, get some speed going. Wave-wheels are easier if you're moving pretty quickly.

2. As you come up one wave, get a modified rocket-move going. To initiate, use a big forward sweep on one side, and edge toward that stroke in order to sink the stern a bit. If you're taking a stroke on the right, edge right.

   Here's the key: you don't really want to go vertical. Just try to get a lot of your kayak off the face of the wave—that's where speed will help. The most important thing is that you get your bow up at the end of the wave. That is, don't initiate too early. Timing is everything. Try to get your nose up as late as you can: this will get more of your boat "hanging" off the peak of the wave. You want to get as much of your bow free of the wave as possible so that you can slam it back down.

3. Now that you've freed your bow, it's time to throw it underwater. As your bow shoots off that last wave, try to shift your weight as far forward as possible. You'll want keep your boat edged—and start edging a little harder if you can. The first part of the wave-wheel (steps one through four) are performed with the boat actually balanced on its side. With the boat edged radically, it will be easier to slice

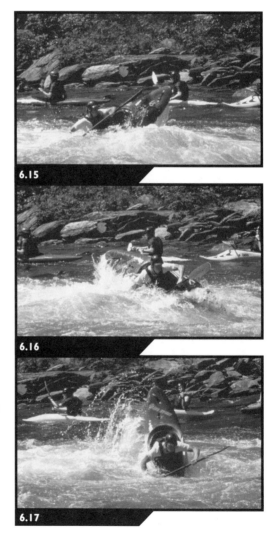

6.15 *Boater lifts the bow up as he gets over the peak of the wave . . .*

6.16 *. . . then slams the bow down in the back of the wave.*

6.17 *The bow goes down . . .*

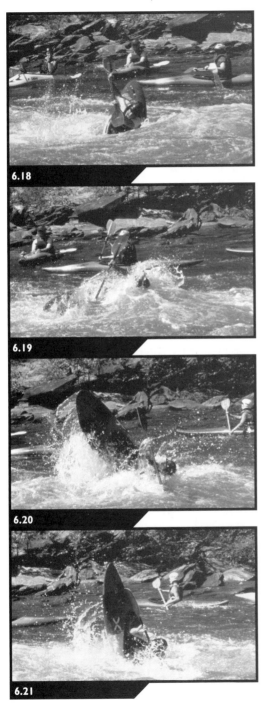

6.18

6.19

6.20

6.21

6.18 – 6.19 *. . . and as the stern starts to fall, the boater starts a forward sweep to bring the stern around and down.*

6.20 – 6.21 *The second point of a wave-wheel. Boater: Aaron Napoleon* the bow down. Be careful not to edge by simply flopping your body over the water—keep your weight centered.

4. As you pass the peak of the wave, you'll turn that forward stroke (to get the bow up) into the cartwheel-initiation stroke (to throw the bow down)—the sweep toward your toes that starts a cartwheel. This cartwheel stroke is used as soon as you're done getting your bow up in that modified rocket move. If all goes well, your bow will slice into the backside of the wave, and you'll get vertical. Poetry in motion.

5. To finish things out, you can also simply throw down the stern again. As you come off the bow point, edge the opposite way you did to initiate the wave-wheel and use a strong forward sweep on that side.

That's all for playing. No more playing—knock it off. I've tried to cover the basic moves involved in playing, as well as some of the more dynamic moves out there. There are still a lot of moves out there that I haven't discussed, like the blunt, blast wheel, mystery move, and the loop. Look for these (and more!) in the sequel. For now, I'm played out. Time to sit in front of the TV for hours, watching old Simpsons episodes and stuffing doughnuts down my throat. Ahhhh—life is good.

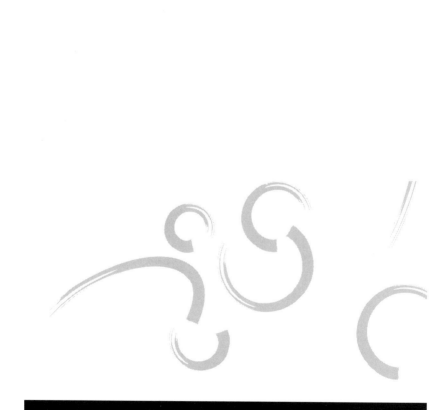

7

Help Yourself:
Whitewater Safety

For most of the year, I have the great fortune to earn my keep as a kayak instructor. The place where I work runs a number of river-rescue clinics each season. These clinics teach all sorts of new skills and techniques for getting out of bad situations, but rescue instructors are quick to point out that, while it's great to know how to set up a **z**-drag using only Powerbar wrappers, gum, and leaves, it's preferable to stay out of trouble in the first place. In other words, time for another kayaking rule:

Rule 6: The better you are, the safer you'll be.

The best way to be a safer kayaker is to be a better kayaker. Usually, a highly skilled boater will be less likely to have a mishap than a novice. Of course, if that highly skilled boater is experimenting with new and exciting moves like running thirty-foot waterfalls upside-down, the rule collapses. The point: a person who understands rivers (and has some modicum of sanity) will tend to be safer than a person who does not. The first thing you should do to be safer is to improve your personal boating skills and your knowledge of the way rivers work. By spending more time on the river, you begin to develop a sixth sense of what moves are riskier than others and where the hazards are, and therefore, you are less likely to get in over your head. You do have to push the envelope to get better, but there is a difference between recklessly throwing yourself into the maelstrom and taking a calculated risk.

There are a number of really great resources about whitewater safety on the market (I've listed some of my favorites in the final section of this book). I urge you to read some of these resources. If you're really serious about learning more about river safety, you may want to take a river-rescue clinic. Nothing can beat hands-on learning. Meanwhile, in this chapter, I cover some basic safety ideas and self-rescue techniques to at least get you started.

Of course, no kayaker, no matter how talented, can completely eliminate risk. Part of the appeal of kayaking is the fact that it's not a totally controlled sport. Anything can happen. If you boat for any length of time, you will eventually have to deal with a potentially dangerous situation. With this frightening idea in mind, this chapter focuses on two ideas:

- Keep dangerous situations to a minimum

- Control dangerous situations as much as possible

RULE 6

The better you are, the safer you'll be.

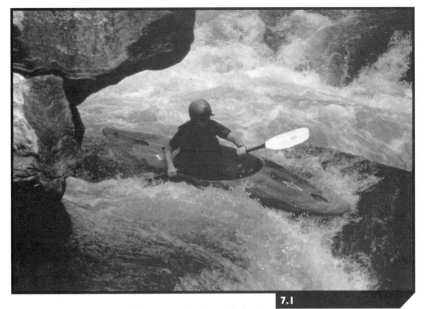

7.1

Just so I can pretend I'm organized, we'll deal with these two topics in turn. First, let's discuss some ways to minimize dangerous situations—how to avoid danger.

7.1 *A solid kayaker is a safe kayaker. Boater: Heather Nagel*

MINIMIZING DANGEROUS SITUATIONS

Hone Your Paddling Skills

Work on your skills. You'll have more fun, you'll be safer, and everyone on the planet will want to boat with you. A better kayaker can run rapids with more control and, just as importantly, can make more informed decisions about how to run.

The best way to improve is to boat more. But don't just go out there and flail around; make the most of your time in the kayak. Be conscious and critical of the way you boat. Watch what others are doing, and try to learn from them. Don't forget to have fun, though.

Instruction can be a big help, too. Instruction can come in a number of forms. You can get formal instruction from an accredited kayak school. You can read various literature out there: books (I know at least one incredibly good book—more of a piece of art, to be honest), articles in magazines, and web sources, to name a few. There are also some really informative videos available. Videos can be very helpful, especially if you're having trouble visualizing a particular move or technique. Check out the list at the end of the book for the names of some great sources.

Bring the Right Stuff!

When you go to the river, you'd feel pretty silly wearing a three-piece suit and water wings while sitting in an old bathtub. I try to save such attire for private moments. Even without the bathtub and suit, you can be just as out-of-place if you have the wrong type of gear. For example, on a really hard creek run in the middle of winter, you wouldn't have a good time in a tiny play-boat, wearing nothing but a short-sleeved paddling jacket for warmth, and using a fragile freestyle paddle.

Clothing. If it's cold, bring plenty of warm layers—there's nothing more miserable than shivering uncontrollably a hundred yards into a six-mile run. And if you've heard it once, you've heard it a hundred times—no cotton! Use the synthetic du jour or the traditional standby—wool. Pogies and skullcaps are nice to have, too. When in doubt, wear too much; you can always take off a layer and stuff it in the back of your boat. If it's hot and sunny, sunscreen, a hat, and a shirt to shield your tender skin are all good ideas.

Boats. In the last few years, rodeo boats have become incredibly popular—the smaller, the better. We all love our funky little play-boats. It's the boat I use most often and the one I feel most comfortable in. And there's nothing as fun as getting that smooth cartwheeling action in a big hole—except when that big hole is a few feet above a gnarly Class V+ rapid. Or when we get that enormous rain, and it's time to hit the steeps, and I'm out there in my creek boat feeling uncomfortable and out-of-control. Not a good thing on those tough rivers. The solution? Force yourself to spend a little more time out of your play-boat. If you get in that other boat just a little more often, you'll thank yourself for it as you go for some huge air. Remember: bring the right boat for the river. While a creek or big-water boat might not be quite as exciting, you'll feel more confident, you'll probably have better lines, and you'll be more inclined to run that crazy drop.

You'll also feel like you're in a lot more control if you take the time to outfit your boat well. For a long time, I didn't bother to outfit any of my boats. Yes, this was because I was a lazy fool. But when I finally got around to it, I was amazed at the difference: you can roll without falling out of the seat! You don't slide forward four inches when you get an ender! Your hips don't hurt after three stern-squirts! Simply incredible. You'll feel better and have more control if you take the time to fit your boat to your body.

Other Gear. This little section might seem boring and obvious. Too bad. You'll read it and you'll enjoy it. I'll be brief:

- Make sure that you or someone else in your group has at least one break-down paddle. There's nothing worse than starting an unplanned six-mile hike up steep, muddy banks while your buds continue downstream whooping it up.

- Make sure your helmet fits comfortably and that it can take a solid hit. Whether or not you believe it, it's nice to have a semi-functional brain. I really enjoy mine.

- Your skirt should fit the boat very tightly. You'll be pissed if you have to swim a Class V rapid because of a blown skirt. You'll probably be pissed no matter what the reason, but that's beside the point. Here's a good test: put your skirt on your boat (without you in it, dummy). If you can pick up the boat by the skirt and swing it around without the skirt popping, you're good to go.

- Elbow pads are nice to have if you're running technical (rocky) rivers—they really do make you feel a lot more secure. I've bashed my elbows enough to really value my pads. A lot of boaters swear by face guards, too. Facial injuries aren't uncommon for kayakers. And they're not too fun. Besides, it's hard to hit on members of the opposite sex when they're not sure if that flattened thing near the center of your face is a nose or a small, mangled rodent.

- Wear a PFD. 'Nuff said.

- Take and drink plenty of water—dehydration is no fun and can be potentially serious. And when you're on a run like the Pigeon or the Reventazon, you're really not going to want to drink right from the river. It's good to have snacks along, too. One hint: in general, stay away from such foods as ice cream, fried chicken, and Jell-O. The best thing about remembering to bring a snack is the pathetic begging from your ill-prepared friends.

Rescue Gear. Good things to carry include carabiners, a river knife, a whistle, a throw rope, prussiks, some kind of first-aid kit, and, of course, duct tape. More about the use of these items in the next section.

Boating People. Kayak with folks you trust. If you swim right above a strainer, do you want

Tom-the-collapsing-crack-addict holding the rope, or a person whom you feel has a pretty good chance of getting you out of trouble? When I run rapids that make my heart rate fly, I like to be with at least two other people whom I trust. You never know. As they say in the boating video, *Wet Ones*, "Sometimes the best piece of rescue equipment is a well-trained friend."

One of the big rules in boating—Never Go Alone! That said, I'll be honest. I kayak alone sometimes. I've done it for years, and I will probably keep doing it (until I end up knocking myself out and drowning in a Class II). But it's not a good idea. I know this, and I accept the risks. I also want to emphasize that I would never run really challenging rapids alone. I know, I know—accidents can happen on even the most innocuous-looking rivers. But I could seriously injure myself on a stroll in the park, yet I don't stay in the house until I can find a walking partner.

I was really hesitant to write about the fact that I sometimes kayak alone. I don't at all want to encourage it. But I want to face the facts that people do go alone. If you sometimes boat without others along, please don't push it. Be extra conservative. If for no other reason, realize that if anything happens to you, Charlie Walbridge will make you look like a complete moron in his next accident report.

Do Your Homework. One of my favorite things is to head down a river I've never seen. It's a fun challenge to figure out the lines, decide whether to run certain rapids, and, most of all, how to run shuttle without involving major car damage. A "personal first descent" can be very rewarding.

However, it's important to be cautious. Don't throw yourself down a river and over a horizon line without first gathering a little data. The amount of data is up to you. If you want, go only on rivers you know like the back of your hand. Or you can choose to paddle new rivers as long as you're with someone who knows the run well. Or, you can opt to do some exploring. Most people's boating involves all three types of trips. There are definitely times when I need my hand held, when I want someone to point out the line and all the possible hazards. There are also times when I like to discover a river for myself. Just exercise common sense. Knowledge can't hurt. The goal of boating isn't to set up a *Mission Impossible* situation every time you get in your kayak.

When I'm on a river, I usually like to have a pretty good idea about a few things:

- The length of the run. It's nice to finish before dark. It's also nice to have enough energy to move during the last few miles.

- The general type of rapids on the river. The difficulty of rapids will dictate a lot—from what boat I'll use to how much I'll scout to whether or not I want to be there in the first place.

- Any major dangers lurking out there. If there is a huge log all the way across the river, it's nice to know about it before you're taking hysterical evasive action.

- The shuttle. This isn't always the most enthralling piece of information. But it's not much fun driving around on some semi-existent road two hours before sunset looking for the two crooked trees that mark the take-out trail. Get directions!

- Finally, it's very important to be aware of the water level. A normally tame run can become way too exciting with a lot more volume. A section can easily change from Class IV to Class V with some rain. Don't assume that just because you aced "White Hot Screaming Death" at 20 CFS, you're ready to throw yourself down it at 2000 CFS.

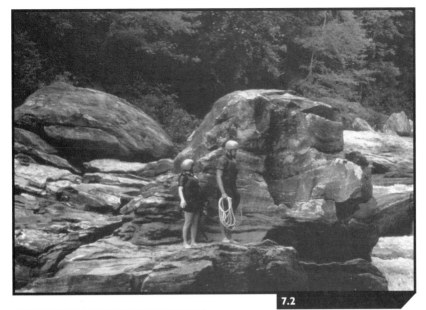

7.2

CONTROLLING DANGEROUS SITUATIONS

When we paddle whitewater that really pushes our abilities, we usually act a little differently than on easier runs. On an easy run, a few of us might head down river, eddying out every so often to play and shoot the breeze. We're aware of what other boaters are doing, but we're not overly vigilant. We might get out of our boats every so often to get a snack or to stretch our legs. We typically run rapids without setting up safety ahead of time. We'll just head on down when we're ready.

On tougher water, we take more time and are much more aware of where each person is. Above particularly hard rapids, we'll eddy out to review the desired line and make sure we know the order in which we'll go. At some points, we might even get out and look at a rapid to make sure we know exactly what we're getting ourselves into. And, importantly, we'll set up safety within difficult rapids. This safety might be a

7.2 Boaters set up safety below a rapid. Safety crew: Dan Pilver and Heather Nagel

boater eddied out at the bottom, or we might get more elaborate and set up safety ropes. There's no perfect recipe for setting up a rapid. Just make sure that safety people have the best chance possible to get to a boater in trouble.

Unfortunately, no matter how ready you are, things won't always go perfectly. Let's talk about how to deal with runs that aren't proceeding according to plan—how to control those dangerous situations.

RULE 7

Thou shalt be cool.

Over the years, I've been in a number of bad spots, and I've seen others who haven't had the best of luck. Getting pinned, trashed in a hole, or swimming down a big, unfriendly drop might not be the most fun moment in your boating career, but if you kayak long enough, you'll find trouble eventually—and it's good to know how to reduce risk.

There is one vital rule to keep in mind when a run turns out a little strange. I'm sure you've heard this idea before, but too bad—it's important:

Rule 7: Thou shalt be cool.

In other words, don't panic. No matter what happens, you'll generally fare better if you're not a hysterical, hyperventilating mess. Relax and be ready to react. Chances are, you'll be OK.

Again, I don't plan on discussing all the possible dilemmas you might encounter in your exciting life as a kayaker, but I will briefly cover some major topics and general ideas as to how to deal with problems. Check out the list of safety references at the end if you want to learn much more about these topics.

Obstructions

Without rocks, trees, and other monsters, we wouldn't have rapids. We love obstructions. However, these river features can make things difficult at times. Let's discuss what to do about obstructions that just refuse to act friendly.

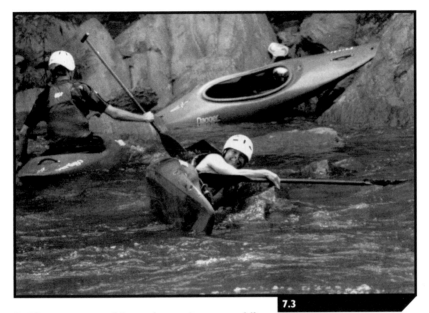

7.3

1. If you see something ugly coming up, paddle away from it!

2. Uh-oh. Despite all your efforts, you're still heading toward that rock. If the rock is small enough so that you might be able to drive your boat up on it, go for it. Try for a little boof. Chances are you'll be more in control than if you slowly drift into the rock. In general, try to hit the rock straight on, not sideways.

3. For some strange reason, you've decided you do want to hit that rock sideways. You're a weird person, but don't worry. Just edge your boat toward that rock, then hug it like it's your pal. While you're there, you can thank it for creating rapids.

   By edging into the rock, the water flowing downstream moves under your boat, keeping you

7.3 Lean into those rocks. Paddler: Barbara Beran

....

Advanced Tip

   A fine point here. If you lean into the rock right before you're about to hit it, you'll probably end up upside-down anyway. How infuriating! You followed my incredibly wonderful advice, and you're pinned upside-down against a rock. The problem is that most rocks have pillows, a small pile of water where the water pushes against the upstream face of a rock. A pillow reacts to your boat a lot like a rock. So if you're moving sideways into a rock, you'll need to lean into the pillow a few important seconds before you hit the rock. It's all about anticipation.

....

upright and happy as a clam. Just make sure you don't lean upstream, away from the rock (a pretty natural reaction); the current will catch your upstream edge and you'll be upside-down against a rock—eek! Just remember to lean into that rock—you'll be golden.

4. So you're sideways against the rock. Don't fret. You're actually not in a terrible position. Ninety-nine percent of the time, you'll be able to push yourself forward or backward, so that you move around the rock. If this isn't happening, you can even get out and stand on that troublesome rock. If worst comes to worst, you can hang out in your boat and wait for help. You're stable, upright, and doing well.

This plan will work for just about any obstruction, whether it's a rock, a tree, or a semi-submerged VW bus. Be especially careful around those extra-unfriendly places, like undercut rocks or strainers.

However, the story doesn't always resolve itself so easily. Occasionally, boaters find themselves pinned, stuck solid against an obstruction, unable to work loose. If you have the misfortune to find yourself in this type of situation, here are some ideas to keep in mind:

- Keep calm. Thrashing around won't help and can make the situation worse.

- If you are stable and can breathe, you're actually not in too bad a position. Try to relax and not do anything that might make your situation worse.

- Sometimes, you'll realize that you need to get out of your kayak. If this is the case, make things happen quickly. As soon as you pop your skirt, get out of the boat. Once water goes into the boat, the boat will tend to be pinned even more solidly than before.

- When trying to help a person, don't move them in such a way that might make their situation worse. Carefully consider what to do, and act efficiently and decisively.

Whenever you are trying to help another person out, remember:

Rule 8: Don't endanger yourself while helping others in danger.

If a person is caught in a bad place, don't immediately throw yourself into that place, despite your noble intentions. Without any forethought, you probably won't be able to help, and you could get into trouble. It's harder to rescue two people than one.

RULE 8

Don't endanger yourself while helping others in danger.

Holes

Just like any other feature that might not treat you nicely, the first thing to do is to try to stay away from bad holes. Learn to recognize unfriendly holes (check out the chapter on scouting for some hints) and avoid them if you can.

If you are going to go into an ugly hole, hit it straight and with speed. As you hit it, keep your weight forward and paddle hard. Try to time your strokes so that you take a big forward stroke just as your body is in the meat of the hole. Keep paddling for a few strokes, even when you're out of the hole; with a really bad hydraulic, you'll want to make sure you're past the backwash before you thank your guardian angel. With some luck, you'll punch through that sticky hole. Nothing to it.

Sometimes, though, that hole will decide it wants to show you the latest rodeo move. Again, back to Rule 7: Stay calm. Lean downstream and stay loose. Here are some strategies for getting out of holes:

- Work your way toward one of the sides of the hole where the current kicks out. If you can

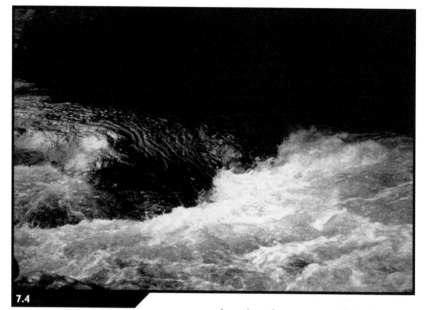

7.4 *Holier-than-thou: a hydraulic.*

get to the edge, the current will kick you so that one end of your boat points downstream. When this happens, paddle your rear end off.

- Move from a side-surf to a front- or back-surf—the hole might ender you out. Paddle hard to get out once you've been endered.

- If all else fails, flip over and hang out upside-down for a few seconds. The current going under the hole might hit your body and wash you out. To help that current, abandon your tuck—let your body dangle so that the current has a target with a large surface area. Some folks even say that you should extend your paddle down to catch the current pushing out. I admit that all these fancy contortions can be tough if you're getting trashed in the hole. No worries.

- If worst comes to worst, you might have to swim. Most holes will kick you out at this point, but if you're still in the hole, relax. Don't fight to stay at the top of the hole for air. Try to go deep to catch those bottom currents. If you ball up, you'll tend to sink better. Another strategy is to try to work your way toward the edge of the hole, just as you would in a boat.

Swimming

The neat thing about being out of that boat is that you really get a chance to feel the incredible power of the river. But there are much more pleasant ways to gain respect for Mother Nature; swimming can be terrifying. So until you drag yourself on shore like a drenched weasel, here are some ideas to keep yourself healthy.

First, back to Rule 7: Don't panic. Think of swimming as a chance for a much-needed bath.

Second, (hopefully, you already know this) don't stand up. We're land-based animals, so whenever things feel a bit out-of-control, we like to get our bearings by planting our feet. But standing in strong current is a terrible idea. Without going into all the gory details, there are all sorts of things on the river bottom (rocks, trees, debris) that are perfectly shaped to snag dangling feet. Once your foot is caught, it's very difficult to keep your head above water. Even a relatively mellow current can easily hold a strong person under. Foot entrapments are scary, awful situations, and rescue is difficult. But the good news is that foot entrapments are easy to avoid—just don't stand up.

Obviously, if you're completely beached, you can go ahead and get on your feet. A general rule of thumb is that it's OK to stand up if the water isn't deeper than your knees. You might get some bruises sliding over shallow rocks, but it's a lot easier to deal with a few black-and-blue spots than a foot entrapment.

Third, be an active self-rescuer. The traditional "safe swimmer" position is on the back, with the feet downstream. This position is great if you're heading down a rapid and you don't feel the slightest inclination to get to a different place in the river, but if you're floating on your back toward the lip of that unrunnable drop, your life is about to get a little too exciting. It's perfectly acceptable to turn over on your belly and swim aggressively toward a safe-looking eddy. If you see a better place to go than where you're headed, swim for it.

Finally, there can be times when you will end up out of your boat in a place you don't want to be. This can be scary. Some ideas:

- If you wind up going over a vertical drop (even a small one), ball up like a cannonball. If you float on your back instead, your feet will end up pointing toward the bottom, creating a chance for foot entrapment—not good. Balling up might be a bit disorienting, but your chances for entrapment will be reduced.

- If you're going to run into something (on the surface), hit it feet first. This should be instinctual. If not, a different sport (Parcheesi?) might be a good idea.

- If you're getting washed into a big obstruction like a strainer (logs or other debris where water can go through but large objects like boats or people can't), try to climb on top. You want to get your body away from the water that's trying to push you into the strainer.

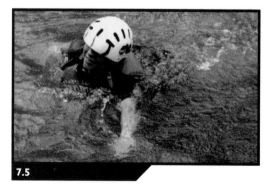

7.5 *Swimmer actively swimming for safety. Swimmer: Barbara Beran*

Safety Equipment

With a few simple tools, every boater can (and should) become a demigod of rescue technology. Knowledge of how to deal with rescue situations can be invaluable, both to yourself and the folks with whom you go boating.

Rope. It's a great idea to bring a rope along whenever you kayak. Ropes are small, easy to carry, and can be really valuable. I rarely have the chance to use my rope, but it's a great comfort to know it's there if I need it. And when it gets time to retire your rope, you can use it for all kinds of things, from a strap to drag your kayak to the put-in to a handy way to tie extra kayaks onto a car.

There are a number of models available, from waist-bags to simple coils of rope to throw-bags. I don't have much of a preference. Just remember a few things:

- Make sure your rope is long enough to be useful. That five-foot rope might pack beautifully into your squirt boat, but it won't be too helpful. I highly recommend seventy-five foot throw-ropes; they're an industry standard and can be found easily.

- Before you leave for each trip, make sure your rope is ready for use—free of tangles, not broken, nicked, etc.

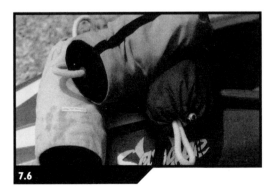

7.6

7.6 *A bevy of throwbags.*

- Keep your rope in a place where it's easy to get to if needed.

- Practice! Every once in a while, go out in your driveway or backyard and work on your accuracy. Not the most fun thing in the world, but still more exciting than Must-See-TV. And your pal will be so happy when you rope him in right before that undercut. You might even get some free beer out of it.

More Rope-Throwing Tips. There are a number of perfectly fine ways to throw a rope—underhand, overhand, or sidearm. Find one method that's most comfortable for you and stick with it. (Hint: the spinning-discus style might look cool, but you won't usually have great results.)

When you do chuck that rope, make sure that you don't throw all seventy-five feet of line to your friend who's drifting ten feet away. She'll be impressed with your arm, but probably a little saddened by the fact that she's only thirty feet from the edge of that crazy Class V+ you wouldn't even think about going down with a kayak.

You'll often find that it's tough to pull a swimmer to the side of the river, especially if the swimmer is downstream of you. No sweat—you can pendulum them into shore pretty easily. Just make sure you're not swinging them into a worse place, like another strainer or an undercut even more gnarly than the one you pulled them away from in the first place.

The force of a swimmer on a rope can be considerable, especially in strong current. To combat the force, you can walk downstream with them. This is called a "dynamic rescue." The dynamic rescue works because you're no longer fighting against the entire force of the river. Walk carefully; you won't help your friend too much if you fall in with him.

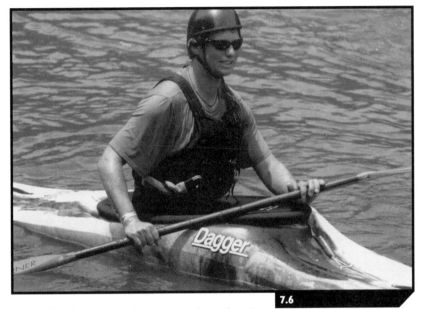

7.6

Finally, when you are being towed in (phew!), relax and enjoy the ride. It will help if you turn over on your back, so that you're not being pulled face-first like a water-skier who won't let go of the tow-line.

7.6 *A typical rescue vest. Boater: Matt Jennings*

Carabiners and Prussik Loops. Sometimes, a boat can get so stuck you'll need a little extra help. Carabiners and short loops of strong webbing or rope can be very useful for setting up fancy pulley systems in order to get a boat unpinned. Biners are also great for more mundane purposes, like clipping gear together. For more information on setting up safety systems, check out some of the recommended reading in the list of resources later on.

River Knives. Mostly for spreading peanut butter. A river knife can be a useful tool, but is one of those items that's usually just a comfort to have. However, whenever you're using ropes, it's good to have a river knife handy, just in case.

Whistles. Another item you might never need. But it's good to be able to alert folks if you need their attention in a hurry.

Rescue PFDs. Many companies make "rescue jackets," PFDs that are specially designed for rescue situations. These PFDs can be very useful, but make sure that if you wear one, you know how to use it! A rescue jacket can be very dangerous if not handled correctly.

First-Aid Kits. It's a good idea to have a first-aid kit along whenever you paddle. But, realistically, you won't always have room or feel that you need one. On shorter or easier trips, a first-aid kit won't always be absolutely necessary (hopefully). If you are going to bring a kit, think about essentials. Items like band-aids for small scratches are good to have, but do you need them? Stick to articles that are really tough to do without in an emergency, items that are tough to improvise easily. Some include:

- A bee-sting kit (a must if people are known to be allergic).

- Portable splints (you can use a stick, but it's a real pain).

- Cravats—for a sling. The most common injury in kayaking is shoulder dislocation. You could rip up your fancy paddling jacket, but why bother?

Duct Tape. The best thing to hit kayaking since water-flow and gradient, duct tape can be used for at least a billion things, from splints to paddle repairs to a way to shut up that guy bragging about his last run. A must-have in any kind of multi-day trip, and a good idea any time you're on the river.

I hope that this too-short gloss of some whitewater safety ideas has been helpful. I've tried to discuss some common sense ideas that are central in ensuring personal safety. I have not gone into much detail at all about some of the rescue techniques that can be used. Hopefully, you'll take the time to look at the more in-depth books on safety. Another great way to learn about safety is to take a swiftwater rescue clinic offered by your local outdoor center. Safety isn't always the most fun or exciting part of boating. But it is definitely the most important.

A

Appendix A:
Sources of Further Learning

So you didn't get everything you needed to
know from my book? Hey, that's OK. The following is a list of some resources that could help
you with your boating. I've listed a few of my
favorites, followed by my obnoxious comments.

Instructional Schools:

Endless River Adventures
14157 HWY 19 West, Box 246
Bryson City, NC 28713
(828) 488-6199
A small but top-notch school with great instructors.

Instructional Schools (continued):

Nantahala Outdoor Center
13077 Hwy. 19 W
Bryson City, NC 28713
(704) 488-2175
    One of the oldest and best kayaking schools in the country.

Sundance Expeditions and Kayak School
14894 Galice Rd.
Merlin, OR 97532
(541) 479-8508
    A beautiful and excellent kayaking center in the West.

Zoar Outdoor
Mohawk Trail
Charlemont, MA 01339
(800) 532-7483
    A top kayaking school in the Northeast.

Instructional Books:

    Kayak! A Manual of Intermediate & Advanced Technique. William Nealy. Menasha Ridge Press, 1986.
    Lots of classic Nealy cartoons provide excellent visual explanations.

    Kayaking: Whitewater and Touring Basics (A Trailside Guide Series). Steven M. Krauzer. W.W. Norton & Co., 1995.
    A good book for beginners. Written with a sense of humor.

    Kayaking Essentials. Bob Beazley. Menasha Ridge Press, 1995.
    A quick introduction to boating.

    Whitewater Handbook. Bruce Lessels. Appalachian Mountain Club, 1994.
    Great explanations by a superb instructor.

Videos:

Essential Boat Control. Tom DeCuir.
Tons of information about just about every aspect of kayaking. Very entertaining.

Grace Under Pressure. Tom DeCuir and Kathy Bolyn.
A very amusing and helpful look at the roll. Contains a great "roll loop" showing perfect rolls from all angles.

Kayak 101. Joe Holt.
Explains kayaking basics very clearly.

Retendo. Kent Ford.
Does a great job demystifying playboating - perfect for visual learners.

Searching for the "Gee" Spot. Corran Addison.
A Cutting-edge freestyle video.

Safety Resources:

Whitewater Rescue Manual. Charlie Walbridge and Wayne A. Sundmacher, Jr. McGraw Hill, 1995.
Lots of in-depth coverage about river safety.

River Rescue. Les Bechdel and Slim Ray. Appalachian Mountain Club, 1997.
Another terrific safety resource.

Whitewater Self-Defense. Kent Ford.
A video on whitewater safety.

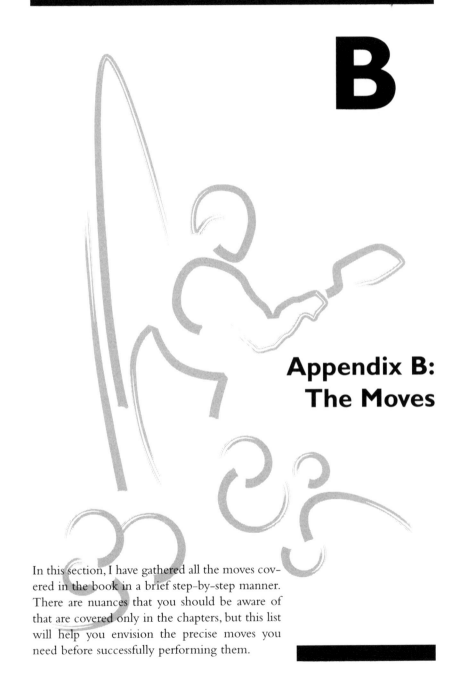

B

Appendix B:
The Moves

In this section, I have gathered all the moves covered in the book in a brief step-by-step manner. There are nuances that you should be aware of that are covered only in the chapters, but this list will help you envision the precise moves you need before successfully performing them.

From **Pushing the Limits (Chapter 3):**

Ledge Boofs

1. Approach the ledge with plenty of momentum.

2. Lean forward as you near the lip and hook your paddle over the ledge. The paddle should be vertical and close to the front of the boat.

3. Shift your weight back and pull your knees to your chest in order to pull the bow up.

4. You should be leaning back as you finish the stroke and go over the drop.

5. Land with your weight forward and continue paddling.

Boofing Rocks

1. Approach an appropriate drop with plenty of momentum.

2. Drive the front of your boat partly onto one of the rocks that border the slot.

2. Lean forward as you near the lip and hook your paddle over the ledge. The paddle should be vertical, close to the front of the boat, and even with the downstream edge of the rock.

3. Shift your weight back and pull your knees to your chest in order to pull the bow up.

4. You should be leaning back as you finish the stroke and go over the drop.

5. Land with your weight forward and continue paddling.

From **Getting Fancy (Chapter 4):**

360-Surfing

1. Start by side-surfing in an appropriate hole, facing the hole's edge. Always keep your eyes on the hole.

2. Move your boat slowly toward the hole's edge while edging downstream.

3. As you reach the edge, the current will grab the bow of your boat and swing it downstream.

4. As the bow swings downstream, lean forward and take a big backstroke on your downstream side to stay in the hole.

5. Don't forget to switch edges.

6. Move the back of your boat slowly toward the hole's edge.

7. The current will grab the stern of your boat and swing it downstream.

8. Take a few strokes to stay in the hole if needed.

Stern-Squirting

1. Approach an eddy line with some speed. Keep your eyes glued to the stern.

2. Hit the eddy line close to the obstruction that creates it.

3. The boat's angle should be a bit upstream of perpendicular to the current.

4. As you cross the eddy line, the current will swing the bow of your boat downstream.

5. Simultaneously sink into your upstream butt cheek (that J-lean again) so that your boat is edged upstream and twist your body toward the stern on the downstream side, planting a big reverse sweep.

6. As you begin to go vertical, keep looking at the stern and keep your blade in the water.

Spinning on a Stern-Squirt

1. Initiate a stern-squirt.

2. As you begin to go vertical, your boat will start to turn. Look over your shoulder in the direction you are rotating.

3. To prolong the spin, slice your paddle from the reverse-sweep position to the bow draw position.

4. Continue bow drawing to keep spinning.

The Screw-up

1. Initiate a stern-squirt.

2. As you begin to go vertical, your boat will start to turn. As you begin to flip over, start a roll on the side that will allow you to keep the momentum of your rotation going.

Splatting

1. Paddle toward an appropriate rock at about a 45-degree angle.

2. Just before you hit the rock, sink into your upstream butt cheek and use a big forward sweep on your upstream side.

3. As your bow rides up on the rock, stop edging so that your kayak lands on the rock flat.

Blasting Holes

1. Approach an appropriate hole from one side.

2. Initiate the move close to the hole: use a big forward sweep on your downstream side, and edge toward that stroke to go vertical.

3. Keep your weight back and use your paddle to keep you from falling toward either side.

Rocket Moves

1. Head downstream on a wave train.

2. As you get to the wave's crest, take a strong forward sweep and edge your boat toward that stroke.

From **Still More Playing Techniques (Chapter 5):**

Enders

1. From the eddy, place your boat right on the edge of the hole.

2. Paddle forward, keeping your kayak parallel to the flow of the water.

3. Lean forward as you enter the hole.

4. To go all the way over (past vertical), keep leaning forward.

5. To keep your boat less than vertical, lean back once you begin the ender.

Pirouette

1. To begin, intitiate an ender.

2. As you start to get vertical, lean back with your back against the deck of your boat.

3. At the same time, rotate (don't lean) your head in the direction you want to spin.

4. You can help the pirouette by using a reverse-sweep on the side toward the direction you want to spin as you start to go vertical.

5. For a more dynamic move, use a crossbow draw to get the spin going: rotate your upper body and plant the stroke before you initiate the ender; keep your body weight over the center of your boat and begin the stroke as you start to go vertical.

Cartwheel

1. Initiate the ender as before.

2. As you initiate, perform the second half of a reverse sweep, starting wide at your side and pushing toward your toes on the side the hole is pushing to.

3. As you rotate, make sure you look at the hole!

4. As the stern lands in the hole initiate another ender.

5. As you begin to go vertical, plant the first half of a forward sweep on the other side of the reverse sweep (do this stroke early).

6. Go back to step 1 and continue throwing down points!

The Back-Deck Roll

1. Start by planting a duffek.

2. Lean back a bit and rotate toward the water on the side that you've set the stroke.

3. Cock the top wrist all the way back.

4. As you start to flip, look back over the shoulder to the side you're flipping toward.

5. Rotate as far as possible. When you flip, your chest should hit the water first.

6. Hold this position as you roll; your body will pass under the boat.

7. Start the actual roll before your body comes all the way to the surface.

8. Leaving your nonworking hand low and relaxed, pull your working blade from the back to the front of your boat.

9. Bring your body forward with the paddle, while dropping your head toward the working shoulder.

Flat Spins

1. Choose an appropriate boat (preferably short, flat-bottomed, and hard-chined) and an appropriate wave (big and steep).

2. Start by front-surfing on the crest of the wave.

3. When ready, slide down into the trough with a little angle in the direction you plan to spin.

4. Initiate the spin as soon as you start down: keep your weight forward and use a wide, powerful reverse sweep on the side to which you're spinning.

5. Keep the boat nice and flat; if you edge, your spin will be way too slow.

6. As you reach a back-surfing position, use a big forward sweep on the opposite side of the initial reverse sweep to keep the spin going and finish the 360.

From **Tear the Roof Off (Chapter 6):**

Rock Spins

1. As usual, find an appropriate rock.

2. Using strong forward strokes, drive your boat onto the rock until the rock is under your butt (which will act as a pivot point).

2. As you drive onto the rock, point the boat in the direction you want to spin. If you have a lot of angle as your butt gets up on the rock, you've already performed a good bit of the spin.

3. An instant before you are on the rock, rotate your head in the direction of the spin. This will wind up your body and help the spin get going.

4. Now throw in a big reverse sweep on the upstream side.

5. As your bow comes around to face upstream, throw your weight forward in order to slice your bow underwater.

6. To keep that spin going, use a forward sweep on the other side and keep looking in the direction of the spin.

Eddy-Line Cartwheel

1. Start in an eddy and get some momentum, aiming near the top of the eddy and pointing a few degrees downstream of parallel with the current.

2. Just before you cross the eddy line, edge your boat hard and take a powerful forward sweep in order to lift your bow up.

3. As you cross the eddy line, slam the bow down by pushing your paddle from wide at your side in toward your toes, and throw your body weight forward. Keep the boat edged hard.

4. Make sure your strokes stay toward the front of your boat and keep your eyes on your feet, not looking downstream.

5. When your bow starts to resurface, use a strong sweep stroke on the opposite side, while edging toward that stroke. This second stroke will pull the stern under.

6. If you want to get tons of points and have no trouble getting your bow down, edge your boat downstream (instead of upstream) as you initiate the move and take a powerful forward sweep on the downstream side.

Wave-Wheels

1. Head down the middle of a big wave train and get some speed going.

2. Just before you reach the peak of the wave, use a big forward sweep and edge toward that side in order to lift the bow a bit and hang off the peak of the wave.

3. As your bow shoots off the peak, shift your weight forward and keep your boat edged as far as possible.

4. As you pass the peak of the wave, turn the forward stroke into a reverse sweep, helping your bow to slice into the backside of the wave.

5. To continue, as you come off the bow point, use a strong forward sweep on the side opposite the first reverse sweep.

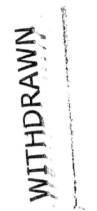